Hearing Conservation:
In Occupational, Recreational,
Educational, and Home Settings

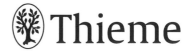

Hearing Conservation: In Occupational, Recreational, Educational, and Home Settings

Vishakha Waman Rawool, PhD
Professor
Department of Speech Pathology and Audiology
West Virginia University
Morgantown, West Virginia

Thieme
New York · Stuttgart

Thieme Medical Publishers, Inc.
333 Seventh Ave.
New York, NY 10001

Acquisitions Editor: Emily Ekle
Managing Editor: Elizabeth D'Ambrosio
Editorial Assistant: Chris Malone
Editorial Director, Clinical Reference: Michael Wachinger
Production Editor: Katy Whipple, Maryland Composition
International Production Director: Andreas Schabert
Senior Vice President, International Marketing and Sales: Cornelia Schulze
Vice President, Finance and Accounts: Sarah Vanderbilt
President: Brian D. Scanlan
Compositor: Maryland Composition
Printer: Sheridan Press

Library of Congress Cataloging-in-Publication Data

Rawool, Vishakha.
  Hearing conservation : in occupational, recreational, educational, and home
settings / Vishakha Rawool. — 1st ed.
     p. ; cm.
  Includes bibliographical references.
  ISBN 978-1-60406-256-4 (pbk.)
  1. Deafness, Noise induced—Prevention. 2. Ear—Protection. 3.
Noise—Physiological effect. 4. Industrial noise—Health aspects. I.
Title.
  [DNLM: 1. Hearing Loss, Noise-Induced—prevention & control. 2. Ear
Protective Devices. 3. Noise—prevention & control. 4. Noise,
Occupational—adverse effects. WV 270]
  RF293.5.R39 2011
  617.8—dc23
                                        2011025259

Important note: Medical knowledge is ever-changing. As new research and clinical experience broaden our knowledge, changes in treatment and drug therapy may be required. The authors and editors of the material herein have consulted sources believed to be reliable in their efforts to provide information that is complete and in accord with the standards accepted at the time of publication. However, in view of the possibility of human error by the authors, editors, or publisher of the work herein or changes in medical knowledge, neither the authors, editors, nor publisher, nor any other party who has been involved in the preparation of this work, warrants that the information contained herein is in every respect accurate or complete, and they are not responsible for any errors or omissions or for the results obtained from use of such information. Readers are encouraged to confirm the information contained herein with other sources. For example, readers are advised to check the product information sheet included in the package of each drug or device they plan to administer or use to be certain that the information contained in this publication is accurate and that changes have not been made in the recommended dose or in the contraindications for administration. This recommendation is of particular importance in connection with new or infrequently used drugs.

Some of the product names, patents, and registered designs referred to in this book are in fact registered trademarks or proprietary names even though specific reference to this fact is not always made in the text. Therefore, the appearance of a name without designation as proprietary is not to be construed as a representation by the publisher that it is in the public domain.

Printed in United States
978-1-60406-256-4

Contents

Preface

This textbook is written for all professionals who are interested in saving hearing of workers who are exposed to either hazardous noise and/or ototoxins in the workplace. A review of the effects of noise on hearing and health, a discussion of the effects of ototoxins on hearing, and an outline of the key elements of a hearing conservation program are included in Chapter 1. Chapters 2, 3, and 4 are dedicated to the key elements of hearing conservation specified by the Occupational Safety and Health Administration including noise measurements, noise control, and audiological monitoring. Chapter 4 also includes a discussion of audiological monitoring for individuals exposed to ototoxic drugs. Chapter 5 includes procedures for comprehensive audiological, tinnitus, and auditory processing evaluations for workers who need such evaluations based on the results of audiological monitoring tests, subjective complaints, and/or exposure to ototoxic substances in the workplace. Detailed information about current hearing protection and enhancement devices, related regulations, procedures for selecting and fitting the devices, and for training workers in the use of hearing protection devices are included in Chapter 6. Chapter 7 provides a discussion of the education and training aspects of the hearing conservation program. Procedures for evaluating the effectiveness of hearing conservation program are discussed in Chapter 8. Hearing conservation procedures for musicians and treatment strategies for music-induced hearing loss are discussed in Chapter 9. Employees can be exposed to hazardous noise levels in nonwork settings. Therefore, strategies for conserving hearing in nonoccupational settings are detailed in Chapter 10. Information included in Chapter 10 is expected to be useful to all individuals who are interested in saving their hearing and minimizing other effects of noise. Workers who have already suffered from occupational hearing loss may be eligible for worker's compensation, which is discussed in Chapter 11. Workers with hearing loss and tinnitus need to be supported in the workplace and should be provided with appropriate treatment to continue to be efficient employees. Strategies for support and treatment for workers with hearing loss are discussed in Chapter 12. Hearing conservation needs to begin early so that individuals entering the workforce are already familiar with hearing conservation procedures and have adopted healthy hearing habits. Therefore, hearing conservation in educational settings is discussed in Chapter 13. Chapter 14 provides a discussion of future trends in hearing conservation including the use of antioxidants and gene therapy.

V. W. Rawool

Dedication

This book is dedicated to my parents and Dr. David Goldstein. My parents did their best in ensuring a great educational foundation. My father, Waman, ensured a multilingual vocabulary to enhance the ability to gain knowledge from several resources. My mother, Shobha, encouraged me to write and publish at a very young age. Both of them emphasized self-discipline, which has been very valuable in completing this and other similar projects. Dr. David Goldstein, one of my mentors from Purdue University, was highly instrumental in my acquisition of the doctoral degree and was influential in ensuring a path of clinical research to guarantee high-quality services to individuals with hearing loss.

Chapter 1

Introduction to Ototoxins and Hearing Conservation

Because hearing loss can be acquired by a variety of factors, there are various ways of conserving hearing. Although aging is a major risk factor for hearing loss (Dobie, 2008), many factors can contribute to the development of hearing loss, including certain nutritional deficiencies (Durga, Verhoef, Anteunis, Schouten, & Kok, 2007; Shargorodsky, Curhan, Eavey, & Curhan, 2010); medical conditions such as high cholesterol, increased blood pressure, hyperlipedemia (Chang, Yu, Ho, & Ho, 2007), and diabetes; smoking; heat; vibrations (Soliman, El-Atreby, Tawfik, Holail, Iskandar, & Abou-Setta, 2003; Sutinen, Zou, Hunter, Toppila, & Pyykkö, 2007); solvents; noise; medications; and genetic factors including degree of pigmentation. Individuals who are not exposed to hazardous noise, have healthy diets, and follow a relatively stress-free lifestyle can be expected to have better hearing compared with populations that are exposed to noise, have poorer diets, and higher stress levels (Goycoolea, Goycoolea, Farfan, Rodriguez, Martinez, & Vidal, 1986; Rosen, Bergman, Plester, El-Mofty, & Satti, 1962). Potential basic strategies for hearing conservation are outlined in **Fig. 1.1** and **Table 1.1**. Two of the major preventable reasons for acquired hearing loss are exposure to hazardous noise and other ototoxins. Thus, noise and other ototoxins can be targeted to reduce acquired hearing loss.

Genetics appears to play an important role in age-related hearing loss (Christensen, Frederiksen, & Hoffman, 2001; Karlsson, Harris, & Svartengren, 1997; Unal, Tamer, Doğruer, Yildirim, Vayisoğlu, & Camdeviren, 2005; Viljanen, Era, Kaprio, Pyykkö, Koskenvuo, & Rantanen, 2007). There is an association between maternal family history and moderate to severe hearing loss in women and paternal family history and moderate to severe hearing loss in men. Thus genetic counseling (McMahon, Kifley, Rochtchina, Newall, & Mitchell, 2008) and, possibly in the future, gene therapy may provide a means to reduce some age-related hearing loss. Potential future trends for hearing conservation are presented in Chapter 14.

◆ Auditory System

Students enrolled in doctor of audiology and other relevant programs are often required to take one or more courses to study the delicate structures of the ear and the auditory pathways and their function. The detailed anatomy and physiology of the auditory system is out of scope of this text. However, all individuals who are interested in hearing conservation efforts should familiarize themselves with the anatomy and physiology of the ear. Several online courses are available for this purpose. The courses can be supplemented by additional available materials. For example, a video curriculum package titled "The anatomy, physiology, and diseases of the human ear" is available from the Council for Accreditation in Occupational Hearing Conservation (CAOHC) at www.caohc.org. For basic understanding of the anatomy and physiology of the cochlea, the Website devised by Remy Pujol called "Promenade 'round the Cochlea" can also be viewed (www.neuroreille.com/promenade/english/). Animated illustrations of the physiology of the ear are also available from the Department of Neurophysiology at the University of Wisconsin (www.neurophys.wisc.edu/~ychen/auditory/fs.auditory.html).

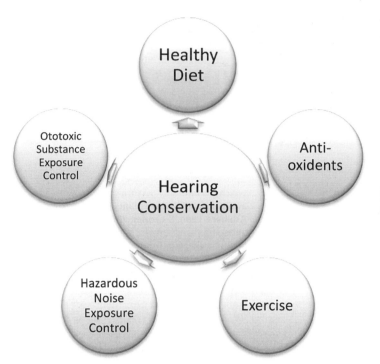

Fig. 1.1 Basic strategies for hearing conservation.

◆ Effects of Noise on the Outer Ear

The key structures of the outer ear include the auricle, the external auditory canal or meatus, and the outer side of the tympanic membrane (**Fig. 1.2**). The eardrum can rupture and bleed with extremely high noise exposure such as blast injuries (Kerr & Byrne, 1975). One of the U.S. Army hospitals in Germany treated 564 troops between March 2003 and May 2004. Among them, 327 suffered from sudden blast exposures. Perforated eardrums were noted in 104 of these individuals (Teufert-Autrey, 2004). Up to 60% of the population with clinically significant blast injuries may suffer from tympanic membrane perforations (DePalma, Burris, Champion, & Hodgson, 2005) depending on the type of bomb and distance from the blast explosion.

◆ Effects of Noise on the Middle Ear

The key structures of the middle ear include the inner side of the tympanic membrane and the three ossicles called the malleus, incus, and stapes. The footplate of the stapes is attached to the oval window (**Fig. 1.3**). With excessive noise exposure such as blast injuries, dislocation of ossicles can occur (Sudderth, 1974).

◆ Effects of Noise on the Cochlea

The key structures of the cochlea are shown in **Fig. 1.4**. In the presence of hazardous low-level noise exposure over relatively shorter time periods, the stereocilia on the top of hair cells may swell, fuse, or have a distorted shape (Stopp, 1982). Other changes related to sensory hair cells include increase in intracellular calcium (Fridberger & Ulfendahl, 1996) and significant decrease in the stiffness of the stereocilliary bundles and outer hair cells. Cochlear histopathological changes that are associated with temporary threshold shifts include buckling of pillar bodies (Nordmann, Bohne, & Harding, 2000), distortion of hair cells (Liberman & Dodds, 1987), edema in the stria vascularis, and vasoconstrictions in the spiral ligament (Hawkins, 1971). If hair cell injury is minimal, hair cells can recover, and the auditory threshold shift is only temporary.

In the presence of hazardous but moderate-level noise exposure, damage is apparent in mammalian ears in the organ of Corti, stria

Table 1.1 Potential Strategies for Reducing Age-Related Hearing Loss in Humans

Rationale	Strategy	Treatment
Creation of toxic-free radicals or reactive oxygen species (Jiang, Talaska, Schacht, & Sha, 2007) due to increase in metabolic activity and/or aging can cause hearing loss.	Improve the cochlea's antioxidant defense system	Create augmented acoustic environment or stimulation with clearly audible but not hazardously loud complex background noise (Tanaka, Bielefeld, Chen, Li, & Henderson, 2009) Administer antioxidant supplements
Caloric restriction can delay or reduce age-related hearing loss (Seidman 2000; Sweet, Price, & Henry, 1988; Willott, Erway, Archer, & Harrison, 1995) possibly due to reduction in metabolic rate, upregulation of the sirtuin pathway, decrease in oxidative stress and glucoregulation, decrease in dietic fat, and maintenance of protein turnover rate.	Restrict consumed calories	Restrict caloric intake by adopting diets that contain foods that are low in calories such as vegetables and certain types of fish Stimulate the effects of calorie restriction with reseveratrol (trans-3,5,40-trihydroxystibene), which is a naturally occurring phytoalexin available from various plants (Burns, Yokota, Ashihara, Lean, & Crozier, 2002) and is a known antiaging (Barger, Kayo, Vann, et al., 2008) agent. It may also reduce noise-induced hearing loss (Seidman, Babu, Tang, Naem, & Quirk, 2003)
Regular exercise improves cardiovascular health and blood supply to the cochlea and thus slows down some forms of age-related declines including hearing loss. It can also lead to faster recovery from noise-induced temporary threshold shifts (Ismail, Corrigan, MacLeod, Anderson, Kasten, & Elliott, 1973; Kolkhorst, Smaldino, Wolf, et al., 1998).	Regular exercise	Adopt a regular exercise routine including muscle training and cardiovascular exercises (Cristell, Hutchinson, & Alessio, 1998; Hutchinson, Alessio, Hoppes, Gruner, Sanker, & Ambrose, 2000)
Exposure to hazardous levels of occupational and nonoccupational noise can cause or augment hearing loss.	Avoid exposure to hazardous noise levels	Monitor and control noise and ensure proper use of hearing protection devices in occupational and nonoccupational settings when noise control strategies are ineffective
Exposure to hazardous levels of other ototoxic substances can cause or augment hearing loss.	Avoid exposure to ototoxic substances	Control abuse of prescription and nonprescription ototoxic drugs In occupational settings, monitor and control exposure to ototoxic substances When ototoxic medications are necessary, supplement with antioxidants

vascularis, spiral ligament, and the afferent neurons. In the presence of extremely high-level exposures approximating 125–130 dB sound pressure level (SPL), the hair cell loss increases rapidly due to mechanical damage to the reticular lamina, disruption of the endolymphatic compartment including the organ of Corti, and mechanical damage to hair cells (Hamernik, Turrentine, & Wright, 1984). For impulse or impact noises, extensive damage may occur at lower sound levels (Qiu, Davis, & Hamernik, 2007). Some of the possible mechanisms for outer hair cell loss include metabolic exhaustion (Lim & Dunn, 1979), ischemia (Hawkins, 1971; Quirk & Seidman, 1995), elevated levels of potassium, and generation of free oxygen radicals (Yamane, Nakai, Takayama, Iguchi, Nakagawa, & Kojima, 1995).

◆ Effects of Noise on the Auditory Nerve

Intense sound stimulation can cause excessive release of the neurotransmitter glutamate by inner hair cells into synapses of the auditory nerve fibers. This can produce swelling and loss of auditory neuron terminals. Swelling of afferent nerve fibers is associated with temporary

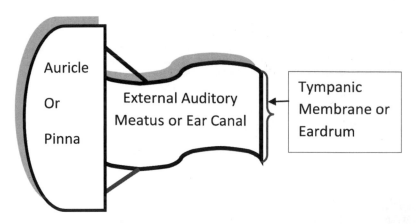

Fig. 1.2   Schematic of outer ear.

threshold shift (Robertson, 1983). Degeneration of the cochlear nerve can continue after acute loss of afferent nerve terminals following hazardous noise exposure associated with moderate reversible loss of hearing sensitivity (Kujawa & Liberman, 2009).

◆ Effects of Noise on the Central Auditory System

The central auditory system can show tonotopic reorganization and neural hyperactivity due to reduced output from the cochlea. When a region in the cochlea is dead or silent following loss of outer and inner hair cells, the subset of neurons that correspond to the particular region or frequencies do not receive any stimulation. After a few weeks these neurons begin to respond to frequencies that are associated with cochlear regions surrounding the damaged area. Such tonotopic reorganization is apparent in the cochlear nucleus (Kaltenbach, Czaja, & Kaplan, 1992), inferior colliculus (Salvi, Wang, & Powers, 1996), and auditory cortex (Robertson & Irvine, 1989; Willott, Aitkin, & McFadden, 1993). One possible mechanism for this reorganization is functional

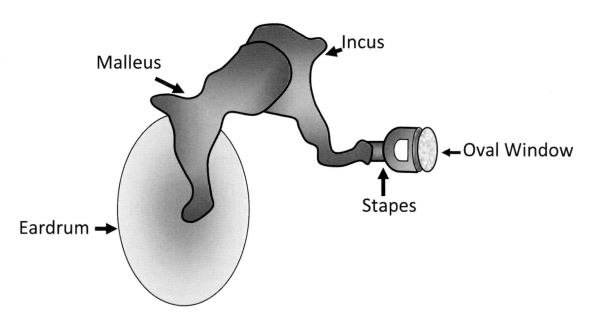

Fig. 1.3   Schematic of the structures in the middle ear.

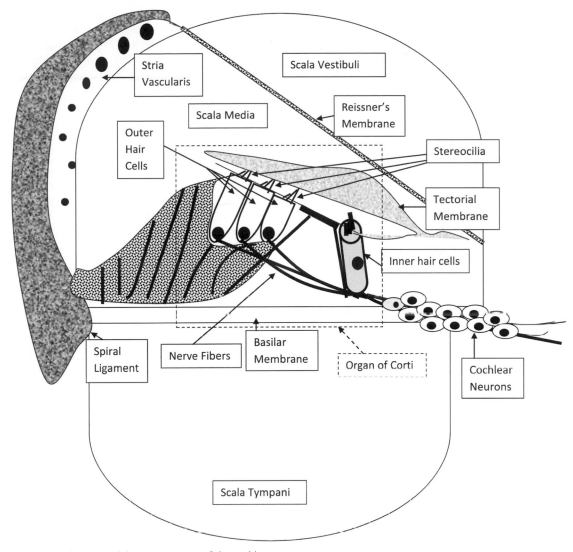

Fig. 1.4 Schematic of the cross-section of the cochlea.

activation of pre-existing excitatory synapses with a potential for being tuned to several different frequencies (Wang, Caspary, & Salvi, 2000).

The central auditory system also appears to compensate for the reduced cochlear output due to noise-induced hearing loss (NIHL) by increasing the gain or by becoming hyperactive. One reason for the hyperactivity may be the loss of gamma-aminobutyric acid–mediated inhibition (Salvi, Wang, & Ding, 2000; Szczepaniak & Møller, 1995). Other excitatory and inhibitory neurotransmitters may also be involved in increasing the gain (Suneja, Potashner, & Benson, 1998).

◆ Effects of Hazardous Noise on Hearing Function

Reduced Audibility

When individuals are exposed to hazardous levels of noise and cochlear structures are exhausted or damaged, the auditory sensitivity can change. The different types of changes in auditory sensitivity that can occur and the associated terms are shown in **Table 1.2**. The presence of high levels of noise can interfere with speech communication on the job, and

Table 1.2 Types of Changes in Auditory Sensitivity Following Noise Exposure

Term	Description
Noise induced threshold shift	Worsening of auditory thresholds due to exposure to hazardous noise levels.
Temporary threshold shift	Temporary change in auditory sensitivity with return of the auditory thresholds to prenoise exposure levels.
Permanent threshold shift	Auditory thresholds remain worse after the noise exposure or do not show any recovery over time.
Compound threshold shift	Auditory thresholds show some recovery but continue to be worse than those obtained prior to the noise exposure. Thus, the threshold shift after noise exposure has a temporary and a permanent component.

hearing loss can worsen the communication difficulties.

Tinnitus or Ringing

Exposure to loud noise and or other ototoxic substances can cause tinnitus. There is a consistent noise dose-dependent relationship between noise exposure and tinnitus in the presence of a hearing loss (Rubak, Kock, Koefoed-Nielsen, Lund, Bonde, & Kolstad, 2008). Tinnitus might be more persistent than hearing loss following occupational noise exposure and may occur even after the use of stricter hearing protection regulations (Mrena, Savolainen, Kiukaanniemi, Ylikoski, & Mäkitie, 2009).

Diplacusis

When a tone of a specific single frequency is presented to the two ears, the pitch perception of that tone can be very different in the two ears for some individuals. This is referred to as *diplacusis* and can interfere with music perception (see Chapter 9).

Hyperacusis

The term *hyperacusis* is used to describe discomfort or annoyance associated with sound levels that are not considered uncomfortable by most other individuals with normal hearing. It is often associated with hearing loss. The most common cause of hyperacusis appears to be exposure to loud sounds and more specifically exposure to loud music (see Chapter 9; Anari, Axelsson, Eliasson, & Magnusson, 1999).

Distortion

Distortion can be defined as pure tones, overtones, and/or harmonics that are not perceived in their original form but seem to be distorted, unclear, fuzzy, and/or out of tune (Kähärit, Zachau, Eklöf, Sandsjö, & Möller, 2003). Some individuals also perceive distortion of speech sounds.

◆ Factors Increasing the Risk of Noise-Induced Hearing Loss

There is considerable variability in susceptibility to noise due to several factors including age, gender, race, genetics, high blood pressure, high cholesterol, smoking, heat, vibration, and white fingers (see case-history form in the Appendix of Chapter 4). For workers who have fewer than two confounding factors out of four key factors (use of analgesics, blood pressure, cholesterol levels, smoking), occupational noise exposure primarily determines the development of NIHL. As the number of confounders increases, other factors become prominent in causing hearing loss (Toppila, Pyykkö, & Starck, 2001). In addition, genetic mutations may increase the susceptibility of some individuals to hearing loss from exposure to noise (Konings, Van Laer, Wiktorek-Smagur, et al., 2009; Lin, Wu, Shih, Tsai, Sun, & Guo, 2009; Sliwinska-Kowalska, Noben-Trauth, Pawelczyk, & Kowalski, 2008). Exposure to other substances such as asphyxiants (carbon monoxide), drugs (prescriptive or nonprescriptive), metals (arsenic), and solvents (xylene) can cause hearing loss and/or augment NIHL. As an example of the effects of ototoxic substances and noise exposure, **Fig. 1.5** shows the audiogram of a 33-year-old man with opiate abuse. **Figure 1.6** shows the audiogram of a 38-year-old man with a history of opiate addiction and occupational noise exposure, and

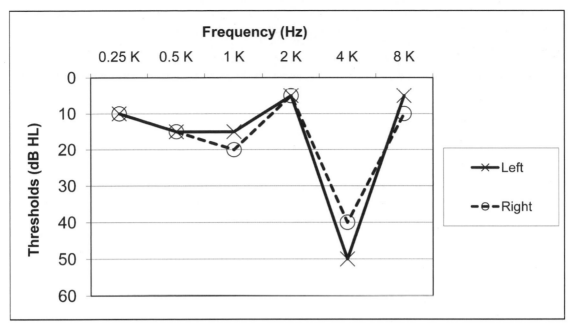

Fig. 1.5 Air conduction thresholds of a 33-year-old man with opiate abuse.

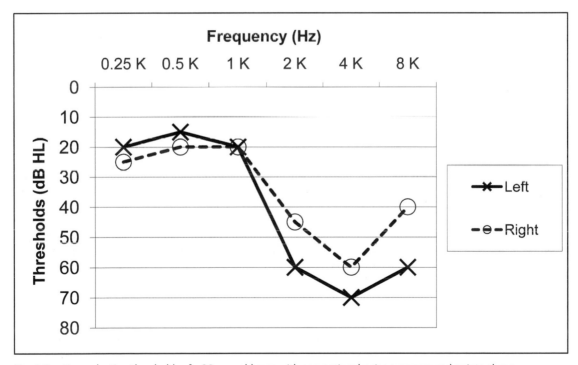

Fig. 1.6 Air conduction thresholds of a 38-year-old man with occupational noise exposure and opiate abuse.

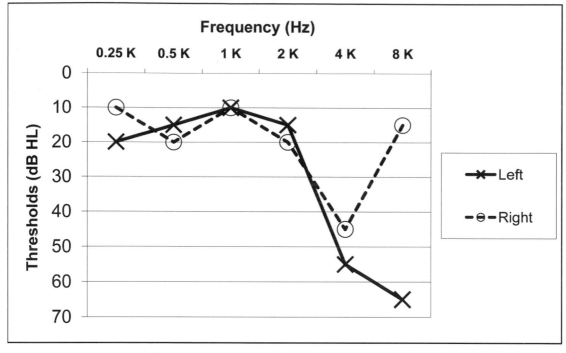

Fig. 1.7 Air conduction thresholds of a 47-year-old man with occupational and recreational noise exposure and opiate abuse.

Figure 1.7 shows the audiogram of a 47-year-old man with a history of recreational noise exposure in addition to occupational noise exposure and opiate addiction. Three of the factors that increase susceptibility to NIHL are discussed in greater detail subsequently.

Age

When workers are matched for blood pressure, cholesterol, smoking, use of analgesics, and noise exposure levels, older individuals appear to be more susceptible to NIHL than younger individuals (Toppila, Pyykkö, & Starck, 2001). Also, older individuals are more susceptible to other risk factors for hearing loss such as smoking (El Zir, Mansour, Salameh, & Chahine, 2008). Part of the greater susceptibility to NIHL in older individuals may be related to lower rate-induced facilitation of acoustic reflex thresholds at higher stimulus rates compared with younger individuals (Rawool, 1996a). A robust acoustic reflex can provide some protection from impulse types of stimuli, especially to those individuals in whom the reflex is maintained for a longer period without fatigue and in individuals in whom the reflex becomes stronger over a short period (Rawool, 1996b).

Amount of Pigmentation

The pigmentation in humans and animals is determined by melanin; it is present in cells in the cochlear duct, the stria vascularis, Reissner membrane, and the modiolus. Melanin may be able to compensate for the inactivation of dehydrogenase resulting from exposure to hazardous sounds. There is a correlation between the amount of melanin in the inner ear and iris. Thus, the color of the iris may provide an index of vulnerability to NIHL. Among noise-exposed workers, fair-eyed (blue, hazel, green, or gray) workers have significantly worse audiometric thresholds than dark-eyed (black or dark or light brown) workers, while no such differences are apparent in non-noise–exposed workers (Da Costa, Castro, & Macedo, 2008). Similarly, white workers have worse auditory thresholds than non-white workers (Ishii & Talbott, 1998).

Smoking

Some investigators have reported that smoking by itself is not a risk factor for hearing loss, but it can be in combination with other factors such as use of analgesics (Starck, Toppila, & Pyykkö, 1999). However, other studies suggest that workers exposed to occupational noise who smoke are at a greater risk of developing hearing loss than nonsmokers (Agrawal, Niparko, & Dobie, 2010; Mizoue, Miyamoto, & Shimizu, 2003; Wild, Brewster, & Banerjee, 2005). Cruickshanks, Klein, Klein, Wiley, Nondahl, and Tweed (1998) investigated 3753 participants to determine the effects of smoking on hearing loss. Smoking history was obtained through self-report, and hearing loss was defined as a pure tone average (0.5, 1, 2, and 4 kHz) greater than 25 dB hearing level in the worse ear. After adjustments for age and other factors, current smokers were 1.69 times as likely to have a hearing loss as nonsmokers. Cruickshanks et al. (1998) suggested direct ototoxic effects on hair cell function due to the presence of nicotine-like receptors in animal hair cells and also indirect effects affecting the blood supply of the cochlea. Furthermore, tobacco smoke contains hydrogen cyanide, an asphyxiant (European Agency for Safety and Health at Work, 2009) that can impair the function of the stria vascularis under severe exposure.

◆ Nonauditory Effects of Noise

Noise does not only have deleterious effects on the structure and function of the auditory system. It can have several other effects, some of which are described below.

Job Productivity

Exposure to hazardous levels of noise can reduce the job productivity of workers due to various reasons. Noise can interfere with the ability to communicate for both work and social exchange purposes. It can interfere with the ability to concentrate on work, especially when the task is complicated or involves the use of multiple sensory modalities. It can also lead to excessive fatigue and slow recovery from fatigue.

Annoyance

Working in noisy conditions can lead to annoyance or irritability, which in turn may lead to more aggressive behavior or disputes or arguments over trivial matters. Annoyance is not always related to high levels of noise. For example, annoyance from the sound of wind turbines appears to be related to attitude toward wind energy and/or wind turbines in the landscape and to the visibility of a wind farm. In addition, residents who receive economic benefits from wind turbines are generally not annoyed, but residents without any benefits are annoyed by wind turbines more than by similar sound levels generated by other noise sources such as road traffic or air traffic. A nonacoustical measure to reduce noise annoyance in such cases is to involve community residents in the planning of the wind farm and allowing them to share the benefits (van den Berg, 2009).

Accidents

Occupational noise has been associated with worker accidents; the accidents are more likely to occur when workers suffer from hearing loss. Use of hearing protection devices that provide overprotection may interfere with the ability to hear verbal instructions and warnings. Noise levels above 90 dBA time weighted average (TWA) can compromise worker safety, and individuals with poorer average hearing at 3, 4, and 6 kHz due to noise exposure are at greater risks for accidents. Workers with severe hearing loss with 90 dBA or greater TWA are three times more likely to have multiple accidents (Girard, Picard, Davis, et al., 2009). Overall, approximately 12% of accidents may be related to noise exposure above 90 dBA and NIHL (Picard, Girard, Simard, Larocque, Leroux, & Turcotte, 2008).

Other Health Effects of Noise and Solvents

Noise can lead to sleep disturbances and increase in blood pressure and heart rate. Occasionally, impulse types of noises can lead to a perilymph fistula (Kung & Sataloff, 2006) due to rupture of the round or oval window resulting from sudden increase in the middle ear pressure (Goodhill, 1971). Chronic exposure to solvents can lead to chronic solvent encephalopathy (CSE), which is characterized by mild to severe cognitive impairments and diffuse pain and sleeping difficulties.

Neuroradiological techniques have demonstrated dose-related neuropathology in workers with CSE, which is correlated with performance on tasks involving attention and psychomotor speed (Visser, Lavini, Booij, et al., 2008). Some studies suggest that current exposure to some solvent conditions may induce or aggravate sleep disordered breathing (Viaene, Vermeir, & Godderis, 2009).

◆ Ototoxins and Their Interactions with Noise

Substances that can cause hearing loss are referred to as ototoxins. Employers should give specific attention to the interactive effects of work-related ototoxic substances and noise on worker's safety and health in conducting risk evaluations (European Union Directive, 2003) and in providing workers' compensation (Work-Cover Australia, 2001). Ototoxins that show evidence of ototoxicity include asphyxiants (carbon monoxide), drugs (some chemotherapy agents, antibiotics, and aspirin and related medications), metals (arsenic, organic tin, mercury and derivatives, and manganese), and solvents (carbon disulfide, ethylbenzene, n-propylbenzene, toluene, n-hexane, styrene and methylstyrenes, trichloroethylene, and p-xylene) (European Agency for Safety and Health at Work, 2009). Ototoxic chemicals include hydrogen cyanide, diesel fuel, kerosene fuel, jet fuel, jet propellant 8 fuel, organophosphate pesticides, and chemical warfare nerve agents (U.S. Army Center for Health Promotion and Preventive Medicine, 2003). Ototoxins and noise can interact in worsening hearing loss, and the interactions can be synergistic or additive. Additive effects are predictable from the sum of the effects of exposure to noise or ototoxin alone. Synergistic effects are greater than those that can be predicted from the sum of the exposure to each of the agents.

Chemical Asphyxiants

Chemical asphyxiants such as carbon monoxide reduce oxygen delivery to tissues or oxygen use by tissues. The resultant oxidative stress leads to overproduction of unstable and reactive oxygen species that can damage cochlear cells. Excessive glutamate release is apparent in the synapses under the inner hair cells from carbon monoxide ototoxicity (Kanthasamy, Borowitz, Pavlakovic, & Isom, 1994; Liu & Fechter, 1995). Exacerbation of hearing loss beyond that caused by noise alone can occur at exposure levels of 200 ppm (Fechter, Chen, Rao, & Larabee, 2000; Rao & Fechter, 2000). Carbon monoxide poisoning after short-term exposure can cause sensorineural hearing loss with full or partial recovery (Shahbaz Hassan, Ray, & Wilson, 2003; Razzaq, Dumbala, & Moudgil, 2010). Firefighters, foundry workers, miners, toll and tunnel workers, and vehicle mechanics have the potential to be exposed to excessive levels of carbon monoxide (Pouyatos & Fechter, 2007).

Heavy Metals

Some heavy metals have toxic effects on the body, including the auditory system. Ototoxic effects of such metals can occur in both occupational and nonoccupational (see Chapter 10) settings. Some of the ototoxic metals are discussed in the following section.

Lead

Lead is a natural bluish-gray metal. Exposure to lead can occur from breathing workplace air or dust and consuming contaminated water or food (see Chapter 10). Lead is released in the environment through the burning of fossil fuels, mining, and the production of batteries, ammunition, metal products (solder and pipes), and X-ray shielding devices. Lead can damage kidneys and the reproductive system. It is also neuro- and ototoxic (Bleecker, Ford, Lindgren, Scheetz, & Tiburzi, 2003; Discalzi, Capellaro, Bottalo, Fabbro, & Mocellini, 1992; Osman, Pawlas, Schütz, Gazdzik, Sokal, & Vahter, 1999; Wu, Shen, Lai, et al., 2000). Blood lead levels of greater than 7 μg/dL are significantly associated with hearing loss in the 3 to 8 kHz range (Hwang, Chiang, Yen-Jean, & Wang, 2009).

Mercury (Methyl Mercury Chloride, Mercuric Sulfide)

Metallic mercury is a silvery odorless liquid (as seen in thermometers) that changes to a colorless and odor-free gas after heating. Mercury salts (crystals) or inorganic mercury compounds are formed when mercury combines with other elements, such as chlorine, sulfur, or oxygen. Organic mercury compounds are formed when mercury combines with carbon. Exposure to mercury can occur from breathing air contaminated by mercury or from skin contact with mercury. Metallic mercury is used in the production of chlorine gas, caustic soda, thermometers, and mercury batteries. The Occupational Safety and Health Administration (OSHA) limit for organic mercury is 0.1 mg for each cubic meter of workplace air (0.1 mg/m³) and 0.05 mg/m³ of metallic mercury vapor during 8-hour work shifts, assuming a 40-hour work week. High-level mercury exposure can damage the nervous system, kidneys, and developing fetus. Mercury can more easily affect the brain in the methyl mercury and metallic mercury vapor forms, increasing the risk of injury (U.S. Department of Health and Human Services [USHHS], Agency for Toxic Substances and Disease Registry [ATSDR], 1999a). Mercury compounds such as methyl mercury chloride and mercuric sulfide are ototoxic in animals; organic mercury poisoning in humans can also be toxic to the auditory system (Chuu, Hsu, & Lin-Shiau, 2001; Musiek & Hanlon, 1999; Rice, 1998; Rice & Gilbert, 1992). Children who accidentally consumed bread made from seeds that were coated with mercury as a fungicide for plantation showed audiological impairment (Amin-zaki, Majeed, Clarkson, & Greenwood, 1978). Andean children who were exposed to mercury vapor from gold mining operations showed auditory brainstem abnormalities (Counter, 2003). Long-term methyl mercury exposure appears to delay auditory brainstem response (ABR) latencies with incomplete recovery (Murata, Weihe, Budtz-Jørgensen, Jørgensen, & Grandjean, 2004). Potential exposure to mercury in nonoccupational settings is discussed in Chapter 10.

Tin

An acute limbic-cerebellar syndrome including hearing loss has been reported in six industrial workers who had inhaled trimethyltin (Besser, Krämer, Thümler, Bohl, Gutmann, & Hopf, 1987).

Germanium (Germanium Dioxide)

Hearing loss due to degeneration of the stria vascularis and the cochlear supporting cells has been noted in guinea pigs following oral administration of germanium dioxide (100 mg/kg/day for 4 weeks and 0.5% in food for 2 months,

respectively) (Yamasoba, Goto, Komaki, Mimaki, Sudo, & Suzuki, 2006). Brainstem transmission changes are apparent in rats following exposure to germanium dioxide (Lin, Chen, & Chen, 2009).

Organic Solvents

Exposure to organic solvents can occur in various ways as alcohol, in paints and adhesives, and in heating (propane, kerosene) and automotive (diesel, gasoline) fuels. Workers are most frequently exposed to a mixture consisting mainly of xylene, toluene, and methyl ethyl ketone. However, some workers like those in the glass-fiber reinforced plastic industry are exposed to only styrene, and some like those in the rotogravure printing industry are exposed to only toluene (Sliwinska-Kowalska, Prasher, Rodrigues, et al., 2007).

Toxic exposure to solvents can cause pulmonary edema, peripheral and central neural system damage, cancer, and liver and kidney failure (Styger, 2009). Solvent exposure increases the risk of high-frequency hearing loss (Rabinowitz, Galusha, Slade, et al., 2008). Exposure to jet fuel, which contains ototoxins such as n-hexane, n-heptanes, toluene, and xylene, increases the adjusted odds of a permanent hearing loss when it is combined with noise exposure during the first 12 years of exposure. The adjusted odds of hearing loss increase by 70% with 3 years of exposure and by 140% with 12 years of exposure (Kaufman, LeMasters, Olsen, & Succop, 2005). However, under some circumstances, the hearing loss may be mostly dominated by NIHL (Sliwinska-Kowalska, Prasher, Rodrigues, et al., 2007). Although the major damage particularly during coexposure is to the cochlea, solvents may compromise the protective role played by the middle-ear acoustic reflex, thus exposing the inner ear to higher noise levels (Campo, Maguin, & Lataye, 2007; Lataye, Maguin, & Campo, 2007; Maguin, Campo, & Parietti-Winkler, 2009). Solvent exposure can also cause poor performance on the dichotic digits test, suggesting central binaural deficits (Fuente, Slade, Taylor, et al., 2009). Some of the ototoxic solvents are discussed subsequently.

Styrene

Styrene is a colorless, oily liquid that evaporates easily. It has a sweetish aroma; chemicals are usually added to it, causing an unpleasant odor.

It is absorbed through skin or airways and is metabolized mainly as mandelic acid and phenylglyoxylic acid. It can cause damage to several organs including mucosa, liver, kidneys, respiratory system, and the central nervous system. According to the International Agency for Research on Cancer, styrene has the potential to cause cancer in humans. Examples of industries that can expose workers to styrene are plastics, glass-fiber reinforced plastics (e.g., wash basins), synthetic rubber, insulators, and some agricultural products. Exposure to styrene can also occur from breathing air that is contaminated with styrene vapors from building materials, tobacco smoke, use of copying machines, and automobile exhaust. Other means of exposure include drinking or bathing in contaminated water or eating food packaged in polystyrene containers.

According to the U.S. Environmental Protection Agency, lifetime daily exposure to 0.1 ppm styrene is expected to be safe. U.S. Food and Drug Administration regulations do not allow styrene concentration in bottled drinking water exceeding 0.1 ppm. Occupational exposure limits for styrene are usually higher, with 12 ppm in Poland and up to 100 ppm in the United Kingdom (Hoet & Lison, 2008). In the United States, OSHA (1997) has a permissible exposure limit of 100 ppm for an 8-hour work day, 40-hour work week. Campo and Maguin (2007) have proposed a limit of 30 ppm to protect hearing. Workers who are exposed to both noise and styrene have significantly worse auditory thresholds between 2 and 6 kHz compared with those who are exposed to only noise (Morata, Johnson, Nylen, et al., 2002). Workers who are exposed to a mixture of solvents with styrene as the main component and noise are more likely to have a hearing loss than workers who are exposed to only styrene or only noise (Sliwińska-Kowalska, Zamyslowska-Szmytke, Szymczak, et al., 2003). A high frequency hearing loss can occur even in workers who are exposed to both styrene and noise levels that are just within the permissible limits if the exposure occurs for 5 or more years (Morioka, Miyai, Yamamoto, & Miyashita, 2000).

Toluene

Toluene is a colorless liquid with a distinctive smell. Examples of industries/processes where workers can get exposed to toluene include leather tanning and printing, painting, and where lacquers, dyes, and degreasing agents are used. Toluene can be absorbed through airways, skin, and the digestive tract. It can damage the central nervous system and liver and can irritate the respiratory tract. The biological index of toluene exposure is the rate of benzoic acid excretion in the urine at the end of the day (Sliwinska-Kowalska & Zamylslowska-Szmytke, 2007). The permissible exposure limit for toluene in air can be as low as 27 ppm, as in Poland, to 200 ppm, as allowed in the United States (Hoet & Lison, 2008). The odds ratio estimates for hearing loss are 1.76 (95% confidence interval, 1.00–2.98) times greater for each gram of hippuric acid (main toluene metabolite) per gram of creatinine in rotogravure printing workers who are exposed to an organic solvent mixture of toluene, ethyl acetate, and ethanol (Morata, Fiorini, Fischer, et al., 1997). Combined exposure to noise and toluene can be more damaging compared with exposure to either noise or toluene alone (Chang, Chen, Lien, & Sung, 2006; Morata, Dunn, Kretschmer, Lemasters, & Keith, 1993). Stapedius reflex decay (Morata, Dunn, Kretschmer, Lemasters, & Keith, 1993) and auditory brainstem response abnormalities (Vrca, Karacić, Bozicević, Bozikov, & Malinar, 1996) have been noted in workers who are exposed to toluene. Based on repeated monitoring of the German printing industry for 5 years, Schäper, Seeber, and van Thriel (2008) found no effect of toluene on auditory thresholds. The average exposure levels in this study for toluene in the printing area was 25.7 (plus or minus 20.1) and for the end-processing area it was 3.2 (plus or minus 3.1) ppm. Thus, average exposure levels of less than 50 ppm may not be toxic to human hearing.

n-Hexane

n-hexane is a colorless volatile liquid with a disagreeable smell. A very high percentage of n-hexane can be absorbed by inhalation; it is then distributed to tissues and organs rich in lipids such as the brain, peripheral nerves, liver, spleen, kidneys, and adrenal glands. Workers in textile, furniture, printing, and shoe industries can get exposed to n-hexane along with other solvents, especially in the presence of poor air ventilation. Special glues used in the roofing and leather industries, quick-drying glues used in various hobbies, gasoline, and rubber cement contain n-hexane (USHHS ATSDR, 1999b).

Solvents containing n-hexane are used to extract vegetable oils from crops such as soybeans. Chronic low-dose n-hexane exposure such as that apparent in industrial workers can cause axonal loss with sensory impairment. Subacute high-dose n-hexane exposure such as that apparent in glue sniffers is also neurotoxic and can cause swelling of axons with secondary demyelination, peripheral neuropathy, muscle wasting, and weakness (Huang, 2008; Kuwabara, Kai, Nagase, & Hattori, 1999). Workers who receive moderate exposure to n-hexane and toluene are more likely to have hearing loss compared with the nonexposed population. The risk of hearing loss is greater in workers who are exposed to noise in addition to these solvents (Sliwinska-Kowalska, Zamyslowska-Szmytke, Szymczak, et al., 2005). The exposure to n-hexane can affect the auditory nervous system beyond the cochlea (Howd, Rebert, Dickinson, & Pryor, 1983) due to its neurotoxic effects. Auditory brainstem transmission time (wave I–V interpeak interval) is longer in patients with n-hexane neuropathies (Chang, 1987).

Xylene

Xylene is a colorless aromatic volatile liquid that can take three forms or isomers: *meta*-xylene, *ortho*-xylene, and *para*-xylene (*m*-, *o*-, and *p*-xylene). Xylene occurs naturally in petroleum and coal tar. Xylene exposure can occur through inhalation or skin contact. Workers in paint, biomedical laboratories, metal, furniture, and automobile garage industries can be exposed to xylene. The OSHA limit for xylene is 100 ppm for workplace air for 8-hour shifts, but other countries such as Denmark have a lower limit of 35 ppm. The biological marker for xylene exposure is the detection of methylhippuric acid in urine. High exposure levels can cause dizziness and confusion. Draper and Bamiou (2009) reported a patient with xylene exposure with no other risk factors who had normal otoacoustic emissions but absent auditory brainstem response and acoustic reflexes, suggesting auditory neuropathy. The patient's auditory complaints of difficulty hearing in complex surroundings and complex stimuli such as music began following xylene exposure. The prevalence of hearing loss among workers in a liquefied petroleum gas infusion factory can be as high as 56.8% (Chang & Chang, 2009) in the presence of relatively low noise doses.

Minimizing Solvent Exposure

Exploration of the use of less toxic compounds needs to continue in the future as a preventative measure. Other preventative measures include reduction to exposures by engineering controls to reduce environmental concentrations, improving general dilution ventilation or local exhaust ventilation, and reducing the permissible exposure limits. For example, the permissible exposure limit for noise can be reduced to 8-hour TWA of 80 dBA in the presence of simultaneous exposure to organic solvents (Campo & Maguin, 2007). Personal protective equipment such as respirators may be used when engineering controls are not technically feasible or are insufficient and need to be supplemented.

Ototoxic Medications

Several drugs can cause hearing loss (European Agency for Safety and Health at Work, 2009). Thus, workers exposed to noise who are on these medications can suffer additional hearing loss. Hearing loss due to these medications begins at higher frequencies, and with continuous ingestion the loss can progress to lower frequencies. Ingestion of multiple ototoxic medications can lead to more severe damage due to damage to multiple structures in the cochlea. For further details about ototoxic medications, see Chapter 10. As an example, several case reports suggest that some individuals are susceptible to hearing loss from excessive consumption of opioids. A combination of noise and opium exposure is possible in occupational settings, such as military service, or recreational settings. Rawool and Dluhy (2010) evaluated auditory sensitivity of individuals with a history of opium abuse and/or occupational or nonoccupational noise exposure. Twenty three men who reported opiate abuse served as participants in the study. Four of the individuals reported no history of noise exposure, twelve reported hobby-related noise exposure, and seven reported occupational noise exposure, including two who also reported hobby-related noise exposure. Fifty percent (2/4) of the individuals without any noise exposure had a hearing loss, confirming previous reports that some of the population is vulnerable to the ototoxic effects of opioid abuse. The percentage of the population with hearing loss increased with hobby-related (58%)

and occupational noise exposure (100%). Mixed multivariate analysis of variance revealed a significant ear, frequency, and noise exposure interaction. Health professionals need to be aware of the possible ototoxic effects of opioids, as early detection of hearing loss from opium abuse may lead to cessation of abuse and further progression of hearing loss. The possibility that opium abuse may interact with noise exposure in determining auditory thresholds needs to be considered in individuals exposed to noise who are addicted to opiates.

◆ Occupations with Potentially Hazardous Noise Exposure

The National Institute of Occupational Safety and Health (NIOSH) (1998) noted several occupations in which workers are exposed to hazardous noise including agriculture, mining, construction, manufacturing and utilities, transportation, and military. Typically, men are most affected by loud noise during jobs involving agriculture, construction, forestry, manufacturing of metal, and mining. Women are more exposed to medium-level noise in occupations such as education, health care, and call centers. Some of the occupational settings where hazardous noise exposure can occur are discussed in the following section.

Acoustic Shock in Call Center Operators

The term *acoustic shock* describes the physiological and psychological symptoms experienced after being exposed to a sudden, unexpected, and very loud sound referred to as an acoustic incident through a telephone headset or handset (European Agency for Safety and Health at Work, 2005). Noise exposure studies have been conducted on call center operators and telephone operators because of potential exposure to hazardous noise from fax machines or due to acoustic feedback through headsets. The overall risk of hearing loss in call center operators may be relatively low (Patel & Broughton, 2002) depending on the particular setting. In noisy call centers, the telephone operators may have to turn up the volume to be able to conduct conversations. In addition to temporary or permanent loss of hearing, acoustic shock may lead to tinnitus, headaches, fatigue, and anxiety (European

Agency for Safety and Health at Work, 2005; Patuzzi, Millhinch, & Doyle, 2000).

Construction

The estimated percentage of workers exposed to noise within the construction industry (NIOSH, 1998) is shown in **Fig. 1.8**. Some construction workers are exposed to very high levels of noise depending on the tools being used. For example, a power-activated nailer can generate noise levels of as high as 128 dBA (Rawool, 2008). Even during a short period of 3 years of work, recordable loss of hearing function can occur in construction workers who are exposed to an average of 90 dBA noise (Seixas, Goldman, Sheppard, Neitzel, Norton, & Kujawa, 2005). Suggestions for controlling construction noise (Eaton, 2000) are outlined in **Fig. 1.9**. Additional information about construction noise and noise control measures is provided in Chapters 3 and 10.

Forestry and Fishing

Forest workers, more specifically those who operate chain saws, can suffer from significant hearing loss, which is most prominent at 4 kHz (Tunay & Melemez, 2008). Equipment used by fishing vessels can produce hazardous levels of noise (Bowes & Corn, 1990). Fishermen often work for extended hours and can be exposed to high levels of noise (Neitzel, Berna, & Seixas, 2006) even when they are not working due to their presence on fishing vessels.

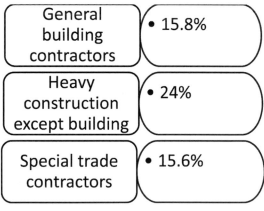

Fig. 1.8   Percentage of construction workers estimated to be exposed to hazardous noise (NIOSH, 1998).

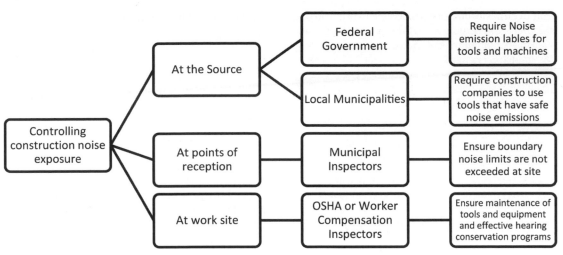

Fig. 1.9 Strategies for controlling construction noise (Eaton, 2000).

Military

Exposure to hazardous noise in the military is significant. Firearms used in the military may produce noise levels of up to 150–180 dB SPL (Ylikoski, Pekkarinen, Starck, Pääkkönen, & Ylikoski, 1995). Hearing loss can occur in the military even with the use of hearing protection devices, and individuals who enter the military with an initial slight hearing loss may have a higher risk of further hearing deterioration either due to greater susceptibility to NIHL or more risky behaviors (Muhr, Månsson, & Hellström, 2006). Individuals may continue to lose hearing after long-term exposure to gunshots, even with the use of dual hearing protection (Wu & Young, 2009). For sailors, time spent on surface warships is more damaging to hearing than that spent performing shore duties. The probability of a standard threshold shift for sailors who spent 15 years of their Navy career aboard a surface warship is 0.48; for those who spent their entire 30-year Navy career in a shore billet, the probability is 0.35 (Trost & Shaw, 2007). Some hearing loss in the military may be unavoidable because of the element of surprise and exposure to other ototoxins such as carbon monoxide. In addition, some noise exposures during war are extremely intense, and in such situations noise can be transmitted to the ears due to skull vibration (Helfer, Jordan, & Lee, 2005). Use of hearing protection devices under such circumstances many increase energy presented to the eardrum due to the occlusion effect.

Manufacturing

According to some estimates, over one-third of all manufacturing workers (5.7 million workers total) are exposed to excessively loud noise (Tak, Davis, & Calvert, 2009). The economic sectors identified under manufacturing are shown in **Table 1.3** (NIOSH, 1998). Twenty five percent of the workers in the manufacturing sector exposed to loud noise may not be using hearing protection devices (Tak, Davis, & Calvert, 2009).

Mining

According to estimates, workers in the mining sector had the highest prevalence of hazardous occupational noise exposure with approximately three out of four workers exposed to hazardous noise between 1999 and 2004 (Tak, Davis, & Calvert, 2009). The mining industry may have the second highest prevalence of hearing loss among all industrial occupations (Tak & Calvert, 2008).

Health Professions

NIHL can occur in health professions. Noise generated by some orthopedic surgical instruments including saws, drills, and hammers can exceed 100 dBA, especially during surgical procedures such as knee replacements. Health professionals such as anesthesiologists,

Table 1.3 Manufacturing Occupations Involving Hazardous Noise Exposure and the Estimated Percentage of Workers (parentheses) Exposed to Hazardous Noise Within Each Economic Sector

Products	Other
Food and kindred (28.9)	Furniture and fixtures (28.3)
Tobacco (54.3)	Printing and publishing (21.4)
Textile mill (42.6)	Primary metal industries (32.7)
Apparel and other finished products (13.9)	Industrial machinery and equipment (14.9)
Lumber and wood (41.3)	Electronic and other electric equipment (8.1)
Paper and allied (33.8)	Transportation equipment (18.2)
Chemicals and allied (33.8)	Miscellaneous manufacturing industries (9.4)
Petroleum and coal (19.9)	
Rubber and miscellaneous (22.8)	
Leather (6.5)	
Stone, clay, and glass (21.5)	
Fabricated metal (29.3)	
Instruments and related (8.7)	

who assist with several orthopedic surgeries in a single day may be at risk for excessive noise dose (Pearlman & Sandidge, 2009). The equipment used by dentists can generate sounds in the range of 60–99 dBA, although brand new equipment appears to be less noisy (Sampaio Fernandes, Carvalho, Gallas, Vaz, & Matos, 2006). Thus, dentists and their assistants in a busy dental clinic may be at risk for hearing loss (Bali, Acharya, & Anup, 2007). The hearing loss is more likely to occur in the left ear of right-handed dentists (Gijbels, Jacobs, Princen, Nackaerts, & Debruyne, 2006; Zubick, Tolentino, & Boffa, 1980).

Large Kitchens

The noise generated by Power Soak dishwashing systems, blenders, and metal-to-metal contact between stainless steel pots, pans, utensils, and metal racks can expose employees in large kitchens to hazardous noise doses. The cooks may be exposed to intermittent impact noise generated by metal-to-metal contact between utensils and industrial-size blenders (Achutan, 2009).

Professional Disc Jockeys

The nightclubs where professional disc jockeys work can range from 93.2–109.7 dBA. Thus, music exposure can lead to temporary threshold shifts, changes in the amplitudes of otoacoustic emissions, and tinnitus (Bray, Szymáski, & Mills, 2004; Santos, Morata, Jacob, Albizu, Marques, & Paini, 2007). For more information about music-induced hearing loss, see Chapter 9.

◆ Noise and Ototoxin Exposure in Nonoccupational Settings

As mentioned previously, exposure to hazardous noise can occur in nonoccupational settings (Rawool, 2008). Recreational noise exposure can worsen hearing loss induced by occupational noise exposure (Agrawal, Niparko, & Dobie, 2010). Ototoxic exposure can also occur in nonoccupational settings. For example, some individuals inhale products (e.g., glues) containing n-hexane because of its euphoric effects, which can cause nerve damage (USHHS ATSDR, 1999b). Noise, ototoxin exposure, and strategies for hearing conservation in nonoccupational settings are discussed in Chapter 10.

◆ Need for Hearing Conservation

Occupational noise exposure is responsible for approximately 16% of disabling hearing loss, with a range of 7 to 21% around the world with greater effects of noise exposure in developing countries (Nelson, Nelson, Concha-Barrientos, & Fingerhut, 2005). Nonoccupational noise exposure (see Chapter 10) can add to this percentage in terms of the number of individuals with hearing loss and severity of hearing loss depending on the type, duration, and degree of nonoccupational noise exposure. Approximately 30 million employees are exposed to dangerous noise levels at work and an additional 9 million workers are at risk for hearing loss from other ototoxins such as metals and solvents (NIOSH, 2004).

According to the U.S. Department of Labor Bureau of Labor Statistics (U.S. Department of Labor, 2009), in 2008 hearing loss was the second most prevalent work-related illness with approximately 22,000 reported cases. The most prevalent service-connected disability for U.S. veterans receiving compensation at the end of fiscal year

2008 was tinnitus (558,232) followed by hearing loss (519,834). Through comprehensive hearing conservation measures the Department of Veterans Affairs saved more than $220 million by decreasing hearing loss disability compensation claims between 1987 and 1997. An additional $140 million was saved by the U.S. Army through reduction of civilian hearing loss compensation between 1986 and 1997 (Ohlin, 1998). One study investigated the effect of stricter hearing protection regulations on tinnitus in the Finnish Defense Forces by comparing subjective symptoms of tinnitus during two periods (before and after stricter hearing conservation regulations). A significantly decreased hazard ratio for constant or disturbing tinnitus was apparent after the initiation of stricter regulations (Mrena, Savolainen, Kiukaanniemi, Ylikoski, & Mäkitie, 2009). When workers suffer from hearing loss due to lack of effective hearing conservation measures, additional cost is associated with treating the hearing loss. Strategies for treating hearing loss and tinnitus are discussed in Chapter 12. If the hearing loss is left untreated, there are several ramifications for the individual, the individual's family, and society.

Effects of Untreated Hearing Loss

Rawool (2008) summarized the effects of untreated hearing loss. Untreated hearing loss is associated with emotional, social, physical, cognitive, and behavioral problems (Mulrow, Aguilar, Endicott, et al., 1990). Individuals with untreated hearing loss are more likely to be tense, irritated, or frustrated during communication and other daily situations. They report feelings of inadequacy in everyday interactions, of being constraining to others, and of being abnormal, prematurely old, or handicapped (Hétu, Jones, & Getty, 1993). Some individuals with hearing loss report experiences of being the object of hurtful jokes or of pity. Because of the feelings of inadequacy and the fear of being ridiculed, older adults with untreated hearing loss may avoid social gatherings. Therefore, hearing loss is associated with reduced socialization and participation in outdoor activities (Gilhome Herbst, Meredith, & Stephens, 1990). Individuals with hearing loss can get physically fatigued when they must ask for repetitions and must pay increased attention when around others who do not have a hearing loss (Hétu, Jones, & Getty, 1993).

Hearing loss can also have an adverse effect on personal safety in nonoccupational settings in addition to occupational settings. Depending on the degree and configuration of hearing loss, some individuals with untreated hearing loss are unable to hear a person walking or riding a bike behind them or a vehicle approaching behind them. While riding a bus, they may not hear the bus conductor announcing the next stop (Hallberg & Barrenäs, 1993). Depending on the severity of the hearing loss, some older individuals may not hear someone entering their home or the telephone or doorbell ringing.

Effects of Untreated Hearing Loss on Significant Others

Hearing loss also affects family and friends. Hétu, Jones, and Getty (1993) reported that untreated hearing loss might cause relationship problems due to misunderstandings arising from not answering questions at all or responding inappropriately. Some significant others may often be required to cope with stressful communication situations by serving as mediators or interpreters and by speaking loudly or closer to the ears (Hallberg & Barrenäs, 1993).

Many individuals with untreated hearing loss need a period of quiet after difficult listening situations to recover from fatigue (Hétu, Lalonde, & Getty, 1987). This can cause the spouse or significant other to feel rejected or misunderstood. Individuals with untreated hearing loss may unconsciously raise their voices, which can be misinterpreted as anger or harsh temperament by family members, acquaintances, or strangers (Hétu, Jones, & Getty, 1993). Any or all these issues can lead to reduction in the frequency of interactions, intimate communications, and everyday companionship. The spouse or significant other may deal with many situations other than communication problems in the relationship. He or she may feel deprived of opportunities to go out or feel isolated during social gatherings. Also, at times the spouse or significant other may feel that he or she must leave early or may even feel embarrassed by the hearing-impaired partner. The spouse or significant other may experience additional stress because of his or her inability to rely on the hearing-impaired person in potentially dangerous situations (Hétu, Jones, & Getty, 1993).

If the hearing-impaired individual denies the hearing loss, it cannot be discussed openly in the family and thus the psychosocial costs for the spouse to adjust to the hearing loss are not acknowledged, leading to frustration and anger (Hétu, Riverin, Lalande, Getty, & St.-Cyr, 1988). Overall, hearing loss in a partner can increase the likelihood of subsequent poorer physical, psychological, and social well-being in partners (Wallhagen, Strawbridge, Shema, & Kaplan, 2004). Symptoms of hearing impairments such as irritability, inattention, and inappropriate responses can sometimes be misinterpreted as symptoms of dementia by caregivers (Corbin, Reed, Nobbs, Eastwood, & Eastwood, 1984).

Effects of Untreated Hearing Loss on Society

Because of the social isolation mentioned previously, individuals with untreated hearing loss may not contribute as much to society as other individuals. They may be less likely to volunteer at hospitals, libraries, or similar places. They are also less likely to go out and spend money at theaters, movies, or restaurants. The impact of untreated hearing loss has been quantified to be in excess of $100 billion annually. Assuming a 15% tax bracket, the cost to the society could exceed $18 billion due to unrealized taxes (Kochkin, 2005).

◆ Effects of Noise on Animals

Animals can also be affected by noise in various ways suggesting that in addition to humans, animals can benefit from noise control. For example, the loudest noises recorded underwater may be generated by seismic air guns used in oil and gas explorations (Nieukirk, Stafford, Mellinger, Dziak, & Fox, 2004), which can cause damage to fish ears at 500 m to several kilometers (McCauley, Fewtrell, & Popper, 2003). Shipping noise can increase secretion of stress hormones in fish (Wysocki, Dittami, & Ladich, 2006) and moderate levels of mid-frequency transient noises generated by military sonar equipment used to obtain information about objects in the sea by underwater sound can lead to death of whales within hours due to stranding or being driven on to the beach. (Fernández, Edwards, Rodríguez, et al., 2005).

◆ Hearing Conservation Programs

The key components of a hearing conservation program (**Fig. 1.10**) in occupational settings include noise monitoring (see Chapter 2), noise

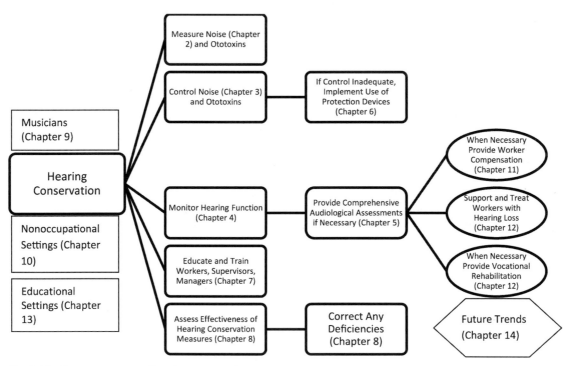

Fig. 1.10   Key components of hearing conservation.

control (see Chapter 3), monitoring of auditory sensitivity (see Chapter 4), detailed audiological evaluations if needed (see Chapter 5), use of hearing protection devices when noise control measures are insufficient (see Chapter 6), education and training of workers and managers (see Chapter 7), and assessment of the effectiveness of the hearing conservation measures and correction of any deficiencies (see Chapter 8). Hearing conservation needs to be also practiced by musicians (see Chapter 9), and it should be implemented in nonoccupational (see Chapter 10) and educational (see Chapter 13) settings. Workers who suffer from hearing loss due to occupational exposure may be eligible

for workers' compensation (see Chapter 11). In addition, they may have to continue to work in the noisy surrounding (e.g., mining) and may continue to be exposed to noise. Attempts should be made to protect their residual hearing. In addition, such workers need special support so that they can continue to be productive and efficient workers (see Chapter 12). Free assistance for implementation of hearing conservation programs is available from OSHA and OSHA-supported state organizations. Related information and materials are available from several websites including those of OSHA, NIOSH, the National Hearing Conservation Association (NHCA), and CAOHC.

Review Questions

1. Outline basic strategies for minimizing hearing loss.
2. Review the effects of noise exposure on the auditory system and hearing.
3. Discuss the key factors that increase the risk of NIHL.
4. Review the nonauditory effects of noise.
5. How can carbon monoxide affect hearing?
6. List and review potentially ototoxic heavy metals.
7. List and discuss organic solvents that are potentially ototoxic.
8. List and review five professions or industries where potentially hazardous noise exposure can occur.
9. Discuss the potential effects of untreated hearing loss.
10. Outline the key components of a hearing conservation program in occupational settings.

References

Achutan C. (2009). Assessment of noise exposure in a hospital kitchen. *Noise Health.* 11(44):145–150.

Agrawal Y, Niparko JK, Dobie RA. (2010). Estimating the effect of occupational noise exposure on hearing thresholds: the importance of adjusting for confounding variables. *Ear Hear.* 31(2):234–237.

Amin-zaki L, Majeed MA, Clarkson TW, Greenwood MR. (1978). Methylmercury poisoning in Iraqi children: clinical observations over two years. *BMJ.* 1(6113):613–616.

Anari M, Axelsson A, Eliasson A, Magnusson L. (1999). Hypersensitivity to sound—questionnaire data, audiometry and classification. *Scand Audiol.* 28(4):219–230.

Bali N, Acharya S, Anup N. (2007). An assessment of the effect of sound produced in a dental clinic on the hearing of dentists. *Oral Health Prev Dent.* 5(3):187–191.

Barger JL, Kayo T, Vann JM, et al. (2008). A low dose of dietary resveratrol partially mimics caloric restriction and retards aging parameters in mice. *PLoS ONE.* 3(6):e2264.

Besser R, Krämer G, Thümler R, Bohl J, Gutmann L, & Hopf HC. (1987). Acute trimethyltin limbic-cerebellar syndrome. *Neurology.* 37(6):945–950.

Bleecker ML, Ford DP, Lindgren KN, Scheetz K, Tiburzi MJ. (2003). Association of chronic and current measures of lead exposure with different components of brainstem

auditory evoked potentials. *Neurotoxicology.* 24(4–5): 625–631.

Bowes SM III, Corn M. (1990). Noise exposure reduction aboard an oceangoing hopper dredge. *Am Ind Hyg Assoc J.* 51(9):469–474.

Bray A, Szymáski M, Mills R. (2004). Noise induced hearing loss in dance music disc jockeys and an examination of sound levels in nightclubs. *J Laryngol Otol.* 118(2): 123–128.

Burns J, Yokota T, Ashihara H, Lean ME, Crozier A. (2002). Plant foods and herbal sources of resveratrol. *J Agric Food Chem.* 50(11):3337–3340.

Campo P, Maguin K. (2007). Solvent-induced hearing loss: mechanisms and prevention strategy. *Int J Occup Med Environ Health.* 20(3):265–270.

Campo P, Maguin K, Lataye R. (2007). Effects of aromatic solvents on acoustic reflexes mediated by central auditory pathways. *Toxicol Sci.* 99(2):582–590.

Chang YC. (1987). Neurotoxic effects of n-hexane on the human central nervous system: evoked potential abnormalities in n-hexane polyneuropathy. *J Neurol Neurosurg Psychiatry.* 50(3):269–274.

Chang SJ, Chang CK. (2009). Prevalence and risk factors of noise-induced hearing loss among liquefied petroleum gas (LPG) cylinder infusion workers in Taiwan. *Ind Health*. 47(6):603–610.

Chang SJ, Chen CJ, Lien CH, Sung FC. (2006). Hearing loss in workers exposed to toluene and noise. *Environ Health Perspect*. 114(8):1283–1286.

Chang NC, Yu ML, Ho KY, Ho CK. (2007). Hyperlipidemia in noise-induced hearing loss. *Otolaryngol Head Neck Surg*. 137(4):603–606.

Christensen K, Frederiksen H, Hoffman HJ. (2001). Genetic and environmental influences on self-reported reduced hearing in the old and oldest old. *J Am Geriatr Soc*. 49(11):1512–1517.

Chuu JJ, Hsu CJ, Lin-Shiau SY. (2001). Abnormal auditory brainstem responses for mice treated with mercurial compounds: involvement of excessive nitric oxide. *Toxicology*. 162(1):11–22.

Corbin S, Reed M, Nobbs H, Eastwood K, Eastwood MR. (1984). Hearing assessment in homes for the aged: a comparison of audiometric and self-report methods. *J Am Geriatr Soc*. 32(5):396–400.

Counter SA. (2003). Neurophysiological anomalies in brainstem responses of mercury-exposed children of Andean gold miners. *J Occup Environ Med*. 45(1):87–95.

Cristell M, Hutchinson KM, Alessio HM. (1998). Effects of exercise training on hearing ability. *Scand Audiol*. 27:219–224.

Cruickshanks KJ, Klein R, Klein BE, Wiley TL, Nondahl DM, Tweed TS. (1998). Cigarette smoking and hearing loss: the epidemiology of hearing loss study. *JAMA*. 279(21):1715–1719.

Da Costa EA, Castro JC, Macedo ME. (2008). Iris pigmentation and susceptibility to noise-induced hearing loss. *Int J Audiol*. 47(3):115–118.

DePalma RG, Burris DG, Champion HR, Hodgson MJ. (2005). Blast injuries. *N Engl J Med*. 352(13):1335–1342.

Discalzi GL, Capellaro F, Bottalo L, Fabbro D, Mocellini A. (1992). Auditory brainstem evoked potentials (BAEPs) in lead-exposed workers. *Neurotoxicology*. 13(1):207–209.

Dobie RA. (2008). The burdens of age-related and occupational noise-induced hearing loss in the United States. *Ear Hear*. 29(4):565–577.

Draper TH, Bamiou DE. (2009). Auditory neuropathy in a patient exposed to xylene: case report. *J Laryngol Otol*. 123(4):462–465.

Durga J, Verhoef P, Anteunis LJ, Schouten E, Kok FJ. (2007). Effects of folic acid supplementation on hearing in older adults: a randomized, controlled trial. *Ann Intern Med*. 146(1):1–9.

Eaton S. (2000). *Construction Noise. Engineering Section Report*. Vancouver, BC: Workers' Compensation Board of British Colmbia.

El Zir E, Mansour S, Salameh P, Chahine R. (2008). Environmental noise in Beirut, smoking and age are combined risk factors for hearing impairment. *East Mediterr Health J*. 14(4):888–896.

European Agency for Safety and Health at Work. (2005). *Noise in Figures*. Luxembourg: Office for Official Publications of the European Communities.

European Agency for Safety and Health at Work. (2009). *Combined Exposure to Noise and Ototoxic Substances. European Risk Observatory Literature Review*. Luxembourg: Office for Official Publications of the European Communities.

European Union Directive (2003). Directive 2003/10/EC of the European Parliament and of the Council of February 6th, 2003 on the Minimum Health and Safety Requirements Regarding the Exposure of Workers on the Risks Arising from Physical Agents (Noise). http://eur-lex.europa.eu/LexUriServ/LexUriServ.do?uri=OJ:L:2003:042:0038:0044:EN:PDF. Accessed June 24, 2011.

Fechter LD, Chen GD, Rao D, Larabee J. (2000). Predicting exposure conditions that facilitate the potentiation of noise-induced hearing loss by carbon monoxide. *Toxicol Sci*. 58(2):315–323.

Fernández A, Edwards JF, Rodríguez F, et al. (2005). "Gas and fat embolic syndrome" involving a mass stranding of beaked whales (family Ziphiidae) exposed to anthropogenic sonar signals. *Vet Pathol*. 42(4):446–457.

Fridberger A, Ulfendahl M. (1996). Acute mechanical overstimulation of isolated outer hair cells causes changes in intracellular calcium levels without shape changes. *Acta Otolaryngol*. 116(1):17–24.

Fuente A, Slade MD, Taylor T, et al. (2009). Peripheral and central auditory dysfunction induced by occupational exposure to organic solvents. *J Occup Environ Med*. 51(10):1202–1211.

Gijbels F, Jacobs R, Princen K, Nackaerts O, Debruyne F. (2006). Potential occupational health problems for dentists in Flanders, Belgium. *Clin Oral Investig*. 10(1):8–16.

Gilhome Herbst KR, Meredith R, Stephens SD. (1990). Implications of hearing impairment for elderly people in London and in Wales. *Acta Otolaryngol Suppl*. 476:209–214.

Girard SA, Picard M, Davis AC, et al. (2009). Multiple work-related accidents: tracing the role of hearing status and noise exposure. *Occup Environ Med*. 66(5):319–324.

Goodhill V. (1971). Sudden deafness and round window rupture. *Laryngoscope*. 81(9):1462–1474.

Goycoolea MV, Goycoolea HG, Farfan CR, Rodriguez LG, Martinez GC, Vidal R. (1986). Effect of life in industrialized societies on hearing in natives of Easter Island. *Laryngoscope*. 96(12):1391–1396.

Hallberg LR, Barrenäs ML. (1993). Living with a male with noise-induced hearing loss: experiences from the perspective of spouses. *Br J Audiol*. 27(4):255–261.

Hamernik RP, Turrentine G, Wright CG. (1984). Surface morphology of the inner sulcus and related epithelial cells of the cochlea following acoustic trauma. *Hear Res*. 16(2):143–160.

Hawkins JE Jr. (1971). The role of vasoconstriction in noise-induced hearing loss. *Ann Otol Rhinol Laryngol*. 80(6):903–913.

Helfer TM, Jordan NN, Lee RB. (2005). Postdeployment hearing loss in U.S. Army soldiers seen at audiology clinics from April 1, 2003, through March 31, 2004. *Am J Audiol*. 14(2):161–168.

Hétu R, Jones L, Getty L. (1993). The impact of acquired hearing impairment on intimate relationships: implications for rehabilitation. *Audiology*. 32(6):363–381.

Hétu R, Lalonde M, Getty L. (1987). Psychosocial disadvantages associated with occupational hearing loss as experienced in the family. *Audiology*. 26(3):141–152.

Hétu R, Riverin L, Lalande N, Getty L, St-Cyr C. (1988). Qualitative analysis of the handicap associated with occupational hearing loss. *Br J Audiol*. 22(4):251–264.

Hoet P, Lison D. (2008). Ototoxicity of toluene and styrene: state of current knowledge. *Crit Rev Toxicol*. 38(2):127–170.

Howd RA, Rebert CS, Dickinson J, Pryor GT. (1983). A comparison of the rates of development of functional hexane neuropathy in weanling and young adult rats. *Neurobehav Toxicol Teratol*. 6:63–68.

Huang CC. (2008). Polyneuropathy induced by n-hexane intoxication in Taiwan. *Acta Neurol Taiwan*. 17(1):3–10.

Hutchinson KM, Alessio HM, Hoppes S, Gruner A, Sanker A, Ambrose J. (2000). Effects of cardiovascular fitness and muscle strength on hearing sensitivity. *Journal of Strength & Conditioning Research.* 14:302–309.

Hwang YH, Chiang HY, Yen-Jean MC, Wang JD. (2009). The association between low levels of lead in blood and occupational noise-induced hearing loss in steel workers. *Sci Total Environ.* 408(1):43–49.

Ishii EK, Talbott EO. (1998). Race/ethnicity differences in the prevalence of noise-induced hearing loss in a group of metal fabricating workers. *J Occup Environ Med.* 40(8):661–666.

Ismail AH, Corrigan DL, MacLeod DF, Anderson VL, Kasten RN, Elliott PW. (1973). Biophysiological and audiological variables in adults. *Arch Otolaryngol.* 97(6):447–451.

Jiang H, Talaska AE, Schacht J, Sha SH. (2007). Oxidative imbalance in the aging inner ear. *Neurobiol Aging.* 28(10):1605–1612.

Kähärit K, Zachau G, Eklöf M, Sandsjö L, Möller C. (2003). Assessment of hearing and hearing disorders in rock/jazz musicians. *Int J Audiol.* 42(5):279–288.

Kaltenbach JA, Czaja JM, Kaplan CR. (1992). Changes in the tonotopic map of the dorsal cochlear nucleus following induction of cochlear lesions by exposure to intense sound. *Hear Res.* 59(2):213–223.

Kanthasamy AG, Borowitz JL, Pavlakovic G, Isom GE. (1994). Dopaminergic neurotoxicity of cyanide: neurochemical, histological, and behavioral characterization. *Toxicol Appl Pharmacol.* 126(1):156–163.

Karlsson KK, Harris JR, Svartengren M. (1997). Description and primary results from an audiometric study of male twins. *Ear Hear.* 18(2):114–120.

Kaufman LR, LeMasters GK, Olsen DM, Succop P. (2005). Effects of concurrent noise and jet fuel exposure on hearing loss. *J Occup Environ Med.* 47(3):212–218.

Kerr AG, Byrne JE. (1975). Concussive effects of bomb blast on the ear. *J Laryngol Otol.* 89(2):131–143.

Kochkin S. (2005). Hearing loss and its impact on household income. *The Hearing Review.* 12(11):16–22.

Kolkhorst FW, Smaldino JJ, Wolf SC, et al. (1998). Influence of fitness on susceptibility to noise-induced temporary threshold shift. *Med Sci Sports Exerc.* 30(2):289–293.

Konings A, Van Laer L, Wiktorek-Smagur A, et al. (2009). Candidate gene association study for noise-induced hearing loss in two independent noise-exposed populations. *Ann Hum Genet.* 73(2):215–224.

Kujawa SG, Liberman MC. (2009). Adding insult to injury: cochlear nerve degeneration after "temporary" noise-induced hearing loss. *J Neurosci.* 29(45):14077–14085.

Kung B, Sataloff RT. (2006). Noise-induced perilymph fistula. *Ear Nose Throat J.* 85(4):240–241, 245–246.

Kuwahara S, Kai MR, Nagase H, Hattori T. (1999). n-Hexane neuropathy caused by addictive inhalation: clinical and electrophysiological features. *Eur Neurol.* 41(3):163–167.

Lataye R, Maguin K, Campo P. (2007). Increase in cochlear microphonic potential after toluene administration. *Hear Res.* 230(1–2):34–42.

Liberman MC, Dodds LW. (1987). Acute ultrastructural changes in acoustic trauma: serial-section reconstruction of stereocilia and cuticular plates. *Hear Res.* 26(1):45–64.

Lim DJ, Dunn DE. (1979). Anatomic correlates of noise induced hearing loss. *Otolaryngol Clin North Am.* 12(3):493–513.

Lin CH, Chen TJ, Chen SS. (2009). Functional changes on ascending auditory pathway in rats caused by germanium dioxide exposure: an electrophysiological study. *Toxicology.* 256(1–2):110–117.

Lin CY, Wu JL, Shih TS, Tsai PJ, Sun YM, Guo YL. (2009). Glutathione S-transferase M1, T1, and P1 polymorphisms

as susceptibility factors for noise-induced temporary threshold shift. *Hear Res.* 257(1–2):8–15.

Liu Y, Fechter LD. (1995). MK-801 protects against carbon monoxide-induced hearing loss. *Toxicol Appl Pharmacol.* 132(2):196–202.

Maguin K, Campo P, Parietti-Winkler C. (2009). Toluene can perturb the neuronal voltage-dependent Ca2+ channels involved in the middle-ear reflex. *Toxicol Sci.* 107(2):473–481.

McCauley RD, Fewtrell J, Popper AN. (2003). High intensity anthropogenic sound damages fish ears. *J Acoust Soc Am.* 113(1):638–642.

McMahon CM, Kifley A, Rochtchina E, Newall P, Mitchell P. (2008). The contribution of family history to hearing loss in an older population. *Ear Hear.* 29(4):578–584.

Mizoue T, Miyamoto T, Shimizu T. (2003). Combined effect of smoking and occupational exposure to noise on hearing loss in steel factory workers. *Occup Environ Med.* 60(1):56–59.

Morata TC, Dunn DE, Kretschmer LW, Lemasters GK, Keith RW. (1993). Effects of occupational exposure to organic solvents and noise on hearing. *Scand J Work Environ Health.* 19(4):245–254.

Morata TC, Fiorini AC, Fischer FM, et al. (1997). Toluene-induced hearing loss among rotogravure printing workers. *Scand J Work Environ Health.* 23(4):289–298.

Morata TC, Johnson AC, Nylen P, et al. (2002). Audiometric findings in workers exposed to low levels of styrene and noise. *J Occup Environ Med.* 44(9):806–814.

Morioka I, Miyai N, Yamamoto H, Miyashita K. (2000). Evaluation of combined effect of organic solvents and noise by the upper limit of hearing. *Ind Health.* 38(2):252–257.

Mrena R, Savolainen S, Kiukaanniemi H, Ylikoski J, Mäkitie AA. (2009). The effect of tightened hearing protection regulations on military noise-induced tinnitus. *Int J Audiol.* 48(6):394–400.

Muhr P, Månsson B, Hellström PA. (2006). A study of hearing changes among military conscripts in the Swedish Army. *Int J Audiol.* 45(4):247–251.

Mulrow CD, Aguilar C, Endicott JE, et al. (1990). Association between hearing impairment and the quality of life of elderly individuals. *J Am Geriatr Soc.* 38(1):45–50.

Murata K, Weihe P, Budtz-Jørgensen E, Jørgensen PJ, Grandjean P. (2004). Delayed brainstem auditory evoked potential latencies in 14-year-old children exposed to methylmercury. *J Pediatr.* 144(2):177–183; Erratum. *J Pediatr.* 2006;149(4):583–584.

Musiek FE, Hanlon DP. (1999). Neuroaudiological effects in a case of fatal dimethylmercury poisoning. *Ear Hear.* 20(3):271–275.

National Institute for Occupational Safety and Health. (1998). *Criteria for a Recommended Standard: Occupational Noise Exposure- Revised Criteria 1998* (Publication No, 98–126). Cincinnati: National Institute for Occupational Safety and Health.

National Institute for Occupational Safety and Health. (2004). Fact Sheet: Work Related Hearing Loss [Department of Health and Human Services Publication No. 2001–103]. www.cdc.gov/niosh/docs/2001–103. Accessed June 24, 2011.

Neitzel RL, Berna BE, Seixas NS. (2006). Noise exposures aboard catcher/processor fishing vessels. *Am J Ind Med.* 49(8):624–633.

Nelson DI, Nelson RY, Concha-Barrientos M, Fingerhut M. (2005). The global burden of occupational noise-induced hearing loss. *Am J Ind Med.* 48(6):446–458.

Nieukirk SL, Stafford KM, Mellinger DK, Dziak RP, Fox CG. (2004). Low-frequency whale and seismic airgun sounds recorded in the mid-Atlantic Ocean. *J Acoust Soc Am.* 115(4):1832–1843.

Nordmann AS, Bohne BA, Harding GW. (2000). Histopathological differences between temporary and permanent threshold shift. *Hear Res.* 139(1–2):13–30.

Occupational Safety & Health Administration. (1997). Occupational Safety and Health Standards. Regulations (Standards –29 CFR). 1910.1000 Table Z-2. [62 FR 42018, August 4, 1997]. www.osha.gov. Accessed June 24, 2011.

Ohlin D. (1998). Let's hear it for our troops. Saving hearing—and money—in the military. *ASHA.* 40(4):50–53.

Osman K, Pawlas K, Schütz A, Gazdzik M, Sokal JA, Vahter M. (1999). Lead exposure and hearing effects in children in Katowice, Poland. *Environ Res.* 80(1):1–8.

Patel JA, Broughton K. (2002). Assessment of the noise exposure of call centre operators. *Ann Occup Hyg.* 46(8): 653–661.

Patuzzi R, Millhinch J, Doyle J.(2000). *Acute Aural Trauma in Telephone Headset and Handset Users.* Paper presented at the Neurootological Society of Australia National Conference, Melbourne. Australia.

Pearlman RT, Sandidge O. (2009). Noise characteristics of surgical space suits. *Orthopedics.* 32(11):825.

Picard M, Girard SA, Simard M, Larocque R, Leroux T, Turcotte F. (2008). Association of work-related accidents with noise exposure in the workplace and noise-induced hearing loss based on the experience of some 240,000 person-years of observation. *Accid Anal Prev.* 40(5):1644–1652.

Pouyatos B, Fechter LD. Industrial chemicals and solvents affecting the auditory system. In: Campbell KCM, ed. *Pharmacology and Ototoxicity for Audiologists.* Clifton Park, NY: Thomson Delmar Learning; 2007:197–215.

Qiu W, Davis B, Hamernik RP. (2007). Hearing loss from interrupted, intermittent, and time varying Gaussian noise exposures: the applicability of the equal energy hypothesis. *J Acoust Soc Am.* 121(3):1613–1620.

Quirk WS, Seidman MD. (1995). Cochlear vascular changes in response to loud noise. *Am J Otol.* 16(3):322–325.

Rabinowitz PM, Galusha D, Slade MD, et al. (2008). Organic solvent exposure and hearing loss in a cohort of aluminium workers. *Occup Environ Med.* 65(4):230–235.

Rao D, Fechter LD. (2000). Protective effects of phenyl-N-tert-butylnitrone on the potentiation of noise-induced hearing loss by carbon monoxide. *Toxicol Appl Pharmacol.* 167(2):125–131.

Rawool VW. (1996a). Effect of aging on the click-rate induced facilitation of acoustic reflex thresholds. *J Gerontol A Biol Sci Med Sci.* 51(2):B124–B131.

Rawool VW. (1996b). Acoustic reflex monitoring during the presentation of 1000 clicks at high repetition rates. *Scand Audiol.* 25(4):239–245.

Rawool VW. (2008). Growing up noisy: The sound exposure diary of a hypothetical young adult. *Hearing Review.* 15(5):30, 32, 34, 39–40.

Rawool VW, Dluhy C. (2010, April). *Can Opiates and Noise Interact in Increasing Hearing Loss?* Podium presentation at the American Academy of Audiology's annual meeting, AudiologyNOW!, San Diego, CA, April.

Razzaq M, Dumbala S, Moudgil SS. (2010). Neurological picture. Sudden deafness due to carbon monoxide poisoning. *J Neurol Neurosurg Psychiatry.* 81(6):658.

Rice DC. (1998). Age-related increase in auditory impairment in monkeys exposed in utero plus postnatally to methylmercury. *Toxicol Sci* 44(2):191–196.

Rice DC, Gilbert SG. (1992). Exposure to methyl mercury from birth to adulthood impairs high-frequency hearing in monkeys. *Toxicol Appl Pharmacol.* 115(1):6–10.

Robertson D. (1983). Functional significance of dendritic swelling after loud sounds in the guinea pig cochlea. *Hear Res.* 9(3):263–278.

Robertson D, Irvine DR. (1989). Plasticity of frequency organization in auditory cortex of guinea pigs with partial unilateral deafness. *J Comp Neurol.* 282(3):456–471.

Rosen S, Bergman M, Plester D, El-Mofty A, Satti MH. (1962). Presbycusis study of a relatively noise-free population in the Sudan. *Ann Otol Rhinol Laryngol.* 71:727–743.

Rubak T, Kock S, Koefoed-Nielsen B, Lund SP, Bonde JP, Kolstad HA. (2008). The risk of tinnitus following occupational noise exposure in workers with hearing loss or normal hearing. *Int J Audiol.* 47(3):109–114.

Salvi RJ, Wang J, Ding D. (2000). Auditory plasticity and hyperactivity following cochlear damage. *Hear Res.* 147(1–2):261–274.

Salvi RJ, Wang J, Powers NL. Plasticity and reorganization in the auditory brainstem: implications for tinnitus. In: Reich G, Vernon G, eds. *Proceedings of the Fifth International Tinnitus Seminar* (pp. 457–466). Portland, OR: American Tinnitus Association; 1996:457–466.

Sampaio Fernandes JC, Carvalho AP, Gallas M, Vaz P, Matos PA. (2006). Noise levels in dental schools. *Eur J Dent Educ.* 10(1):32–37.

Santos L, Morata TC, Jacob LC, Albizu E, Marques JM, Paini M. (2007). Music exposure and audiological findings in Brazilian disc jockeys (DJs). *Int J Audiol.* 46(5):223–231.

Schäper M, Seeber A, van Thriel C. (2008). The effects of toluene plus noise on hearing thresholds: an evaluation based on repeated measurements in the German printing industry. *Int J Occup Med Environ Health.* 21(3):191–200.

Seidman MD. (2000). Effects of dietary restriction and antioxidants on presbyacusis. *Laryngoscope.* 110(5 Pt 1): 727–738.

Seidman M, Babu S, Tang W, Naem E, Quirk WS. (2003). Effects of resveratrol on acoustic trauma. *Otolaryngol Head Neck Surg.* 129(5):463–470.

Seixas NS, Goldman B, Sheppard L, Neitzel R, Norton S, Kujawa SG. (2005). Prospective noise induced changes to hearing among construction industry apprentices. *Occup Environ Med.* 62(5):309–317.

Shahbaz Hassan M, Ray J, Wilson F. (2003). Carbon monoxide poisoning and sensorineural hearing loss. *J Laryngol Otol.* 117(2):134–137.

Shargorodsky J, Curhan SG, Eavey R, Curhan GC. (2010). A prospective study of vitamin intake and the risk of hearing loss in men. *Otolaryngol Head Neck Surg.* 142(2): 231–236.

Sliwinska-Kowalska M, Noben-Trauth K, Pawelczyk M, Kowalski TJ. (2008). Single nucleotide polymorphisms in the cadherin 23 (CDH23) gene in Polish workers exposed to industrial noise. *Am J Hum Biol.* 20(4):481–483.

Sliwinska-Kowalska M, Prasher D, Rodrigues CA, et al. (2007). Ototoxicity of organic solvents - from scientific evidence to health policy. *Int J Occup Med Environ Health.* 20(2): 215–222.

Sliwinska-Kowalska M, Zamylslowska-Szmytke E. Organic solvent exposures and occupational hearing loss. In: Luxon L, Prahser D, eds. *Noise and its effects.* Hoboken, NJ: John Wiley & Sons Ltd; 2007: 477–498.

Sliwiska-Kowalska M, Zamyslowska-Szmytke E, Szymczak W, et al. (2003). Ototoxic effects of occupational exposure to styrene and co-exposure to styrene and noise. *J Occup Environ Med.* 45(1):15–24.

Sliwinska-Kowalska M, Zamyslowska-Szmytke E, Szymczak W, et al. (2005). Exacerbation of noise-induced hearing loss by co-exposure to workplace chemicals. *Environmental Toxicology and Pharmacology.* 19:547–553.

Soliman S, El-Atreby M, Tawfik S, Holail E, Iskandar N, Abou-Setta A. (2003). The interaction of whole body vibration and noise on the cochlea. *International Congress Series*. 1240:209–216.

Starck J, Toppila E, Pyykkö I. (1999). Smoking as a risk factor in sensory neural hearing loss among workers exposed to occupational noise. *Acta Otolaryngol*. 119(3):302–305.

Stopp P.The effect of moderate intensity noise on cochlear potentials and structure. In: Hamernik RP, Henderson D, Salvi R, eds. *New perspectives in noise induced hearing loss*. New York: Raven Press; 1982; 331–343.

Styger PS. (2009). Potential of chemical ototoxicity by noise. *Semin Hear*, 30(1):38–46.

Sudderth ME. (1974). Tympanoplasty in blast-induced perforation. *Arch Otolaryngol*. 99(3):157–159.

Suneja SK, Potashner SJ, Benson CG. (1998). Plastic changes in glycine and GABA release and uptake in adult brain stem auditory nuclei after unilateral middle ear ossicle removal and cochlear ablation. *Exp Neurol*. 151(2):273–288.

Sutinen P, Zou J, Hunter LL, Toppila E, Pyykkö I. (2007). Vibration-induced hearing loss: mechanical and physiological aspects. *Otol Neurotol*. 28(2):171–177.

Sweet RJ, Price JM, Henry KR. (1988). Dietary restriction and presbyacusis: periods of restriction and auditory threshold losses in the CBA/J mouse. *Audiology*. 27(6):305–312.

Szczepaniak WS, Møller AR. (1995). Evidence of decreased GABAergic influence on temporal integration in the inferior colliculus following acute noise exposure: a study of evoked potentials in the rat. *Neurosci Lett*. 196(1–2):77–80.

Tak S, Calvert GM. (2008). Hearing difficulty attributable to employment by industry and occupation: an analysis of the National Health Interview Survey—United States, 1997 to 2003. *J Occup Environ Med*. 50(1):46–56.

Tak S, Davis RR, Calvert GM. (2009). Exposure to hazardous workplace noise and use of hearing protection devices among US workers—NHANES, 1999–2004. *Am J Ind Med*. 52(5):358–371.

Tanaka C, Bielefeld EC, Chen GD, Li M, Henderson D. (2009). Ameliorative effects of an augmented acoustic environment on age-related hearing loss in middle-aged Fischer 344/NHsd rats. *Laryngoscope*. 119(7):1374–1379.

Teufert-Autrey SM. (2004). Duty to serve, opportunity to listen. *Hearing Health*. Fall:20.

Toppila E, Pyykkö I, Starck J. (2001). Age and noise-induced hearing loss. *Scand Audiol*. 30(4):236–244.

Trost RP, Shaw GB. (2007). Statistical analysis of hearing loss among navy personnel. *Mil Med*. 172(4):426–430.

Tunay M, Melemez K. (2008). Noise induced hearing loss of forest workers in Turkey. *Pak J Biol Sci*. 11(17):2144–2148.

Unal M, Tamer L, Dőruer ZN, Yildirim H, Vayisőlu Y, Camdeviren H. (2005). N-acetyltransferase 2 gene polymorphism and presbycusis. *Laryngoscope*. 115(12):2238–2241.

U.S. Army Center for Health Promotion and Preventive Medicine. (2003). *Just the Facts. . . Occupational Ototoxins (Ear Poisons) and Hearing Loss* (Pub No. 51-002-0903). Aberdeen Proving Ground, MD: U.S. Army Center for Health Promotion and Preventive Medicine.

U.S. Department of Health and Human Services, Public Health Service, Agency for Toxic Substances and Disease Registry. (1999a). *Toxicological Profile for Mercury* (CAS No. 7439-97-6). Atlanta, GA: U.S. Department of Health and Human Services, Agency for Toxic Substances and Disease Registry.

U.S. Department of Health and Human Services, Public Health Service, Agency for Toxic Substances and Disease Registry. (1999b). *Toxicological Profile for n-hexane* (CAS No. 110-54-3). Atlanta, GA: U.S. Department of Health and Human Services, Agency for Toxic Substances and Disease Registry.

U.S. Department of Labor. (2009). *Nonfatal Occupational Illnesses by Major Industry Sector and Category of Illness, 2008*. Washington, DC: U.S. Department of Labor.

van den Berg F. (2009). Perspectives on wind turbine noise. *Echoes*. 19(3):1, 3.

Viaene M, Vermeir G, Godderis L. (2009). Sleep disturbances and occupational exposure to solvents. *Sleep Med Rev*. 13(3):235–243.

Viljanen A, Era P, Kaprio J, Pyykkö I, Koskenvuo M, Rantanen T. (2007). Genetic and environmental influences on hearing in older women. *J Gerontol A Biol Sci Med Sci*. 62(4):447–452.

Visser I, Lavini C, Booij J, et al. (2008). Cerebral impairment in chronic solvent-induced encephalopathy. *Ann Neurol*. 63(5):572–580.

Vrca A, Karací V, Boziceví D, Bozikov V, Malinar M. (1996). Brainstem auditory evoked potentials in individuals exposed to long-term low concentrations of toluene. *Am J Ind Med*. 30(1):62–66.

Wallhagen MI, Strawbridge WJ, Shema SJ, Kaplan GA. (2004). Impact of self-assessed hearing loss on a spouse: A longitudinal analyses of couples. *J Gerontol B Psychol Sci Soc Sci*. 59(3):S190–S196.

Wang J, Caspary D, Salvi RJ. (2000). GABA-A antagonist causes dramatic expansion of tuning in primary auditory cortex. *Neuroreport*. 11(5):1137–1140.

Wild DC, Brewster MJ, Banerjee AR. (2005). Noise-induced hearing loss is exacerbated by long-term smoking. *Clin Otolaryngol*. 30(6):517–520.

Willott JF, Aitkin LM, McFadden SL. (1993). Plasticity of auditory cortex associated with sensorineural hearing loss in adult C57BL/6J mice. *J Comp Neurol*. 329(3):402–411.

Willott JF, Erway LC, Archer JR, Harrison DE. (1995). Genetics of age-related hearing loss in mice. II. Strain differences and effects of caloric restriction on cochlear pathology and evoked response thresholds. *Hear Res*. 88(1–2):143–155.

WorkCover Australia. (2001). *WorkCover Guides for the Evaluation of Permanent Impairment*. Sydney, Australia: WorkCover Australia.

Wu TN, Shen CY, Lai JS, et al. (2000). Effects of lead and noise exposures on hearing ability. *Arch Environ Health*. 55(2):109–114.

Wu CC, Young YH. (2009). Ten-year longitudinal study of the effect of impulse noise exposure from gunshot on inner ear function. *Int J Audiol*. 48(9):655–660.

Wysocki LE, Dittami JP, Ladich F. (2006). Ship noise and cortisol secretion in European freshwater fishes. *Biological Conservation*. 128(4):501–508.

Yamane H, Nakai Y, Takayama M, Iguchi H, Nakagawa T, Kojima A. (1995). Appearance of free radicals in the guinea pig inner ear after noise-induced acoustic trauma. *Eur Arch Otorhinolaryngol*. 252(8):504–508.

Yamasoba T, Goto Y, Komaki H, Mimaki M, Sudo A, Suzuki M. (2006). Cochlear damage due to germanium-induced mitochondrial dysfunction in guinea pigs. *Neurosci Lett*. 395(1):18–22.

Ylikoski M, Pekkarinen JO, Starck JP, Pääkkönen RJ, Ylikoski JS. (1995). Physical characteristics of gunfire impulse noise and its attenuation by hearing protectors. *Scand Audiol*. 24(1):3–11.

Zubick HH, Tolentino AT, Boffa J. (1980). Hearing loss and the high speed dental handpiece. *Am J Public Health*. 70(6):633–635.

Chapter 2

Documenting Hazardous Noise Levels and Exposures

Due to the various effects of noise identified in Chapter 1, the first step of an effective hearing conservation program is to document the characteristics of noise.

◆ Purposes of Conducting Noise Measurements

Noise measurements in the context of hearing conservation can be used for the following purposes:

- To determine if noise levels or exposures are hazardous to safety and hearing
- To identify and label areas with hazardous noise in the work setting
- To identify workers who are exposed to hazardous noise levels
- To evaluate if noise levels meet or exceed regulatory standards
- To determine if a hearing conservation program is necessary
- To determine if use of hearing protection by employees is necessary or recommended and, if necessary, the amount of protection needed
- To monitor any changes in noise environment that may require a change in any recommendations related to hearing conservation
- For workers' compensation purposes, to predict if specific hearing loss in employees could result from the noise exposures they received (see Chapter 11)
- To continue to research the relationship between hearing threshold shifts with

or without the use of hearing protection devices and the amount and type of noise exposure
- To continue to research interaction of noise exposure with other exposures (e.g., ototoxins, vibrations) in augmenting hearing loss

◆ Noise

Noise can be defined in a variety of ways, including the following:

- Any audible sound (Noise at Work Regulations, 2005)
- An erratic or statistically random oscillation
- A disagreeable or undesired sound

Oscillation or vibration is the to-and-fro motion of an object. Sound is generated by the oscillation of particles within a medium (air, water, or structure) caused by elastic forces. The accompanying pressure changes produce sound waves emanating away from the turbulent or vibrating sound source (**Fig. 2.1**). Any auditory sensation resulting from the pressure changes is also referred to as sound.

◆ Noise Characteristics Relevant to Hearing

Although other risk factors play a role in noise-induced hearing loss (NIHL), as discussed in Chapter 1, the effect of noise on hearing is partially

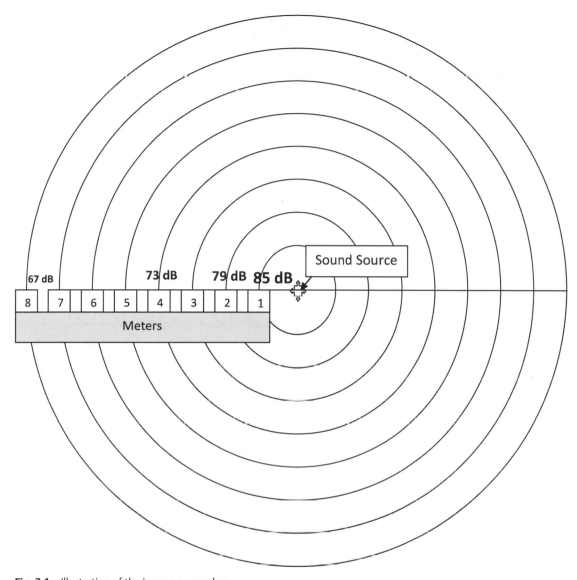

Fig. 2.1 Illustration of the inverse-square law.

dependent on the overall noise exposure, which is determined by the following factors:

- The temporal pattern of noise
- The level of noise
- The frequency content of the noise
- The overall duration of noise exposure

Temporal Pattern

The temporal characteristics of noise partially determine the extent of damage to the auditory system.

Continuous (Steady State or Stationary) Noise

If the noise level is relatively constant or has negligibly small fluctuations in level involving maxima at intervals of 1 second or less, it is considered continuous noise.

Time-Varying (Nonsteady or Nonstationary) Noise

If the noise level varies substantially during the period of observation, the noise can be considered to be time-varying noise.

Intermittent Noise

If the noise exposure has breaks (few seconds to hours) when the noise levels are relatively low, the noise exposure can be considered to be intermittent. If the levels are not too high, this type of noise can allow the ear time to recover from temporary threshold shifts.

Impulse/Impact Noise (Transient Noise)

Impulse and impact noises are often considered similar and are combined in one category. The National Institute for Occupational Safety and Health (NIOSH; 1998) uses the term *impulsive noise* to define both impulse and impact noises and defines impulsive noise as noise with duration of less than 1 second and sharp rise and rapid decay times. The U.S. Department of Defense (DoD, 2004) defines impulse/impact noise as a short burst of acoustic energy consisting of single or multiple impulses. The rise time of such impulses to a 40 dB peak pressure is 1 second or less followed by a somewhat slower, but less-than-1-second decay to ambient pressure. If the interpulse interval is less than 500 milliseconds, the noise is considered continuous, with the exception of short bursts of automatic weapons fire, which are considered impulse noise.

Impulse noise usually results from a very sudden release of sound energy, such as that occurring after an explosion or gunshot, and can produce levels exceeding 140 dB sound pressure level (SPL). Exposure to this type of noise can lead to mechanical damage to hair cells in the cochlea when the peak impulse noise levels are very high. Impulse noises usually occur in military work settings because of the use of weapons. The daily exposure of military workers to impulse noises can be one or a few impulses due to a rocket launch or several hundred impulses from small arms. Impact noise can be characterized by slightly longer rise time than those associated with impulse noise. It usually results from the impact of mechanical objects such as hammers. There is usually some ringing or persistence of noise from the mechanical resonances elicited by the impact. Daily exposure to impacts can be in the range of thousands (Hodge & Price, 1978).

Level of Noise

With higher levels of noise, the possibility of hearing loss increases. Therefore, it is important to document the levels of noise exposure.

Levels of Continuous Steady State Noise

For continuous noise in air or gases, sound levels are usually documented by using sound pressure levels in dB expressed by the following equations:

$$SPL = 10 \log_{10} (p^2/p_{ref}^2) = 10 \log_{10} (p/p_{ref})^2 = 20 \log_{10} (p/p_{ref})$$

where p is the measured sound pressure and p_{ref} is the reference pressure; the most commonly used and assumed reference pressure value is 20 μPa for airborne sounds unless a different reference value is specifically stated.

For sounds in media other than gases, unless a different reference values is specified, reference SPL is 1 μPa.

Maximum Sound Level (Maximum Frequency-weighted Sound Pressure Level)

This is the greatest or maximum SPL recorded during an observation period. The Occupation Safety and Health Administration (OSHA; 1983) has specified that the maximum SPL during work should not exceed 115 dBA.

Levels of Transient Noise

For impulsive noises or noises that have peaks, measures of peak levels are used and expressed as peak sound pressure (P_{peak}), which is the peak value of the instantaneous noise pressure and is usually measured using the "C" frequency weighting with a very fast response characteristic.

Levels of Fluctuating Noise

Fluctuating or intermittent noises are measured in terms of the level of a continuous noise that would have the same (equivalent) total energy as the fluctuating noise, and such measurements are referred to as equivalent SPL.

Changes in Sound Levels with Sound Propagation

In a free sound field (without any reflections or boundaries), the sound radiates in the area uniformly in all directions, as shown in **Fig. 2.1**. As shown in the figure, the level of the sound drops by 6 dB with the doubling of distance. Thus,

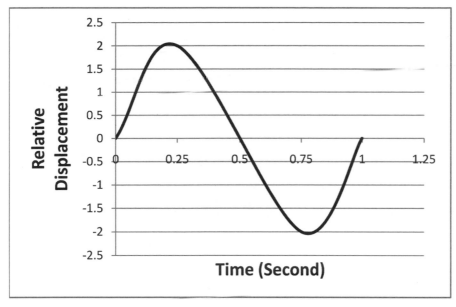

Fig. 2.2 Representation of a sound with a frequency of 1 Hz.

moving workers away from a sound source is one strategy that is often useful in decreasing the noise exposures.

Frequency Content of Noise

As mentioned previously, sound is generated due to the oscillation of particles in a medium. One complete round trip of an oscillating motion is referred to as a *cycle*. Frequency refers to the number of complete cycles or vibrations that occur in one second. It is measured in units of Hertz (Hz) and is plotted on the X-axis on an audiogram (see Chapter 4). A frequency of 1 Hz means that one cycle is occurring per second (**Fig. 2.2**), 2 Hz means that 2 cycles are occurring per second (see **Fig. 2.3**), and 1000 Hz means that 1000 cycles are occurring per second. A high frequency sound is perceived as being higher in pitch. Thus, a sound with a frequency of 500 Hz is perceived as being lower in pitch compared with a sound of 6000 Hz. At a younger age, humans have the ability to hear sounds with frequencies in the range of 20 to 20,000 Hz. With increasing age, the ability to hear higher frequency sound diminishes. Hazardous noise exposure first has a detrimental effect on the ability to hear sounds with frequencies between 3000 and 6000 Hz.

The frequency content of complex sounds or noises can be measured in bands that can vary in width of one octave bands, third octave bands, or in narrower bands. A frequency band is considered to be an octave in width when its upper band-edge frequency (f_2) is twice the lower band-edge frequency (f_1); $f_2 = 2\ f_1$. Each *octave band* is named for the center frequency (geometric mean) of the band, calculated as $f_c = (f_1 f_2)^{1/2}$. For example, an octave band with a center frequency of 1000 Hz has a lower band-edge frequency of 707 Hz and a higher band-edge frequency of 1414 Hz. An octave band with a center frequency of 2000 Hz has a lower band-edge frequency of 1414 Hz and a higher band-edge frequency of 2828 Hz. The bandwidth of an octave band filter is 70.7% of the center frequency and can also be calculated by subtracting the lower band-edge frequency from the upper band-edge frequency. Thus, the bandwidth of an octave band with a center frequency of 1000 Hz is $1000 \times 70.7\% = 707$ Hz or $1414 - 707 = 707$ Hz. A frequency band whose upper band-edge frequency (f2) is the cube root of two times the lower band-edge frequency (f1) or ($f_2 = (2)^{1/3} f_1$) is referred to as *one-third octave band*.

An effective procedure for considering the frequency content of the noise is to add the energy at all frequencies present in the noise to arrive at

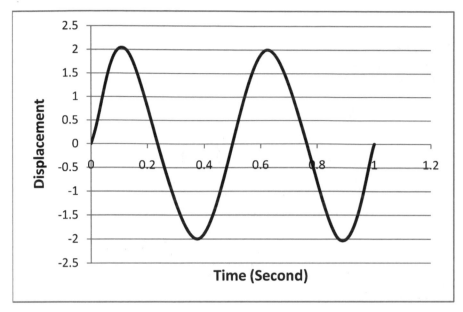

Fig. 2.3 Representation of a sound with a frequency of 2 Hz.

a single sound level. The following formula can be used for combining octave-band levels into an overall SPL:

$$L = 10 \log \sum_{i=1}^{n} 10^{\,Li/10}$$

where L = combined level in dB SPL, n = number of bands being combined, i = the ith band, and Li = the octave band level of the ith band.

The human ear is more sensitive to middle frequencies than lower frequencies. This difference in sensitivity was demonstrated by Fletcher and Munsen (1933) through the equal loudness curves. These curves were created by presenting a reference tone of 1000 Hz at various SPLs and asking listeners to adjust the SPLs of tones of various frequencies so that the reference tone of 1000 Hz and the presented tones of various frequencies sound equal in loudness.

Frequency Weighting

In measuring the level of continuous noise, various frequency weighting options can be used including A, B, and C shown in **Fig. 2.4**. Most modern sound level meters (SLMs) and dosimeters provide automatic readouts of A- and C-weighted SPLs.

A-Weighted Sounds Level [dBA or dB(A)]

In this case, the energy is summed to allow simulation of the frequency response of the human ear at relatively low but clearly audible sounds.

$$L = 10 \log \sum_{i=1}^{n} 10^{\,Li + Ki/10}$$

Note that this formula is similar to the formula for combining overall sound levels in various bands, except for the fact that the level in each band is corrected (Ki) to simulate human auditory sensitivity, which is less for lower frequencies. The applied corrections for each frequency band are shown in **Table 2.1**. For example, if the SPL in the octave band with a center frequency of 250 Hz is 78.6 dB, then the corrected value will be 78.6 + (− 8.6, Ki) = 70 dB. Such corrections were applied in creating the curves shown in **Fig. 2.4**.

The A frequency weighting is usable over a much wider range of SPLs and is used frequently in the context of hearing conservation. It gives good estimation of the threat to human hearing. Thus, OSHA and other regulatory bodies require the use of dBA levels when measuring most of the occupational and environmental noise exposure.

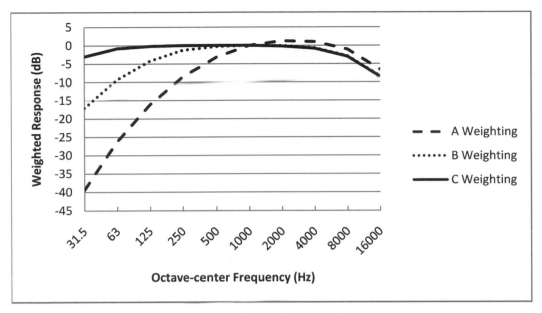

Fig. 2.4   Relative frequency response of A-, B-, and C-weighting networks.

B-Weighted Sound Level [dBB or dB(B)]

This curve approximates the sensitivity of the human ear at medium SPLs. B-weighted sound levels are generally not used in the context of hearing conservation.

C-Weighted Sound Level [dBC or dB(C)]

The curve for C-weighted sound levels approximates human sensitivity at high SPLs. In this case, the energy at all frequencies in the noise is summed fairly equally, yielding a relatively flat frequency response. This weighting scale is often recommended for measuring peak SPLs of high-level impulse sounds because the response of the human ear is nearly flat at high listening levels. C-weighted sound level measurements can be used along with dBA levels to determine if a sound has predominantly low frequency components. In the presence of significantly low frequency components, the dBC levels can be

expected to be higher than the dBA levels; in the absence of significantly low frequency, contributions to the overall noise levels the dBA and dBC readings are similar. When the difference in the dBA and dBC readings is more than 15 dB, the noise is considered to have an intense low frequency component (U.S. Navy and Marine Corp Public Health Center [NMCPHC], 2008).

D-Weighted Sound Level [dBD or dB(D)]

The D-scale provides an overall indication of perceived loudness for sounds such as those generated by aircrafts.

Duration of Exposure

The duration of exposure has a significant effect on the amount of hearing loss that can occur from hazardous levels of exposure. For example, exposure to 95 dBA SPLs over 8 hours on a daily

Table 2.1   Corrections to be Applied to Linear Octave Band Levels for Summing Overall Sound Levels in Various Bands into a Single dBA Level

Center frequency of the octave band (Hz)	31.5	63	125	250	500	1000	2000	4000	8000
dBA weighting	−39.4	−26.2	−16.1	−8.6	−3.2	0	1.2	1.1	−1.1

basis is much more damaging than exposure to the same level over 1 hour.

Equal Energy Principle and Exchange Rate

The total amount of noise a person is exposed to over time can be reported in terms of overall energy, which is determined by the SPL of the noise and the duration over which the exposure occurs. According to the equal energy principle, the amount of biological damage caused by noise exposure is determined by the total amount of energy. Thus, equal amounts of sound energy are expected to produce equal damage regardless of how the exposure is distributed over time. For example, a noise exposure level of 85 dBA over a period of 8 hours is expected to cause the same damage as an exposure level of 88 dBA over a period of 4 hours or a level of 91 dBA over a period of 2 hours (**Table 2.2**). This time-intensity relationship is most

commonly referred to as "exchange rate," but it is also referred to as the "time-intensity tradeoff," "trading ratio," or "doubling rate." The equal energy principle may not necessarily apply to impulse types of noises (Clifford & Rogers, 2009).

More specifically, the term *exchange rate* can be defined as an increase in dB exposure levels that requires the halving of exposure time or a decrease in dB exposure levels that allows doubling of the exposure time. The term *doubling rate* can be used when the exchange rate is 3 dB, as in the previous example, because an increase of 3 dB results in doubling of sound energy. However, several different exchange rates have been proposed, including 3 (NIOSH, 1998), 4 (DoD, 2004), or 5 dB (OSHA, 1983). With a 5 dB exchange rate, an exposure level of 90 dBA over a period of 8 hours is assumed to cause the same damage as the exposure level of 95 dBA over a period of 4 hours (**Table 2.2**).

Criterion Exposure Duration

Criterion exposure duration (TC) is used as a basis for determining an employee's noise exposure or dose and is usually considered over 8 hours.

Table 2.2 Duration Limits for Selected Exposure Levels

Exposure level, L (dBA)	Reference Duration, T	
	Required by OSHA (1983). Calculated by using equation T (hours) = $8/(2^{(L-90)/5})$	Recommended by NIOSH (1998). Calculated by using equation T (hours) = $8/(2^{(L-85)/3})$
85	16	8 h
88	10.6 (10 h 36 min)	4 h
90	8	2 h 31 min
91	7	2 h
94	4.6 (4 h 36 min)	1 h
95	4	47 min 37 s
97	3	30 min
100	2	15 min
103	1.3 (1 h 18 min)	7 min 30 s
105	1	4 min 43 s
106	0.87 (52 min 12 s)	3 min 45 s
109	0.57 (34 min 12 s)	1 min 53 s
110	0.5 (30 min)	1 min 29 s
112	0.38 (22 min 48 s)	56 s
115	0.25 (15 min)	28 s
118	0.16 (9 min 36 s)	14 s
120	0.125 (7 min 30 s)	9 s
121	0.11 (6 min 36 s)	7 s
124	0.072 (4 min 19 s)	3.5 s
125	0.063 (3 min 47 s)	3 s
127	0.047 (2 min 49 s)	1.75 s
130	0.031 (1 min 52 s)	0.88 s
140	0.0078 (28.1 s)	Less than 0.1 s

NIOSH, National Institute for Occupational Safety and Health; OSHA, Occupational Safety and Health Administration.

◆ Criterion Sound Level

Criterion sound level (LC) is the constant sound level in dB which, if continued for the TC (usually 8 hours), will result in a 100% noise dose, which is 100% of a worker's allowable noise exposure. The criterion sound level recommended by NIOSH (1998) is 85 dBA, whereas OSHA (1983) has specified a level of 90 dBA for a period of 8 hours.

◆ Allowed Exposure Time (Reference Duration, Exposure Duration Limit)

The allowed exposure duration or exposure duration limit or reference duration (*Ti*) is based on a specified LC (e.g., 85 dBA), TC (e.g., 8 hours), and exchange rate (Q; e.g., 3 dB). The relationship between the variables is expressed as follows:

$$Ti = TC/(2^{(L-LC)/Q})$$

where L is the measured A-weighted sound level. The reference duration limits in **Table 2.2** are calculated using this formula.

National Institutes for Occupational Safety and Health Recommended Exposure Limit

NIOSH (1998) has recommended a criterion exposure limit of 85 dBA for 8 hours; exposures at or above this level are considered hazardous. Using this recommendation and an exchange rate of 3 dB, the occupational noise exposure should be controlled in such a way so that the duration (Ti) at a particular exposure level (L) is *below* the duration (Ti) as calculated by the following formula:

$$Ti\,(\mathrm{min}) = 480/(2^{(L-85)/3})\ \text{or}\ Ti\,(\mathrm{hours}) = 8/(2^{(L-85)/3})$$

For example, if a worker is exposed to 91 dBA, the recommendation is to keep the daily exposure time below 120 minutes or 2 hours as shown here:

$$Ti\,(\mathrm{min}) = 480/(2^{(91-85)/3}) = 480/2^{(6/3)} = 480/2^2 = 480/4 = 120\ \text{minutes}$$

$$Ti\,(\mathrm{hours}) = 8/(2^{(91-85)/3}) = 8/2^{(6/3)} = 8/2^2 = 8/4 = 2\ \text{hours}$$

Exposure duration limits for various exposure levels are presented in Table 1.1 of the NIOSH criterion document (NIOSH, 1998). Exposure duration limits for selected exposure levels are presented in **Fig. 2.5** and the last column of **Table 2.2**.

Occupational Safety and Health Administration Exposure Limit

OSHA (1983) requires an LC exposure limit of 90 dBA 8-hour time weighted average (TWA) with an exchange rate of 5 dB. Thus, the equation for computing the OSHA reference duration is as follows:

$$Ti\,(\mathrm{hours}) = 8/(2^{(L-90)/5})$$

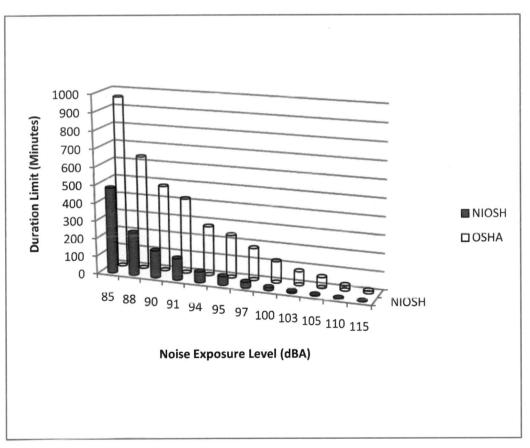

Fig. 2.5   Exposure duration limits (minutes) for selected exposure levels.

Thus for an exposure level of 91 dBA, the exposure time should be below 7 hours or 420 minutes, as shown in the following calculation:

$$Ti \text{ (hours)} = 8/(2^{(L-90)/5})$$
$$Ti = 8/(2^{(91-90)/5}) = 8/2^{(0.2)} = 7 \text{ hours}$$

Exposure duration limits (reference durations for each exposure level) are presented in Table G-16 of the OSHA standard (OSHA, 1983). When exposures *exceed* those listed in Table G-16, feasible administrative or engineering controls are required; if the controls are insufficient in reducing sound levels within the levels of Table G-16a, personal hearing protection devices are required to reduce sound levels within the levels of the table. The duration limits for selected exposure levels are presented in **Fig. 2.5** and the middle column of **Table 2.2**.

◆ Factors Used in Determining Criterion Noise Levels

The recommended (e.g., 85 dBA) or required (e.g., 90 dBA) LCs established by various agencies vary depending on the following criteria:

- ◆ The amount of hearing loss that can be predicted at specified audiometric frequencies in a given percentage of the people exposed over a specific duration (Tonndorf, von Gierke, & Ward, 1979): Based on field and laboratory data, scientifically rigorous relationships have been established between the amount of noise exposure and the related shifts in auditory thresholds. The international (International Organization for Standardization, 1999-1990) and national (American National Standards Institute [ANSI], 1996b) standards are based on these types of data.
- ◆ The particular frequencies at which NIHL is expected to have a significant impact: Hearing loss at 0.5, 1, and 2 kHz can be considered important, as these are the most important frequencies for speech communication. The protection goal is focused on preserving hearing for speech discrimination (American Academy of Ophthalmology and Otolaryngology, 1959; American Conference of Governmental Industrial Hygienists

[ACGIH], 1969). If the effects of noise on speech understanding are to be considered, then hearing loss at 3 (American Academy of Otolaryngology & American Council of Otolaryngology, 1979) and/or 4 kHz (U.S. Environmental Protection Agency [EPA], 1974) can also be considered. If hearing of other sounds such as music (see Chapter 9) is considered important, hearing loss at additional frequencies can also be considered significant.
- ◆ The degree of NIHL that is acceptable: The acceptable degree of hearing loss can vary from none (EPA, 1974) to 25 dB hearing level at 0.5, 1, and 2 kHz (ACGIH, 1969).
- ◆ The percentage of population targeted for preventing NIHL: This percentage can vary from 50% (ACGIH, 1969) to 90–96% (EPA, 1974). As shown in **Table 2.3**, limiting daily noise exposure to 90 dBA TWA over a 40-year duration can limit NIHL to approximately 21 or 29% of the population or prevent NIHL in 71 to 79% of the population. Limiting the daily noise exposure to 80 dBA TWA can limit NIHL to 0 to 5% of the exposed population or prevent NIHL in 95 to 100% of the population.
- ◆ Acceptable procedures for measuring noise exposure: Procedural variations can result in measured noise exposures.
- ◆ Costs of noise control: A strict damage criterion such as that proposed by EPA (1974) can be perceived as expensive. Monitoring, enforcement, and control of hazardous noise

Table 2.3 Estimated Risk of Developing an Average of More than 25 dB Hearing Level NIHL at 0.5, 1, and 2 kHz as a Function of Average Daily Noise Exposure over a 40-year Period (NIOSH, 1998)

Average daily noise exposure (dBA)	Estimated risk (%) in an occupational noise–exposed population after subtracting the percentage that would have such impairment from causes other than noise exposure		
	ISO (1971)	EPA (1973)	NIOSH (1972)
90	21	22	29
85	10	12	15
80	0	5	3

EPA, U.S. Environmental Protection Agency; ISO, International Organization for Standardization; NIOSH, National Institute for Occupational Safety and Health.

to protect the hearing of most of the population can significantly increase the expense of employers and production costs.

- Practical feasibility of limiting personal noise exposure: In some situations, such as war settings, complete noise control is not always feasible. In addition, all of the workers do not use hearing protection, for a variety of reasons.
- Acceptable procedures for determining audiometric thresholds and the percentage of individuals with higher susceptibility to NIHL that can be identified early based on audiological monitoring.

◆ Noise Dose

Many workers may operate different types of equipment or different types of production processes during the day. Thus, the noise exposure can be different over different segments of the workday. The amount of noise exposure for such employees can be calculated using the concept of noise dose, which is a measure of noise exposure presented as a percentage. More specifically, noise dose is the amount of noise exposure experienced by the worker relative to the amount of allowable exposure. A dose of 100% and/or above represents hazardous exposures. The noise dose is calculated using the following formula:

$$D = [C1/T1 + C2/T2 + ...Cn/Tn] \times 100$$

where Cn = total time of noise exposure at a specified noise level and Tn = exposure (reference) duration at or above which noise becomes hazardous.

The reference durations are shown in Table G-16a of OSHA (1983) standard or Table 1.1 of the NIOSH (1998) recommendations. This reference duration can also be calculated using the previously specified equation [Ti = TC/ $(2^{(Li-Lc)/Q})$]; some reference durations are presented in **Table 2.2**.

◆ Thresholds Used in Integrating Noise Levels

When sound levels are integrated, the lowest levels to be integrated are specified. These levels are sometimes referred to as threshold.

If an employee is exposed to levels below the specified threshold, the noise dose is zero. For example, OSHA (1983) requires integration of noise levels from 80 to 130 dBA (**Table 2.4**) to determine if any action in the form of implementation of hearing conservation is necessary. The threshold in this case is 80 dB and thus, during the integration process, all levels below 80 dBA are ignored and are not integrated in the final reading. For the determination of permissible exposure limit (PEL), OSHA requires integration of noise levels from 90 to 140 dBA, which means that the threshold in this measurement is set at 90 dBA and the integrating process will ignore any noise below 90 dBA. If the PEL of 90 dBA is exceeded, implementation of feasible engineering and administrative noise controls is required. If compliance with OSHA PEL is being determined, the noise dose calculation shown in the middle column of **Table 2.5** will change as follows because the exposure of 85 dBA will be ignored, which is below the threshold of 90 dBA.

$$D = [C2/T2 + C3/T3] \times 100$$
$$D = [3/3 + \frac{1}{2}] \times 100 = 150\%$$

◆ Time Weighted Average Exposure

The calculation of overall exposure by considering different exposure levels over various durations during an exposure period is referred to as TWA. It can be calculated by using the previously shown noise dose, which considers any variations in exposure levels during different periods of the work shift, thus assigning different weights based on exposure levels to different exposure durations.

Eight-Hour Time Weighted Average or Personal Daily Noise Exposure Level

The 8-hour TWA average sound level ($L_{TWA(8)}$) can be calculated using the following formula (ANSI, 1996a):

$$L_{TWA(8)} = (Q/Log_{(10)}2) \times [log_{10}(D/100)] + LC = (Q/0.3) \times [log_{10}(D/100)] + LC$$

where Q = exchange rate, D = noise dose, and LC = criterion exposure limit.

Table 2.4 Sound Level Parameters to be Used for Monitoring Noise*

| Agency | Range of sound levels to be integrated | | Measurement parameters | | |
	For determining compliance with exposure limit	For determining compliance with action level	Exchange rate	Impulse/impact noise measures to be made using the "peak" option	Ceiling limits (maximum allowable noise levels in dBA)
OSHA (1983)	90 to 140 dBA (levels above 90 dBA TWA require noise controls and hearing protector use)	80 to 130 dBA (levels at or above 85 dBA TWA require hearing conservation program)	5 dB	Should not exceed 140 dB peak SPL to be integrated with measurements of all other noises	No unprotected exposure above 115 dBA
MSHA (2000)	90 to at least 140 dBA (levels above 90 dBA TWA require noise controls and hearing protector use; levels above 105 dBA require dual hearing protection)	80 to at least 130 dBA (Levels at or above 85 dBA TWA require hearing conservation program)	5 dB	Integrate with all other noise measures	No protected or unprotected exposure above 115 dBA
FRA (2008)	80 to 140 dBA		5 dB	Same as OSHA	No exposure greater than 115 dBA except exposures above 115 dBA and up to 120 dBA are allowed if the exposure is less than or equal to 5 s
DoD (2004)	80 to 130 dBA; exposure limit is 85 dBA; when workers are exposed to steady-state noise, including impulse noise below 130 dB peak SPL, with simultaneous exposure to impulse noise above 130 dB peak SPL, the hazard criteria are applied separately		Should not be greater than 4 dB; 3 dB is strongly recommended	The noise monitoring instrument should be capable of measuring peak SPLs exceeding 140 dB	Not applicable
NIOSH (1998)	80 to 140 dBA; recommended exposure limit is 85 dBA		3 dB	Not to exceed 140 dBA; integrate with all other noises	No protected or unprotected exposure to any sounds above 140 dBA

* Continuous and intermittent noise levels should be measured using "A" weighting, with a "slow" meter response.
DoD, U.S Department of Defense; FRA, Federal Railroad Administration; MSHA, Mine Safety and Health Administration; NIOSH, National Institute for Occupational Safety and Health; OSHA, Occupational Safety and Health Administration; SPL, sound pressure level.

Table 2.5   Example of Calculation of Noise Dose (D) for a Hypothetical Worker Whose Sound Exposure Level Varies Through the Entire Work Shift of 8 Hours

Steps	OSHA (1983) for determining compliance with action level	NIOSH (1998)
Step 1. Measure and record the employee exposure level and associated duration of exposure	85 dBA for 4 h(C1), 97 dBA for 3 h (C2), and 100 dBA for 1 h (C3)	
Step 2. Locate the reference duration for each exposure level or calculate it using previously specified equation [Ti = TC/ $(2^{(Li-Lc)/Q)}$] Use the equation D = [C1/T1 + C2/T2 + C3/T3] × 100	Use Table G-16a (OSHA, 1983) Reference duration for 85 dBA is 16 (T1) h, for 97 dBA it is 3 (T2) h, and for 100 dBA it is 2 (T3) h D = (4/16 + 3/3 + 1/2) × 100 = (0.25 + 1 + 0.5) × 100 = 175%	Use Table 1.1 (NIOSH, 1998) Reference duration for 85 dBA is 8 (T1) h, for 97 dBA it is 0.5 (T2) h, and for 100 dBA it is 0.25 (T3) h D = (4/8 + 3/0.5 + 1/0.25) × 100 = (0.5 + 6 + 4) × 100 = 1050%

NIOSH, National Institute for Occupational Safety and Health; OSHA, Occupational Safety and Health Administration.

Eight-Hour Time Weighted Average (NIOSH, 1998)

When the exchange rate is 3 dB, $(Q/Log_{(10)}2)$ = (3/0.3) = 10. Thus when the criterion exposure limit is 85 dBA, the TWA can be calculated using the following equation:

$$TWA = 10 [log_{10}(D/100)] + 85$$

Example: For a dose of 400%, shown in the last column of **Table 2.6**:

$$TWA = 10 [log_{10}(D/100)] + 85 =$$
$$10 [log_{10}(400/100)] + 85 = 10 (log 4) + 85 =$$
$$10 (0.6) + 85 = 91 dBA$$

Eight-Hour Time Weighted Average (OSHA, 1983)

When the exchange rate is 5 dB, $(Q/Log_{(10)}2)$ = (5/0.3) = 16.61. Thus, considering the exposure

limit of 90 dBA specified by OSHA, TWA can be calculated using the following equation:

$$TWA = 16.61 [log_{10}(D/100)] + 90.$$

Example: For a dose of 114% shown in the middle column of **Table 2.6**:

$$TWA = 16.61 [log_{10}(D/100)] + 90 -$$
$$16.61 [log_{10}(114/100)] + 90 =$$
$$16.61 [log_{10}(1.14)] + 90 =$$
$$16.61 (0.06) + 90 = 91 dBA$$

Thus when an employee is exposed to a single level throughout the 8-hour work shift, the 8-hour TWA is equal to the exposure level.

Weekly Noise Exposure Level ($L_{EX,8h}$ dBA)

This is the TWA of the daily noise exposure levels for a nominal week of five 8-hour working days.

Table 2.6   Example of Calculation of Noise Dose (D) for a Hypothetical Worker Whose Sound Exposure Level is Constant (91 dBA) Through the Entire Work Shift of 8 Hours

Steps	OSHA (1983)	NIOSH (1998)
Step 1. Measure and record the employee exposure level	91 dBA	
Step 2. Locate the reference duration (T) for the exposure level of 91 dBA or calculate it using previously specified equation [Ti = TC/ $(2^{(Li-Lc)/Q)}$]	Use Table G-16a (OSHA, 1983) T = 7 h or 420 min	Use Table 1.1 (NIOSH, 1998) T = 2 h or 120 min
Step 3. Use the equation D = (C/T) × 100; in this case C is 8 h due to constant exposure through the work shift	D = (8/7) × 100 = 114%	D = (8/2) × 100 = 400%

NIOSH, National Institute for Occupational Safety and Health; OSHA, Occupational Safety and Health Administration.

This measure is recommended by the European Parliament and Council (2003) for those circumstances where daily noise exposure varies considerably from one working day to the next depending on the duties assigned to the worker, provided that the weekly noise exposure does not exceed the exposure limit value of 87 dBA and suitable procedures are in place to minimize hearing loss.

◆ Ceiling Limit (Maximum Allowable Level)

This is the maximum level of exposure that is permitted in dBA (not TWA). Ceiling limits specified by different agencies are shown in the last column of **Table 2.4,** and most specify a limit of 115 dBA. However, the Federal Railroad Administration allows exposures to continuous noise greater than 115 dBA and equal to or less than 120 dBA if the daily duration of such exposures does not exceed 5 seconds. Using NIOSH recommendations, the exposure duration for 116 dBA (above the maximum limit of 115 dBA specified by OSHA) has to be under 23 seconds, and for 119 dBA (allowed by FRA) the duration has to be under 12 seconds.

According to NIOSH, exposure to continuous, varying, intermittent, or impulsive noise should not exceed 140 dBA. Henderson, Subramaniam, Gratton, and Saunders (1991) showed that the critical level for chinchillas is between 119 and 125 dB. By adjusting this level for humans by 20 dB to account for the differences in susceptibility to NIHL between chinchillas and humans, the critical level for humans is estimated to be between 139 and 145 dB (NIOSH, 1998). Based on the 85 dBA exposure limit and 3 dB exchange rate recommended by NIOSH, the allowable exposure time is less than 0.1 second or 100 microseconds for the ceiling limit of 140 dBA, as shown in **Table 2.2**.

◆ Exposures Requiring Implementation of Hearing Conservation Programs

OSHA (1983) requires and NIOSH (1998) recommends implementation of hearing conservation programs for exposures equal to or above 8-hour TWA of 85 dBA, as shown in **Table 2.4**. The European Commission Directive 2003/10/EC is more stringent and recommends that hearing protectors should be made available at 8-hour TWA of 80 dBA or where peak levels are at 112 Pa or 135 dBC (European Parliament and Council, 2003).

◆ Applicable Standards for Implementing Noise Monitoring

There are some similarities and differences in the conditions and procedures required for noise monitoring among different regulating bodies. Relevant regulations should be carefully and thoroughly reviewed before implementing noise monitoring procedures.

Occupational Safety and Health Administration (OSHA, 1983; 29 CFR 1910.95)

Employers are required to develop and implement a noise monitoring program in the presence of information indicating that any of the employees' exposure may equal or exceed an 8-hour TWA of 85 dB or the maximum SPLs exceed 115 dBA or the peak SPLs may exceed 140 dB. Where area monitoring is inappropriate due to high worker mobility, significant variations in sound level, or a significant component of impulse noise, representative personal sampling is required unless the employer can show that area sampling yields equivalent results. Repetition of noise measures is required whenever a change in operations, equipment, processes, or controls increases noise exposure in such a way that additional employees may be exposed to hazardous noise levels or the attenuation provided by hearing protection devices used by employees becomes insufficient.

Mine Safety and Health Administration (1999; 30 CFR Part 62)

Each mine operator is required to establish a monitoring system for evaluating each miner's noise exposure to determine compliance with the noise standard.

Federal Railroad Administration (71 FR 63123, Oct. 27, 2006, as amended at 73 FR 79702, Dec. 30, 2008)

The Federal Railroad Administration requires the measurement of noise under typical operating conditions. Requirements for repeating noise measures are similar to those specified by OSHA (1983).

U.S. Department of Defense (Instruction 6055.12, DoD Hearing Conservation Program, March 5, 2004)

The DoD requires measurement of SPLs in all work areas with potentially hazardous noise levels (8-hour TWA of greater than 84 dBA; impulse noises with peak SPLs equal to or greater than 140 dB; upper sonic and ultrasound acoustic radiation exposure). In addition, measurements of TWA noise levels are required for all civilian employees and military personnel working in areas where noise levels are hazardous. Area monitoring can be used to determine worker exposure. In the presence of high worker mobility, significant variations in noise levels, or a significant component of impulse noise, representative personnel sampling is required. The measurements should be performed at least once or within 30 days of any changes in operations that can affect noise levels.

◆ Personnel Responsible for Conducting Noise Measurements

An industrial hygienist, audiologist, safety specialist, exposure monitor, noise control engineer, or others who have received appropriate training in conducting noise measures can perform noise measurements. Appropriate training may be specified by each agency. For example, the U. S. Navy specifies "appropriate training" as the Exposure Monitoring course or other training approved by the NMCPHC (2008).

◆ Frequency of Noise Measurements

Noise measurements should be performed at least once at the beginning of noisy operations and at the beginning of the employment of new employees. In addition, noise measurements should be repeated within 30 days (DoD, 2004) or within 3 months (NIOSH, 1998) following any alterations (e.g., equipment, process, production, personnel, restructuring of the noisy area) that can potentially affect noise levels or when significant threshold shifts are apparent in workers. In addition, periodic noise monitoring should be conducted at least once in 2 years in areas with noise exposure levels higher than 95 dBA and at least once in 5 years where noise levels are less than 95 dBA. This type of periodic noise monitoring will allow identification of changes in noise levels due to aging or poorly maintained equipment, or other undocumented process changes (NIOSH, 1996).

◆ Equipment for Noise Measures

The commonly used instruments for noise sampling are an SLM, a noise dosimeter, octave band analyzers, and acoustic calibrators. Some standards have specific requirements about the types of equipment that can be used under specific conditions. For example, the Mine Safety and Health Administration (MSHA) requires that instruments used in underground coal operations that are used in a return air course must have MSHA 2G approval. The DoD requires that instrumentation used for noise surveys must meet or surpass requirements for type 2 SLM, in ANSI Standard S1.4–1983 (revised in 1985 and reaffirmed in 2001). The Federal Railroad Administration has similar requirements but also allows the use of an integrated SLM meeting, at least the requirements of ANSI S1.43–1997 (ANSI, 1997; reaffirmed in 2002) for noise dosimetry. The Federal Railroad Administration requires that any noise dosimeter should at least conform to the requirements of ANSI S1.25–1991 (ANSI, 1991; reaffirmed in 2002). When purchasing equipment, it is beneficial to review specific standards to ensure that the equipment meets the criterion and will allow use of measurement parameters specified by the standards.

Sound Level Meter

An SLM contains a microphone, a preamplifier, an amplifier with an adjustable calibrated gain, filters for frequency weighting, meter response circuits, and a reading meter. SLM readings can be useful in documenting noise exposures from specific machines or sources, evaluating area noise levels, and calibrating audiometers. The SLM indicates the SPL in decibels by measuring sound pressure, then amplifying and scaling it. Many SLMs offer different weighting options including "A" or "C" and different response speeds including "fast" and "slow." Many new SLMs also integrate energy and can calculate the daily noise dose. Some of the additional options available in modern SLMs include time-history data-logging, acoustic spectral curves, reverberation, and speech intelligibility measurements. Speech intelligibility measures can be useful in ensuring clear recognition of messages delivered by voice-actuated fire alarms, mass communications, and public address systems in the workplace.

Types of Sound Level Meters

ANSI (1983) includes the following levels of classifications for SLMS:

♦ Type 0 is a laboratory standard SLM
♦ Type I is an SLM useful for precision measurements in the field
♦ Type II is an SLM useful for general purpose measurements. An SLM meeting at least the Type II meter classification (**Fig. 2.6**) is often required in the field for noise evaluation purposes and has an accuracy of ± 2 dB.

Sound Level Meter Microphones

Microphones are specially designed for use in particular environments across a specific range of SPLs and frequencies. In addition, microphones can also have different directionality. Some are intended to be pointed directly at the sound and others are designed to measure sounds from a "grazing" angle of incidence. It is important to follow the instructions provided in the manufacturer's manual to ensure accurate use of microphones. It is also important to avoid shielding of the microphone by persons or objects (ANSI, 1996a).

Some noise measurement systems incorporate multiple microphones (collecting data at slightly different angles) built for special purposes such as measurement of aircraft noise near airports. Such microphones can be used in all weather conditions and have a built-in heater, a built-in sound source for automatic calibration,

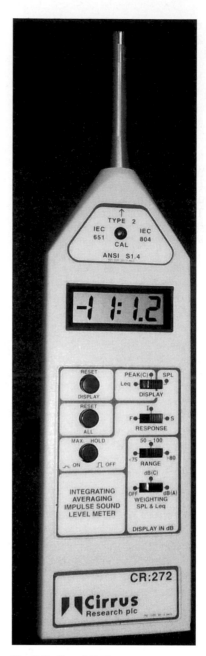

Fig. 2.6   Type II SLM.

and special windscreens with spikes on them to keep away birds.

Time Constants of Exponential Time Averaging

An SLM can average SPLs using a faster or slower time-constant. A shorter 125-millisecond time constant is referred to as fast, and a longer 1-second time constant is considered slow. The meter indicator shows the average SPL measured by the meter during the fast or slow period selected. The meter dynamics are such that the meter reaches 63% of the final steady state reading within one time constant. With a fast response time, the meter can closely follow the fluctuations in sound levels. In most occupational settings, the meter fluctuations are less when using a slow time constant compared with a fast time constant. Although a slow response is more sluggish, it allows easier averaging of fluctuating sound levels. Thus for most occupational noise measurements, a slow time constant is used. Meters that are set to integrate or average sounds typically sample SPLs many times each second.

Peak and Impulse Response

Some sound level meters provide "impulse" and "peak" response options for monitoring transient sounds. The impulse response is an integrated measure, while the peak value is the maximum value of the waveform. OSHA (1983) requires that the peak SPLs not exceed 140 dB. While making measurements to ensure compliance with this limit, the "peak" response option should be selected. For impulse measurements, the DoD (2004) specifies the use of an SLM or instrument that has a peak hold circuit, a rise time not exceeding 35 microseconds, and capability of measuring peak SPLs exceeding 140 dB.

Octave Band Analyzers

An octave band analyzer is usually integrated in a type I or precision SLM. The function of the octave band analyzer is to separately measure noise levels in different frequency bands. Depending on the type, octave band analyzers can filter the sampled noise spectrum into 9 or 10 octave bands into one-third octave bands, or they can provide even more detailed analysis. Such information can be used in the following ways:

◆ Identifying frequency bands with the highest levels of noise that can be targeted for noise control by using different approaches for reducing noise at various frequencies
◆ Selecting attenuation characteristics for hearing protectors to allow maximum

attenuation at frequencies where noise levels are high
◆ Monitoring room noise levels during audiological testing (see Chapter 4)
◆ Checking calibration of audiometers (see Chapter 4)

Sound Intensity Analyzers

Most SLMs provide information about the SPLs but not the direction from which the sound is coming. Such information can be obtained by using a sound intensity analyzer. Sound intensity or sound power intensity is the rate of sound energy transmitted in a specified direction at a point through a unit area and is represented by the unit watt/meter^2 (w/m^2). Thus, sound intensity is a measure of both the magnitude and direction of the sound energy. With an intensity analyzer, noise sources can be identified and ranked according to sound power. The analyzer is helpful in pinpointing noise sources, targeting sources for noise control, and determining suitable engineering controls.

Sound intensity analyzers usually incorporate more than one microphone for the identification of sound sources. For example, aircraft noise measurements near airports are often conducted using four microphones. These acoustic measurements can be combined with the radar signals transmitted by aircrafts to identify the sound source.

Noise Dosimeter/doseBadge/Sound Exposure Meter

A noise dosimeter allows measurements of personal noise exposure for each worker and is recommended by agencies such as MSHA to determine compliance with their noise standards. It consists of a microphone and a microprocessor-controlled monitor (**Fig. 2.7**). The dosimeter continuously monitors, integrates, and records the sound energy a worker is exposed to and calculates the daily noise dose. Specific measurement parameters can be selected on a noise dosimeter, including exchange rate (3, 5, etc.), frequency weighting (A or C), fast or slow response, criterion exposure level, and threshold. Most dosimeters can perform all functions of SLMs, including recording the highest sound levels to indicate if these levels exceed the maximum levels (ceiling limit) allowed by the noise standards. It is convenient to use a dosimeter that can integrate sound levels for two separate ranges (e.g., 80 to

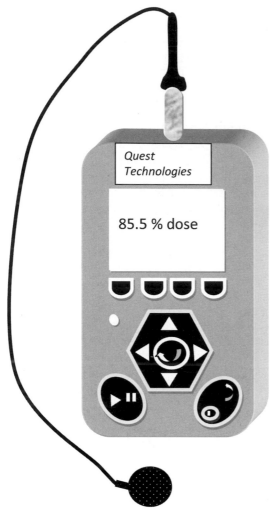

Fig. 2.7 Schematic of a dosimeter from Quest Technologies.

130 dBA and 90 to 140 dBA) to check compliance with OSHA and other standards. Cable-free noise dosimeters referred to as doseBadges (**Fig. 2.8**) are less restrictive to workers and may be safer to use in certain situations. An optional vibrating alarm can be added to some noise dosimeters. The requirements for operating and maintaining noise dosimeters specified in the equipment manuals should be carefully followed.

Acoustic Calibrator

Acoustic calibrators (**Fig. 2.9**) are used to check the calibration of SLMs and dosimeters before and after each measurement. The calibrator applies a

known SPL to the microphone of the instrument, and the SLM can be adjusted to read the proper level using the manufacturer's instructions. The acoustic calibrator must be accurate to within ± 1 dB and must undergo a complete factory electroacoustic calibration every year (DoD, 2004).

Maintenance of Noise Monitoring Equipment

Instructions provided in the manual for equipment should be carefully followed for proper operation and maintenance of the equipment. In general, the following precautions can be helpful:

◆ Do not kink, stretch, pinch, or otherwise damage any cables attached to the microphones.
◆ Use of a microphone windscreen is useful in most industrial operations, especially when the areas are dusty or dirty or the equipment is being used outdoors.
◆ Protect meters from extreme heat and humidity.
◆ Do not use any other type of covering such as a plastic wrap or bag on the microphone to protect it from moisture. Such materials will distort the noise entering the microphone, yielding invalid readings. Do not clean the microphone, particularly with compressed air, as this can damage the microphone.
◆ When the equipment is being stored for more than a few days, remove the batteries.

◆ Determination of the Need for Noise Measures

Noise monitoring is necessary only if noise levels may be hazardous because of (or "from") following indicators:

◆ Employees complain of diminished hearing at the end of the day and/or tinnitus.
◆ Employees perceive several sounds or some sounds to be too loud or extremely loud.
◆ Difficulty conducting normal conversations: In general, if it is necessary to speak very loudly, the noise levels can be expected to be above 80 dBA; if it is necessary to shout to carry on a conversation, the noise levels can be expected to be above 85 dBA.
◆ There are loud noise emissions from specific machines.
◆ Results of informal or formal workplace noise measures suggest hazardous noise levels.

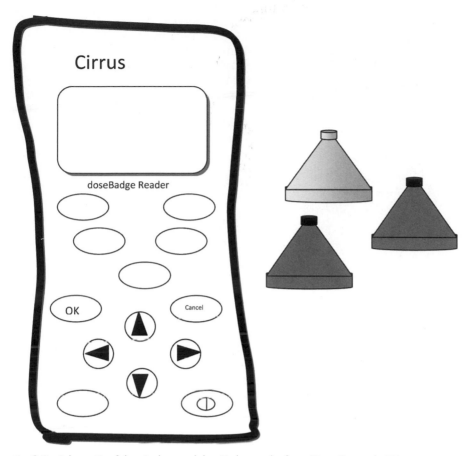

Fig. 2.8 Schematic of doseBadges and doseBadge reader from Cirrus Research, UK.

◆ Walkaround Noise Survey

An initial survey obtained by observing work processes and machines and by listening to noises generated within work areas can be used to see if additional noise measurements or monitoring is necessary. The following general approach is recommended by OSHA for a walkaround survey:

♦ Tour the facility with someone who is knowledgeable about the general operations and potential noise sources. Make relevant notes on the floor plan of the facilities.
♦ Note if it is necessary to speak very loudly or shout, suggesting noise levels exceeding 80 or 85 dBA.
♦ Measure the noise levels using an SLM; make notes about which machines are on or off during such measurements.

♦ Estimate worker exposures by the noise levels and the time spent in different noise levels.
♦ If the results suggest that noise exposures exceed 80 dBA TWA, then detailed noise monitoring should be performed.

◆ Type and Amount of Noise Sampling

A noise monitoring protocol should be established for the workplace, and noise exposure assessments should be done in a typical work setting during typical production cycles. If noise exposures vary significantly during different phases of production cycles, then measurement of noise exposures separately for each phase (NIOSH, 1996) can be useful in targeting noise control measures for phases with maximum noise exposures.

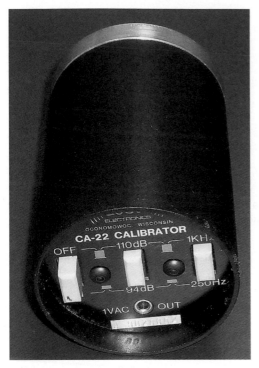

Fig. 2.9   An acoustic calibrator.

Area Noise Monitoring

During area noise monitoring, an SLM is used to take several measurements at different locations where the workers work. The obtained SPLs can be drawn on maps of the different areas of the workplace or different machines in the workplace (**Fig. 2.10**). By using this type of noise level map and information about worker locations throughout the day, individual noise exposure levels can be estimated. This method of estimating noise exposures is referred to as *area noise monitoring*. Area noise monitoring is useful when the noise levels are relatively constant and workers do not change their locations frequently.

Personal Noise Monitoring

When noise levels fluctuate over time or employees move around in several locations, personal noise monitoring yields more accurate estimates of noise exposure than area noise monitoring. Personal noise monitoring is conducted by asking the worker to wear a dosimeter that measures and integrates noise levels at all locations where the employee works. The microphone of the dosimeter is placed on the shoulder of the employee, and the dose and TWA can be read at the end of the work shift. An integrating SLM can also be used for personal monitoring by positioning it near the head of the exposed worker at each location used by the employee.

It is not always necessary to sample the noise exposure of each worker. Instead, careful evaluation of the work site and sampling of exposures of representative employees from each job classification that may be exposed to hazardous noise levels may be sufficient. The analyses of exposure of

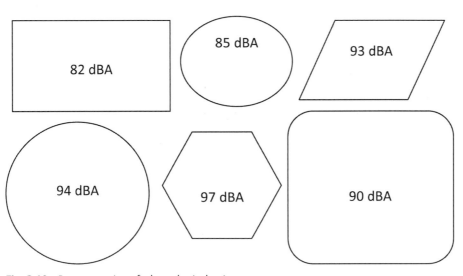

Fig. 2.10   Representation of a hypothetical noise map.

these workers can provide guidance in determining if it is necessary to measure exposure levels of additional workers or workers in additional areas or noise levels emitted by specific machines.

◆ Procedures for Noise Measurements

Notifying the Workers about Noise Measures

Workers and their representatives (e.g., union leaders) should be notified about the day and time when noise exposure will be monitored so that they have an opportunity to observe the measurements.

Equipment Calibration and Calibration Checks

All SLMs, dosimeters, octave band analyzers, and acoustic calibrators should be serviced and calibrated annually by sending them to the manufacturer.

In addition, each noise-measuring device should be calibrated before and after each noise sample using the calibrator that is suitable for each device. SLMs and noise dosimeters can be purchased with a calibrator intended for specific use with the particular equipment. The external calibrators can be either a pistonphone or a multifrequency acoustic calibrator. The pistonphone provides a continuous tone of 124 dBSPL at 250 Hz. A high-frequency calibrator provides the options of 94 and 114 dBSPL at 1000 Hz. Multifrequency calibrators provide calibration levels at 94, 104, and 114 dBSPLs and at discrete frequencies from 31.5 Hz to 16 kHz.

Routine calibration of a noise sampling device is performed by placing the microphone into the opening of the calibrator, with the supplied coupler. The dosimeter is set on the SLM function. Both the SLM and dosimeter should read at the sound level intensity ± 1 dB. For example, if the calibrator is set at 94 dB SPL, the SLM reading should be between 93 to 95 dB SPL. If the level is not within ± 1 dB, then the instrument must be recalibrated according to the manufacturer's instructions before performing any noise measures.

Instructions to Workers on Noise Monitoring Day

On the day of monitoring, the workers who will be wearing noise dosimeters should be well informed about the equipment, the procedures, and the purpose of monitoring. They should also be informed that they should operate all equipment and perform their daily tasks as usual during the monitoring of noise exposure. The worker needs to understand the importance of working in a usual manner and not removing the dosimeter unless it is absolutely necessary to do so. The worker should be discouraged from making unusual noises that can be picked up by the microphone including whistling, shouting, or tapping on the microphone. The windscreen (**Fig. 2.11**) on the microphone

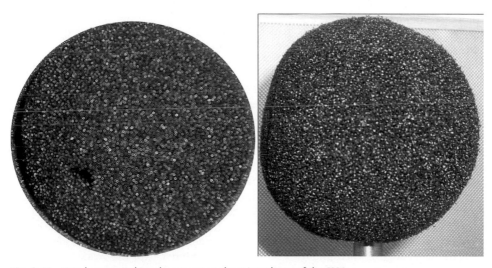

Fig. 2.11   Windscreen and its placement on the microphone of the SLM.

should be on but the microphone should be left uncovered. The dosimeter should not be bumped, dropped, or abused. The worker should understand that the microphone placement and the dosimeter would be monitored periodically during the day. The worker should be informed about when and where the dosimeter will be removed.

Steps for Monitoring Noise

The following guidelines are partially based on those provided by the MSHA (2000).

Noise Sampling with a Dosimeter/doseBadge/ Sound Exposure Meter

1. Insert the battery, turn on the dosimeter, and check the "battery OK" indicator. If necessary, change the battery, considering the fact that the battery needs to last for the entire workday. Always carry spare fresh batteries.
2. Save any previous data and delete any previous readings from the dosimeter.
3. Set all parameters as required by the specific standard that applies to the worker and as required by the purpose of the measure. For most measurements, "A" weighting and "slow" response is used. The setup parameters required or recommended by different agencies are shown in **Table 2.4**. For example, MSHA requires integration of SPLs from 80 to at least 130 dBA to evaluate if a hearing conservation program needs to be in place. However, for evaluating the PEL and the level where dual hearing protection will be required, sound energy is integrated from 90 to at least 140 dBA. Thus it is convenient to use a dosimeter that can integrate sound levels for both ranges. Otherwise, two dosimeters are necessary, with one set to measure sound levels from 80 to 130 dBA and another set to measure levels from 90 to 140 dBA. As shown in **Table 2.4**, NIOSH (1998) has recommended integration of all continuous, varying, intermittent, and impulsive sound levels from 80 to 140 dBA in conducting noise measurements.
4. Check the calibration and record the dosimeter number and results of the calibration.
5. Place the windscreen on the microphone if necessary. Place the doseBadge or microphone of the dosimeter on the top of the shoulder, at

midpoint, facing upward. If the noise is primarily on one side of the worker, the microphone should be located on the shoulder on the side of the noise source. In case of dosimeters with cables, the casing of the meter and the cables should be hidden under clothing whenever possible.

6. Turn the dosimeter on and record the time when it was turned on.
7. It is important to check the microphone's position and battery indicator periodically during the shift. Some workers admit to hiding the microphone in the lunch box to record lower exposure because of fear of losing their jobs due to closure of the mine as a result of a lack of compliance with the noise standard.
8. Full-shift sampling is recommended when worker's tasks and exposures vary over time. During the sampling period, record all pertinent data or observations in writing.
9. At the end of the sampling period, remove the doseBadge or dosimeter from the worker, recheck the battery indicators, and record all of the final readings provided by the dosimeter, including the time at the end of the sampling period.
10. Recheck the dosimeter's calibration. If the dosimeter fails the battery or calibration checks, the results are considered invalid.
11. Save any data as necessary, turn off the dosimeter, and store appropriately.
12. Explain the results to the worker with reference to relevant standards and distribute cards, fact sheets, or handouts on noise sampling, importance of implementation and maintenance of any noise controls, effects of hazardous noise levels, and importance of audiological monitoring.

Noise Sampling with a Sound Level Meter

1. Set the SLM on the "A" weighting network, slow meter response, for all measurements.
2. Check the calibration using equipment manual and note the results in writing.
3. Place the windscreen on the microphone (**Fig. 2.11**) if necessary. The microphone of the measuring equipment should be held at arm's length, avoiding any obstruction in the path of the noise. Depending on the purpose of the measurement, the microphone should be positioned within 1 ft of the worker's most exposed ear to the best possible extent or within

1 ft of any noise-generating equipment. Use the manufacturer's instructions to determine the correct microphone orientation (perpendicular or pointed toward the source).

4. Observe any readings for approximately 30 seconds before recording. Ignore any momentary fluctuations that may occur.

5. Take several readings for each activity the worker performs during the work shift with the goal of finding the highest sound levels at each work site or of any equipment or noisy areas.

6. Record the sound level reading or range of sound levels and worker exposure duration for each sound level. Also, record other pertinent information including the time, location, specific activity performed by the worker, identification number of any equipment operated by the worker, whether doors/windows are open, and any noise controls in place.

7. Make a sketch or area map (**Fig. 2.10**) illustrating where the various readings were recorded; this can be helpful for future identification and determination of alterations at the work site.

8. Recheck the calibration. If the SLM fails the calibration checks, the results are considered invalid.

9. Save any data as necessary, turn off the SLM, and store appropriately.

10. Explain the results to the worker or workers with reference to relevant standards and distribute cards, fact sheets, or handouts on noise sampling, importance of implementation and maintenance of any noise controls, and effects of hazardous noise levels.

◆ Unique Noise Exposures

In some settings, such as those encountered by individuals in the military or aboard ships, unusual noise exposure is possible. Special attention should be paid in measuring noise and recording relevant observations when any of the following conditions appear to exist:

◆ Greater than 16 hours of continuous or intermittent noise exposure per day: The TWA exposures should be less than 80 or 81 dBA for such longer duration of exposures (NIOSH, 1998).

◆ Intense low-frequency noise with a greater than 15 dB difference between the C-weighted and A-weighted values: In the presence of high-level low-frequency noise, the dBA SPL readings may underestimate the resulting changes in auditory sensitivity (Cohen, Anticaglia, & Carpenter, 1971).

◆ High-intensity noise above 140 dBA SPL.

◆ Impulse/impact noise above 150 dB peak SPL.

◆ High-frequency noise above 10 kHz.

◆ Infrasonic Acoustic Radiations

Infrasonic sounds have lower frequencies than the normal range of human auditory sensitivity and can be generated by air conditioning systems, some industrial processes, and wind turbines. Even though these sounds are inaudible, outer hair cells in the cochlea can be stimulated by such sounds. Workers with conditions such as asymptomatic endolymphatic hydrops, Meniere disease, or superior canal dehiscence can be hypersensitive to infrasounds (Salt & Hullar, 2010), and hearing loss caused by audible noises in animals can become worse in the presence of infrasounds (Harding, Bohne, Lee, & Salt, 2007).

◆ Upper Sonic and Ultrasound Acoustic Radiation

Ultrasonic sounds have higher frequencies than the normal audible range. Although ultrasonic sounds are inaudible, they can still damage hearing and have other health effects. In addition, some noises made by ultrasonic sources such as welders or cleaners are audible because of the presence of subharmonics (10 kHz) of the ultrasonic frequencies (20 kHz) generated by the machines.

The DoD (2004) has specified special limits to upper sonic and ultrasonic acoustic radiation. To the best possible extent, noise with high and ultrasonic frequencies should be controlled to stay within the limits shown in **Fig. 2.12**. When ultrasound is present and hearing protection is not already used for the audible noise components, the possible impact of ultrasonic noise should be evaluated, and hearing protection devices should be provided if sound levels exceed

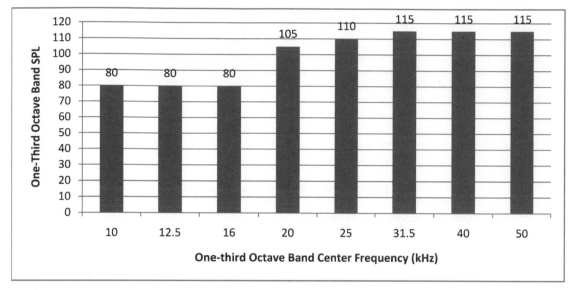

Fig. 2.12   Exposure limits for high-frequency and ultrasonic acoustic radiations above which hearing protection is required by the DoD.

those shown in **Fig. 2.12**. The limits specified for inaudible frequencies above 20 kHz in the figure are necessary to protect hearing at subharmonic levels of the inaudible frequencies (ACGIH, 2006). Measurement and evaluation of ultrasonic acoustic radiations may require consultation with appropriate DoD component technical centers.

◆ Noise Exposure of Employees Wearing Sound-Generating Headsets

More than 3 million workers, including aircraft pilots and other cockpit personnel, air traffic controllers, emergency personnel, disc jockeys, and telephone operators are required to wear communication headsets to perform their duties. Some headsets have maximum SPL limits incorporated in the headsets and are capable of liming noise levels below OSHA permissible exposure limits. Other headsets do not have any limiting capabilities and can cause hazardous noise exposure exceeding the limits specified by OSHA. Noise exposure monitoring is necessary for individuals wearing such headsets (see www.osha.gov/dts/osta/otm/noise/exposure/evaluating_headsets.html).

Probe microphones and similar devices allow sound levels to be measured inside the ear between the eardrum and the headset. However, placement of probe microphones for an entire 8-hour work shift can be uncomfortable, and the probe may move during activities such as talking, yawning, and chewing. In addition, in the absence of carefully trained and experienced service providers, there is some potential for ear drum damage.

OSHA has developed a method of monitoring noise exposure without invading the ear canal. This sampling method evaluates the noise dose that an employee receives during the actual workday while wearing an insert-type headset, a monaural or binaural muff, or a monaural or binaural foam headset.

The first step in determining noise exposure using the OSHA method is to send the actual headset or an identical model of the headset used by the employee to the OSHA Salt Lake Technical Center for calibration. The calibration procedure involves placement of the headset on an ear and head simulator to simulate the acoustic response of a median human ear. White noise is presented through the headset, and the transfer function for the headset is determined at all frequencies over the range of human hearing. The transfer function of the specific headset is saved and preprogrammed into a digitally programmable one-third octave filter set or audio equalizer. The filter accounts for the electrical-to-acoustical conversion effectiveness of the headset and the differences between the sound levels in a median ear canal and the free field. Employee monitoring can then be conducted during a regular work shift. The input to the employee's headset is sent into both the preprogrammed audio equalizer attached to a Brüel & Kjær (Nærum, Denmark) dosimeter and the employee's headset. After the sampling period (usually an 8-hour workday), the employee's noise dose (in percent) can be recorded from the dosimeter.

The method appears to be safe, easy to operate, and convenient for field use. Shortcomings of the procedure include the use of transfer functions based on the median ear canal and head, which has the potential for recording inaccurate noise doses for exceptionally small or large ear canals and the need for having to mail each type of headset to a specific site in the United States.

◆ Record Dissemination and Retention

For SPL readings, the real-time SPL readings in dBA must be recorded along with dBC levels with clear identification of the area, processes, or equipment that was measured. For representative noise dosimetry, the 8-hour TWA with the exchange rate (3, 4, or 5) specified by the relevant regulation must be recorded. For individual noise dosimetry, the records should contain the name of the worker, identification number, job code, job specification, department, the current noise exposure level, the date of the last exposure measurement, noise exposure history, the procedures used for making the measurements, and the name of the individual responsible for making the measurements (NIOSH, 1996). Some agencies require use of specific forms for recording noise measures. For example, the U.S. Navy requires the use of Industrial Hygiene Noise Survey Form or the Industrial Hygiene Noise Dosimetry Form, which can promote systematic data collection and records.

Noise exposure data and analysis must be provided to the worker(s), all members of the hearing conservation team including the team members assessing program effectiveness, the supervisors, the managers, the command leaders, and any other individuals providing medical surveillance. The noise level data, including any area noise maps, should be posted at appropriate points with high visibility for a minimum of 30 days. The posting should include sufficient information to permit understanding of the results by all related personnel in the context of the monitored noisy operations or areas. Warning signs directing the use of hearing protectors should be posted in the periphery of noisy areas in English or other languages that are used by workers and in graphic formats for workers who are unable to read (NIOSH, 1998).

OSHA (1983) requires retention of noise exposure records for 2 years, while NIOSH (1998) has recommended retention of noise records for at least 30 years.

◆ Monitoring of Ototoxins in the Worker Environment

Ototoxins such as toluene can be monitored by collecting vapors in an absorption tube with subsequent desorption of toluene with carbon disulfide and gas. Use of personal monitoring badges is an efficient and cost-effective way of monitoring ototoxins in the worker environment. They are easy to use, require minimal training and experience, are small and lightweight, and are not likely to interfere with worker productivity. As an example, the mercury vapor badge from ChemExpress (Shanghai, China) allows monitoring of mercury vapor emitted from mining operations and fluorescent lamps. The collection of mercury vapor is accomplished through a thin, ultra high–purity layer of gold. The badge allows monitoring of low levels of mercury with a detection limit of 0.0002 ppm over an 87-hour period. Each badge is equipped with a screen that prevents particles containing mercury from entering the sampler during monitoring, thus preventing biased or erroneous results. The analysis of elemental mercury is performed by cold vapor atomic absorption.

Single or multiple gas detection monitors that sense and measure gases such as carbon monoxide are available commercially. A schematic of a single gas monitor from Quest Technologies (Oconomowoc, WI) is shown in **Fig. 2.13**. With this monitor, carbon monoxide

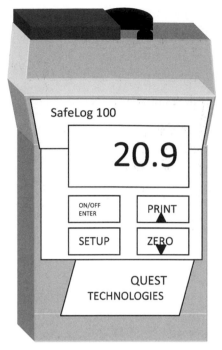

Fig. 2.13 Graphic representation of a single-gas monitor from Quest Technologies.

within the range of 0 to 999 ppm can be detected with a resolution of 1 ppm with a response time less than or equal to 25 seconds. The associated data management and analysis software (Quest-Suite for Windows – Gas Applet) allows graphic comparisons of synergistic gas and noise exposure and selection and charting of critical peak exposure data.

◆ Assessment of Interactions of Noise Exposure with Other Agents

Whenever possible, an assessment of the following interactions that can have a direct or indirect negative impact on health and safety should be conducted (European Parliament and Council, 2003):

- ◆ Noise and ototoxins
- ◆ Noise and vibrations
- ◆ Noise and warning signals or other sounds that have the potential to augment the risk of accidents

Review Questions

1. List the purposes of conducting noise exposure measurements.
2. List and describe characteristics of noise that are relevant to hearing conservation.
3. Explain the concept of exchange rate.
4. Describe the factors that are considered in specifying or recommending criterion noise levels (e.g., 85 or 90 dBA TWA) for 8-hour work shifts.
5. Calculate the exposure duration limit or reference duration (T_i) using a criterion exposure limit of 85 dBA TWA, TC of 8 hours, and an exchange rate of 4 dB for a hypothetical employee who is exposed to noise levels of 91 dBA over the entire work shift of 8 hours. Calculate the noise dose in percentage for this employee and for the hypothetical employee shown in **Table 2.5** using a criterion exposure limit of 85 dBA and an exchange rate of 4 dB.
6. Describe the equipment that is used in monitoring noise exposures and discuss the differences between area and personal noise monitoring.
7. List the steps involved in measuring noise exposures using a dosimeter.
8. List the steps involved in making noise measurements using an SLM.
9. Discuss the procedure for monitoring noise exposures of employees wearing sound-generating headsets.
10. How can other ototoxins be monitored in the worker environment?

References

American Academy of Opthalmology and Otolaryngology. (1959). Guide for the evaluation of hearing impairment. *J Occup Med.* 1(3):167–168.

American Academy of Otolaryngology, American Council of Otolaryngology. (1979). Guide for the evaluation of hearing handicap. *JAMA.* 241(19):2055–2059.

American Conference of Governmental Industrial Hygienists. (1969). *Threshold Limit Values of Physical Agents Adopted by ACGIH fir 1969*. Cincinnati, OH: American Conference of Governmental Industrial Hygienists.

American Conference of Governmental Industrial Hygienists. (2000). *Documentation of the Threshold Limit Values and Biological Exposure Indices*. Cincinnati, OH: American Conference of Governmental Industrial Hygienists.

American National Standards Institute. (1996a). ANSIS12. 19–1996. *American National Standard: Measurement of Occupational Noise Exposure*. New York: American National Standards Institute.

American National Standards Institute. (1996b). ANSI S3.44–1996. *American National Standard Determination of Occupational Noise Exposure and Estimation of Noise Induced Impairment*. New York: American National Standards Institute.

American National Standards Institute . (1983). S1.4–1983 (Reaffirmed 2001). *American National Standard Specification for Sound Level Meters*. New York: American National Standards Institute.

American National Standards Institute. (1991). S1.25–1991 (Reaffirmed 2002). *American National Standard Specification for Personal Noise Dosimeters*. New York: American National Standards Institute.

American National Standards Institute . (1997). S1.43–1997 (Reaffirmed 2002). *American National Standard Specifications for Integrating-Averaging Sound Level Meters*. New York: American National Standards Institute.

Clifford RE, Rogers RA. (2009). Impulse noise: theoretical solutions to the quandary of cochlear protection. *Ann Otol Rhinol Laryngol.* 118(6):417–427.

Cohen A, Anticaglia JR, Carpenter P. (1971). Temporary threshold shift in hearing from exposure to different noise spectra at equal dBA level. *J Acoust Soc Am.* 51(2): 503–507.

European Parliament and Council. (2003). *Directive 2003/10/EC on the Minimum Health and Safety Requirements Regarding the Exposure of Workers to the Risks Arising from Physical Agents (Noise)*. (Seventeenth individual Directive within the meaning of Article 16(1) of Directive 89/391/EEC). *Off J Eur Union.* L42/38–L42/44.

Federal Railroad Administration. (2008). 71 FR 63123, Oct. 27, 2006, as amended at 73 FR 79702, Dec. 30, 2008. Part 227. *Occupational Noise Exposure*. Washington, DC: Federal Railroad Administration.

Fletcher H, Munsen MA. (1933). Loudness: Its definition, measurement, and calculation. *J Acoust Soc Am.* 5:82–108.

Harding GW, Bohne BA, Lee SC, Salt AN. (2007). Effect of infrasound on cochlear damage from exposure to a 4 kHz octave band of noise. *Hear Res.* 225(1-2):128–138.

Henderson D, Subramaniam M, Gratton MA, Saunders SS. (1991). Impact noise: the importance of level, duration, and repetition rate. *J Acoust Soc Am.* 89(3):1350–1357.

Hodge DC, Price GR. (1978). Hearing damage risk criteria. In: Lipscomb DM, ed. *Noise and Audiology*. Baltimore, MD: University Park Press:167–192.

International Organization for Standardization. (1971). *Acoustics–Assessment of Occupational Noise Exposure for Hearing Conservation Purposes* (Reference No. ISO/R

1999 1971(E). 1st ed. Geneva, Switzerland: International Organization for Standardization.

International Organization for Standardization. (1999-1990). *Acoustics—Determination of Occupational Noise Exposure and Estimation of Noise Induced Hearing Impairment*. Geneva, Switzerland: International Organization for Standardization.

Mine Safety and Health Administration. (1999). *Health Standards for Occupational Noise Exposure: Final Rule* (30 CFR Part 62, 64 Fed. Reg. 49548–49634, 49636–49637). Arlington, VA: Mine Safety and Health Administration.

Mine Safety and Health Administration. (2000). *A Guide to Conducting Noise Sampling*. (Instruction guide series, IG32). Arlington, VA: Mine Safety and Health Administration.

National Institute for Occupational Safety and Health. (1972). *Criteria for a Recommended Standard. Occupational Exposure to Noise*. (Publication No. HSM73–11001). Atlanta, GA: National Institute for Occupational Safety and Health.

National Institute for Occupational Safety and Health. (1996). *Preventing Occupational Hearing Loss—A Practical Guide* [DHHS (NIOSH) Publication No. 96–110]. Atlanta, GA: National Institute for Occupational Safety and Health.

National Institute for Occupational Safety and Health. 1998. *Criteria for a Recommended Standard: Occupational Noise Exposure—Revised Criteria 1998*. (Publication No, 98–126). Atlanta, GA: National Institute for Occupational Safety and Health.

Noise at Work Regulations. (2005). *The Control of Noise at Work Regulations*. Milton Keynes, UK: The Stationery Office Limited.

Occupational Safety and Health Administration. (1983). 29 CFR 1910.95. Occupational noise exposure; hearing conservation amendment; final rule, effective 8 March 1983. *Federal Register.* 48:9738–9785.

Salt AN, Hullar TE. (2010). Responses of the ear to low frequency sounds, infrasound and wind turbines. *Hear Res.* 268(1-2):12–21.

Tonndorf J, von Gierke HE, Ward WD. (1979). Criteria for noise and vibration exposure. In: Harris CM, ed. *Handbook of Noise Control*, 2nd ed. New York: McGraw-Hill: 1–14.

U.S. Department of Defense. (2004). Instruction 6055.12. *DoD Hearing Conservation Program*. Washington, DC: Department of Defense.

U.S. Environmental Protection Agency. (1973). *Public Health and Welfare Criteria for Noise*. (Report No. 550/9-73-002). Washington, DC: U.S. Environmental Protection Agency.

U.S. Environmental Protection Agency, Office of Noise Abatement and Control. (1974). *Information on Levels of Environmental Noise Requisite to Protect Public Health and Welfare with an Adequate Margin of Safety* (Report No. 550/9-74-004). Washington, DC: U.S. Environmental Protection Agency.

U.S. Navy and Marine Corps Public Health Center. (2008). *Navy Medical Department Hearing Conservation Program Procedures* (NMCPHC - TM 6260.51.99-2). Portsmouth, VA: U.S. Navy and Marine Corps Public Health Center.

Chapter 3

Noise Control

Noise control is the most effective approach to hearing conservation. Thus, every attempt should be made to reduce noise exposure below hazardous levels. In many cases, regulations require the abatement of hazardous noise.

◆ Applicable Standards/Directives/ Recommendations

Occupational Safety and Health Administration (OSHA; 1983; 29 CFR 1910.95)

When workers are exposed to hazardous noise levels above 90 dBA time weighted average (TWA; 5 dB exchange rate), OSHA requires the implementation of feasible engineering or administrative controls. Impulse or impact noise should be controlled in such a way that it does not exceed 140 dB peak sound pressure level (SPL).

Mine Safety and Health Administration (MSHA; 1999; 30 CFR Part 62)

When workers are exposed to hazardous noise levels (measured by integrating all sound levels from 90 dBA to at least 140 dBA) above 90 dBA TWA (5 dB exchange rate), MSHA requires the use of all feasible engineering and administrative controls to reduce the miner's exposure to the 90 dBA TWA level. Miners should not be exposed to any sounds exceeding 115 dBA with or without hearing protection devices. Thus, all noise exposures should be below 115 dBA TWA.

Federal Railroad Administration (FRA; 2008; 71 FR 63123, Oct. 27, 2006, as amended at 73 FR 79702, Dec. 30, 2008)

FRA encourages railroads to use noise operational controls by reducing the duration of exposure to excessive noise when the noise exposure for workers exceeds an 8-hour TWA of 90 dBA measured by integrating all continuous, intermittent, and impulse sound levels from 80 dB to 140 dB.

U.S. Department of Defense (DoD; Instruction 6055.12, DoD Hearing Conservation Program, March 5, 2004)

DoD specifies that engineering controls incorporating all possible engineering principles should be the primary means of eliminating potentially hazardous noise exposure, and the goal of such controls should be to reduce steady state levels to below 85 dBA regardless of the TWA exposure and to reduce impulse noise to below 140 dB peak SPL.

European Parliament and Council Directive 2003/10/EC (2003)

The European Union Directive has established lower exposure action values of $L_{EX,8h} = 80$ dBA and peaks of 135 dB peak SPL, upper exposure action values of $L_{EX,8h} = 85$ dBA and 137 peak SPL, and exposure limit values of $L_{EX,8h} = 87$ dBA and 140 dB peak SPL. The Union requires elimination or reduction of noise exposure at the source by using all available technical resources. Some of the specified means of noise reduction are as follows:

- Use of alternative working methods that lead to less noise exposure
- Provision of alternative work equipment with least possible noise emission
- Restructuring the layout and design of workplaces and work stations
- Training workers in the appropriate use of equipment aimed at reducing noise exposure
- Using methods such as shields, enclosures, and sound-absorbent materials to reduce airborne noise
- Using methods such as damping and isolation to minimize structure-borne noise
- Adequate maintenance of work equipment, the workplace, and workplace systems
- Scheduling work to reduce the duration and intensity of exposure, including adequate rest periods

WorkSafe Recommendations (Division of the Department of Commerce, the Western Australian State Government Agency in Charge of the Management of the Occupational Safety and Health Act 1984)

For workers who are exposed to other ototoxic substances (e.g., solvents or metals), the recommended limit for daily noisy exposure is 80 dBA or below until revised standards are established.

◆ Individuals Responsible for Noise Controls

For engineering noise controls, noise control engineers may serve as the key personnel. However, collaboration of several professionals, including the workers, is likely to produce the most effective noise control measures. For example, the U.S. Navy requires collaboration between industrial hygienists, command leaders, facilities managers, and safety managers in reducing or eliminating noise.

◆ Economic Efficiency of Noise Control Measures

It is important to assess the economic efficiency of any technically advanced noise measures by considering both benefits and costs. Ineffective noise controls are costly and time-consuming, and they do nothing to save the worker's hearing while creating a false impression of the presence of noise control (Reeves, Randolph, Yantek, & Peterson, 2009). Costs of implementing noise control measures will depend on the targeted reduction in noise exposure levels and the specific noise control procedures used to achieve the target. During this process, the impact of reduced noise on worker safety and work efficiency, as well as the reduction of community noise, should be considered.

OSHA (2010) has proposed an interpretation of the word *feasible* to mean "capable of being done" or to mean that the cost of implementation of such controls will not threaten the viability of the employer's business (Docket No. OSHA-2010-0032; 29 CFR Parts 1910 and 1926). It should be noted that employers' claims of lack of economic feasibility can be rejected in courts. For example, in Manchester Timber Importers (FWM) Ltd v Deary, 1984, an employer claimed that the fitting of acoustic enclosures to noisy woodworking machines would reduce the productivity of the machines and would place the small business at risk for closure. An industrial tribunal in Manchester rejected the claim because it was possible to install the enclosures and still operate the machines without much loss of productivity after the workers became adapted to them (Ping, 1986).

◆ Benefits of Noise Control Measures

Potential Elimination of Costs Related to the Implementation of a Hearing Conservation Program

If application of noise control measures reduces the noise below levels specified by standards (e.g., 80 or 85 dBA TWA) above which implementation of hearing conservation programs is required, then the need for hearing conservation programs and the related costs is eliminated.

Reduction of Noise-Induced Hearing Loss

The degree of noise-induced hearing loss (NIHL) is directly related to the amount of noise exposure. Therefore, reduction in noise levels can be expected to reduce the amount of NIHL.

Reduced Worker Compensation and Related Legal Costs

If fewer workers have compensable hearing loss or if the amount of NIHL is less, then the related worker compensation costs will be reduced accordingly.

Improved Communications

The amount of vocal effort required for speaking and the amount of attention required for listening to speech in noisy backgrounds increases with increase in noise levels. Reduction in noise levels can be expected to improve ease of communication. It can also be expected to reduce miscommunication and the resulting number of production errors, as well as any negative impact on the employer-employee relationship.

Reduction in Absenteeism

High noise exposure levels are associated with increased absence due to sickness (Melamed, Luz, & Green, 1992). Thus, reduction of noise levels has the potential for improving attendance.

Potential for Reduction in Accidents

High noise levels may be associated with higher accident rates by masking warning shouts, sirens, and machinery sounds suggesting dangerous malfunction. Reduction of noise exposure levels through the use of hearing protection devices can result in a significant reduction in the injury rate, suggesting that reduction of noise levels through noise controls may similarly reduce injuries (Schmidt, Royster, & Pearson, 1982).

Potential for Reduction in Coronary Heart Disease

Chronic exposure to hazardous occupational noise is significantly associated with coronary heart disease (Gan, Davies, & Demers, 2011). Thus, noise control has the potential to reduce the incidence of chronic heart disease.

◆ Source, Path, and Receiver Approach to Noise Control

For effective noise control, the source, path, and receiver model (Bolt & Ingard, 1957) is generally used. More specifically, noise exposure can be minimized by reducing noise at the source, by mitigating the propagation of noise toward the workers, and/or reducing noise levels reaching the workers' eardrums.

Reduction of Noise at the Source

Reduction of noise at the source is the most efficient procedure for reducing the noise exposure levels for a large number of workers and to also reduce any community noise. The following measures can reduce noise at the source.

Purchasing Quiet Equipment

For new manufacturing sites, the best strategy to control noise is to purchase quiet equipment. According to the European Union Directive (2006/42/EC), manufacturers have the responsibility to design and construct machinery so as to reduce the risks from the emission of airborne noise to the lowest possible level, using all available means. Some ways of designing quiet machines are as follows (European Parliament and Council Directive, 2003; U.S. Department of Labor, 1980):

- ◆ Selecting nonmetallic (e.g., plastic) materials
- ◆ Adjusting the shape, thickness, and size of components to avoid resonance peaks
- ◆ Damping vibrations through insertion of joints
- ◆ Reducing the height of fall of parts
- ◆ Regulating the flow of compressed air exhaust
- ◆ Selecting power transmission that permits the quietest speed regulation (e.g., rotation-speed–controlled electric motors)
- ◆ Including effective cooling flanges that reduce the need for air jet cooling and related noise
- ◆ Reducing speeds gently between forward and reverse movements
- ◆ Enclosing especially noisy parts of the machine
- ◆ Providing proper transmission loss and seals for doors for machines

One or more of these attempts can reduce noise exposure significantly. For example, purchasing an acoustically treated tractor can reduce the noise exposure of tractor operators through the use of mufflers, quilted sound-absorption materials, antivibration cab mounts, and enclosed cabs. Adding noise protection techniques after the machine has been manufactured is less efficient than designing it to be quiet. Companies could specify a stringent noise purchase specification, such as an 80 dBA noise emission limit at 3 ft. Some major corporations are now requiring project machinery to meet the 80 dBA noise limit at 1 m (Bruce, 2006). The DoD (2004) requires any new equipment to have the least possible sound emission levels that are technologically and economically possible while still performing well in the environments that the equipment will be used.

The National Institute of Occupational Safety and Health (NIOSH) in the United States is leading a national initiative called Prevention through Design (PtD) to design out hazardous noise during the design process of the machines. As an example, a noise control was developed for the conveyor of a Joy Mining Machinery continuous mining machine (Warrendale, PA) by using the PtD approach. More specifically, a chain conveyor with flight bars coated with a heavy duty, highly durable urethane was developed, which minimized the noise generated by metal-to-metal and metal-to-coal contact. The noise control successfully reduced the noise exposure of continuous mining machine operators by 3 dBA (Kovalchik, Matetic, Smith, & Bealko, 2008).

Replacement of Equipment with Alternative Equipment with Lower Noise Emission

Often, other versions of the same equipment generate lower noise levels. For example, fans, gears, motors, and bearings are available in a variety of sizes, shapes, and operating speeds. As another specific example, new printers are quieter because of the use of laser beams or ink-jet drops instead of impacting print heads (Lyon & Bowen, 2007). When buying quiet machines, it is helpful to have clear specifications for noise with the condition that the low noise levels will be validated through measurements and that the machine will

be replaced if the noise levels are not within the specified limits.

Modification of Equipment by Implementing Engineering or Technical Measures

Identify the Noisiest Machines and Machine Parts

In modifying equipment, first the machines that are noisiest should be identified because the noise generated by these machines will contribute most to the noise exposure levels. This can be achieved by turning only one machine on and measuring the sound levels generated by the machine. The processes or parts of the machine that are noisiest should then be identified and targeted for noise control. A machine with a single purpose can have multiple noise sources. Aaberg (2008) described various noise sources from a generator set. These noise sources and the corresponding noise levels from each source are listed in **Table 3.1**.

Identify the Cause of Noise

If the cause of noise can be identified, such as that caused by mechanical impacts, vibration of machine parts, or fluids or air flowing at high velocities, then appropriate modifications can be made to reduce the noise. For example, reducing the distance between impacting parts, changing the pump in hydraulic systems, dynamically balancing rotating equipment, or reducing the force driving the impacting parts can minimize noise caused by mechanical impacts. Damping or isolating different parts can reduce noise caused by vibration of machine parts. For fluids, flow velocities less than or equal to 30 ft/second are recommended. Also, a design that ensures that the downstream pressure of a valve is greater than the vapor pressure of the liquid minimizes the formation of bubbles in the

Table 3.1   Possible Sources of Noise from a Generator Set and Potential Noise Levels Generated by Each Source

Source	Cause	Noise levels measured at 1 m
Engine	Mechanical and combustion forces	100 to 121 dBA; varies with engine size
	Engine exhaust without silencer	120 to 130 dBA
Cooling fan	Air being forced across the engine and through the radiator at high speed	100 to 105 dBA
Alternator	Friction between cooling air and brush	80 to 90 dBA
Induction	Fluctuations in current in the alternator windings	80 to 90 dBA
Structural and mechanical	Mechanical vibrations of various structural parts and components radiated as sound	Varies

Table 3.2   Examples of the Use of Noise Control Principles

Principle	Application	Example
Greater changes in pressure and force produce louder noises	Complete a task or process with smaller force over longer time to reduce noise as opposed to conducting the task with stronger force over shorter time	A quiet way of bending a flat strip of metal is to use pliers as opposed to a hammer
Lowering the height at which objects are dropped can reduce impact noise	When possible, reduce the height from which objects and products are dropped	Use a hydraulic system for raising or lowering the conveyer belt so that the height at which objects are dropped in a bin is reduced
Use of sound-absorbing materials can reduce impact noise	Whenever possible, use sound-absorbing materials	The bin in the previous example can be made of soft rubber or plastic and can further be lined with sound-absorbing material to reduce noise
Resonance increases noise but it can be damped	Damp vibrating surfaces; sometimes damping only part of the vibrating surface can reduce noise	Clamp a urethane rubber coating to a saw blade to reduce intense resonance sound.

Source: U.S. Department of Labor, 1980.

fluid, which can cause cavitation noise when they collapse. In the example in **Table 3.1**, the most efficient way to implement noise control will be to use a silencer for the engine exhaust.

The U.S. Department of Labor (1980) has identified several noise control principles, including those shown in **Table 3.2**, that can be used to identify problems and mitigate noise. **Table 3.3** provides a list of materials and systems that can be used for controlling noise.

Silencers/Mufflers

Use of silencers, which are devices inserted in the path of a flowing medium such as air,

is an effective way of reducing the levels of the sounds propagating through the medium. As an example, a good muffler has the potential to reduce noise levels of an exhaust pipe as close as 1 ft to the operator's ear by 3 dBA for diesel tractors and 6 dBA for gasoline tractors. There are different types of silencers, as described subsequently.

Dissipative or Absorptive Silencers

These types of silencers attenuate sound by use of porous sound-absorbing materials such as fiberglass. Typically, such silencers are arranged to create a parallel baffle (**Fig. 3.1**). The thickness

Table 3.3   Materials and Systems Used for Controlling Noise

Purpose	Materials	Systems
Sound absorption	Felts, foams, glass fiber, mineral fiber, perforated sheet metal, spray-on coatings	Ceiling systems, noise cancellers, panels, unit absorbers, wall treatments
Sound barrier	Pipe lagging, plain and mass-loaded plastics, sealants and sealing tapes, sheet glass, and plastic	Curtains, doors, operable partitions, panels, seals, transportation noise barriers, walls, windows
Sound absorption and barrier composites	Barrier/fiber composites, barrier/foam composites, masonry units	Curtains, enclosures, partitions, panels, quilted composites, roof decks
Vibration dampers/ isolators	Active dampers, adhesives, constrained-layer composites, coatings, sheets, tapes	Active and cable isolators, bases, elastomeric, floating floors, machinery mounts, pipe connectors, pneumatic, steep springs

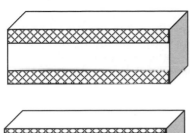

Thick absorbents on the wall with a large space in between provides more low frequency attenuation.

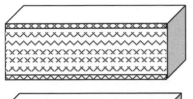

Thin absorbing baffles with small spaces in between provide more high frequency attenuation.

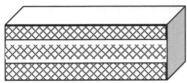

Thick absorbing baffles with small spaces in between provide both high and low frequency attenuation.

Fig. 3.1 Absorptive silencers.

of acoustical linings or baffles should be selected to dissipate the sound levels in the predominant frequency of the noise. The noise reduction provided by dissipative silencers varies across the frequency range, with usually more reduction apparent in the 1000 to 4000 Hz range. As an example, dissipative silencers are used in heating, ventilation, and air conditioning duct systems.

Reactive or Reflective Silencers

These use large impedance changes and sound reflection properties to reduce noise in a pipe or duct. The primary sound attenuation is accomplished through multiple expansion chambers. The inlet pipe of the silencer often has several tiny perforations, and the sound waves flow from the inlet tube into the expansion chamber. When the sound waves expand into the larger cavity, the waves reflect off the sides of the silencer shell and interfere with incoming sound waves; the interference causes noise reduction (**Fig. 3.2**). In addition, bends are also

incorporated in reactive silencers to allow a long flow path through the silencer while maintaining relatively compact length. Reactive silencers are more efficient in reducing low-frequency sounds and are commonly used to reduce the exhaust noise generated by internal combustion engines.

Combination Silencers Incorporating Dissipative and Reactive Elements

Addition of a layer of fiberglass or other absorptive material to the outer shell of a reactive silencer can provide more efficient noise reduction across the frequency range. However, their applications may be limited in the presence of high temperature or contaminated air streams.

A variety of silencers are available for specific applications including duct silencers, electric motor silencers, fan silencers, filter silencers, general industrial silencers, high-pressure exhaust silencers, intake and exhaust silencers, and splitter/louvre silencers.

Fig. 3.2 Example of a reactive muffler.

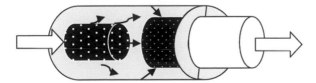

Selection of Silencers

Silencers are usually selected for specific applications using the following criteria:

- Any physical constraints in fitting the silencers in terms of the size, shape, and weight
- The aerodynamic considerations to minimize flow interference and satisfy back pressure requirements
- Acoustical performance of the silencer in terms of insertion loss: Octave-band SPLs and corresponding dBA sound level measures of the pipe or duct are necessary to select the most appropriate silencer. Higher insertion loss leads to higher pressure drop, so it is important to select a silencer only for the amount of needed attenuation.

Active Noise Cancellation

This is usually used in combination with standard passive silencers to capitalize on the advantages of both procedures. The pressure loss caused by active noise cancellers is usually negligible compared with that caused by passive silencers. In addition, active noise cancellers provide excellent low-frequency attenuation, eliminate pure tones, and work well in moisture- or particle-laden air. Active noise cancellation can reduce the level of pure tones radiating from exhaust stacks and ducts, thus reducing the nuisance to community residents. The limitations are that active noise cancellers are ineffective for sounds containing frequencies above 1000 Hz and that their components require periodic maintenance.

The first component within a noise canceller is a sensor microphone, which picks up the sound and conveys it to a controlling unit. The controller evaluates the sound, determines the anti-phase signal required to cancel the sound wave, and sends it to a loudspeaker located downstream. The loudspeaker then emits a signal that is equal in level but 180 degrees out of phase to the original signal, causing cancellation or minimization of the original sound. A second sensor microphone picks up any remaining processed signal and sends it back to the controller for further cancellation.

Acoustic Pipe Lagging

When the wall of a pipe radiates most of the acoustic energy and an inline silencer is not feasible, acoustical pipe lagging can be used. In pipe lagging, the exterior surface of the pipe is wrapped with a sound absorption material; the absorptive material is then covered with a barrier material with high sound transmission loss properties (**Fig. 3.3**). If vibratory energy is being

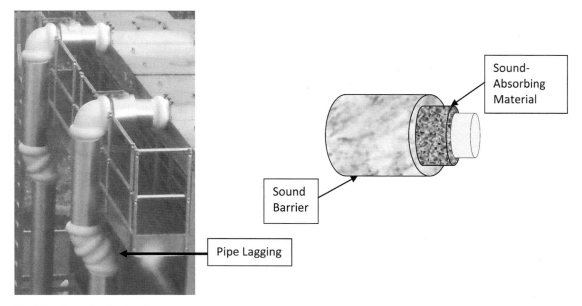

Fig. 3.3 Acoustic pipe lagging.

transferred to pipe supports (e.g., clamps), then vibration isolators at each support point may be necessary.

Reducing Noise Due to Equipment Vibration

Vibrations can be reduced by:

1. Mounting the equipment on vibration isolators such as rubber pads or springs
2. Attaching or spraying vibration damping materials on vibrating surfaces
3. Adding noise damping rubber joints between parts within a machine

Vibration Control Efficiency

In improving the efficiency of vibration, damping the amount of resonance of the surface should be considered. Vibration damping is efficient for surfaces that have resonant ringing or buzzing. Large vibrating plates often have low-frequency resonance, which is difficult to damp. However, if the plate is stiffened, the resonance shifts to a higher frequency, allowing easier damping.

Vibration Damping

Vibration damping can be achieved by using either extensional damping or constrained layer damping.

Extensional damping: In this case, the damping material is sprayed or brushed directly on the surface that is targeted for damping.

Constrained layer damping: In this case, the damping material is sandwiched between the treated panel and an additional cover material that can be the same material as the treated panel. The constraining layer is usually thinner than the treated panels. An example of constrained layer damping is a safety glass with a plastic core between sheets of hardened glass.

Device for Controlling Vibration, Noise, and Deflections in Composite Structural Beams and Panels

The National Aeronautics and Space Administration's Langley Research Center has developed a low-cost piezoelectric device called macrofiber composite for controlling vibration, noise, and deflections in composite structural beams and panels.

Acoustic or Audio Shock Limiters

The term *acoustic shock* describes the physiological and psychological symptoms that individuals can experience after hearing a sudden, unexpected, loud sound or acoustic incident through a telephone headset or handset. Such noises can travel over telephone communication equipment through electronic feedback oscillations, fax modems, alarm signals, signaling tones, or malicious callers who use devices such as whistles. People using a handheld telephone can limit their sound exposure to less than a second by quickly removing the phone from their ear. However, workers such as call center operators use a headset that is not as easy to move away from the ear, and this can cause noise exposure for a longer period.

One way to reduce the shocks caused by feedback oscillations is to always maintain the equipment properly. Use of sound shields to filter narrowband tones such as feedback or noises caused by whistles might also reduce the levels of acoustic shocks (European Agency for Safety and Health at Work, 2005). Use of acoustic shock limiters is another way of reducing the acoustic shock. In the United Kingdom, major manufacturers have incorporated an acoustic limiter in the telephone headsets to ensure that sounds above 118 dB are not transmitted through the headsets. This type of limiting does not differentiate among speech and non-speech signals and can cause speech output to be distorted or masked. Such distortions can increase stress levels of call center operators because of the required extra listening effort. New algorithms incorporating the combination of compression and limiting technology (similar to that used in hearing aids) have been proposed to reduce the level and distortion of speech during shock onset (Soltani, Hermann, Cornu, Sheikhzadeh, & Brennan, 2004).

Ensuring Proper Use of Equipment

Training workers to use equipment correctly and informing them about how incorrect use can increase noise levels can reduce noise levels in some cases. For example, high-velocity air from compressors and pneumatic devices such as air cylinders and air valves can generate excessive noise. Machine operators may increase the air pressure in an attempt to deliver more power, which does not necessarily improve production. If the manufacturer's specifications for the air regulators (per square inch gauge) are followed, the noise levels can be reduced significantly. Another example is the use of proper operating speed. Running equipment at lower speeds than those specified by the manufacturer can reduce noise.

Reduction of Noise Along the Path Reaching Workers

Vibration control is an important means of controlling noise reaching workers. However, the sound from a source can reach a worker either directly or indirectly through reflections. Reflections from walls, floors, and ceilings can increase the sound levels generated by a source. There are several ways of controlling the noise/vibrations reaching the worker (**Fig. 3.4**).

Acoustic Enclosures/Barriers

Acoustic enclosures (**Fig. 3.5**) can be an effective way of controlling noise reaching a worker for equipment that stays in one place. In building enclosures, required work postures such as sitting, standing, or bending; climate controls for heating and cooling; and optimal lighting should be considered to minimize reduction of work efficiency and quality (Franks, Stephenson, & Merry, 1996). Well-built and well-maintained enclosures can contain the noise generated by a source within the enclosed area. Such enclosures usually have sound-absorbing materials such as foam on the inside and heavy stiff materials such as wood on the outside. The attenuation provided by the enclosure depends on a variety of factors, including the following:

♦ The materials used in the construction of the panels: The efficiency of the material to absorb the sound is described by a sound-absorption coefficient. Absorption coefficients for some common materials are provided in **Table 3.4**. The absorption coefficient in theory varies from 0 to 1 and is the ratio of sound energy absorbed by a surface to the sound energy incident on the surface.

In practice, absorption coefficients of slightly greater than 1 are possible depending on the mounting techniques used during the testing process (NIOSH, 1980). The noise reduction coefficient (NRC) is an arithmetic average of sound absorption coefficients at 250, 500, 1000, and 2000 Hz and is used to indicate the overall ability of a material to absorb sound. For broadband noise sources that contain maximum SPLs in the 250 to 2000 Hz range, the NRC allows comparison of the absorption properties of different materials. However, materials that have similar NRCs can provide different absorption at different frequencies; when the noise has significant frequency-specific components, the frequency specific data should be considered in determining the most effective material. Also, the frequencies of 250 to 2000 Hz include the first few overtones of human speech and thus NRC provides a simple quantification of how well human speech will be absorbed. When absorption of music is required, a broader range of frequencies should be considered. The absorption material should be covered with a light splash barrier such as a thin plastic film to prevent contamination. If necessary, a wire mesh or hardware cloth can be used to maintain the sound-absorption material.

♦ The tightness of seals: All wall joints and openings around pipe penetrations, electrical wirings, etc., should be properly sealed with materials such as silicone caulk.

♦ Isolation of the enclosure from the equipment: This is done to prevent transmission of mechanical vibrations to the enclosure panels. Vibration isolation should be used when necessary.

Ordering Acoustic Enclosures

Ready-made or custom-made acoustic enclosures can be ordered from several manufacturers after providing the following information:

1. Overall noise level and noise levels in octave bands
2. The desired attenuation
3. The size of the equipment and the required clearance for optimal performance of the equipment
4. Any operational and maintenance requirements, including ventilation and lighting

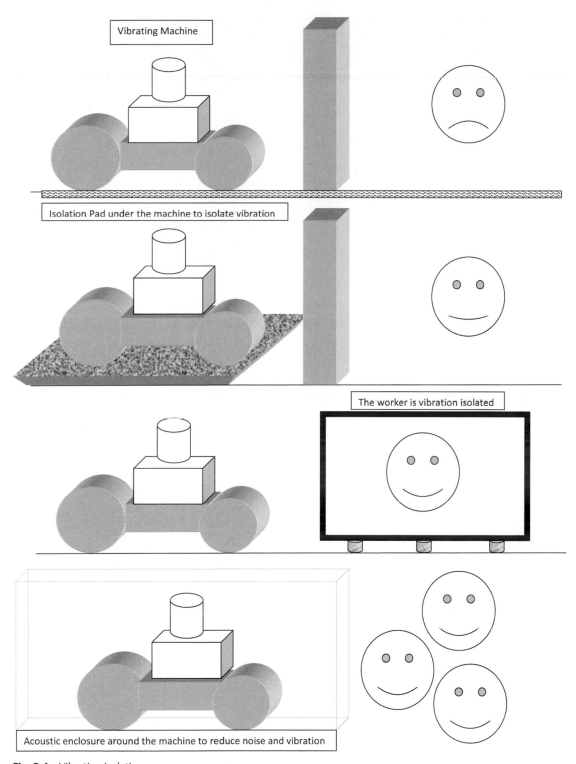

Fig. 3.4 Vibration isolation.

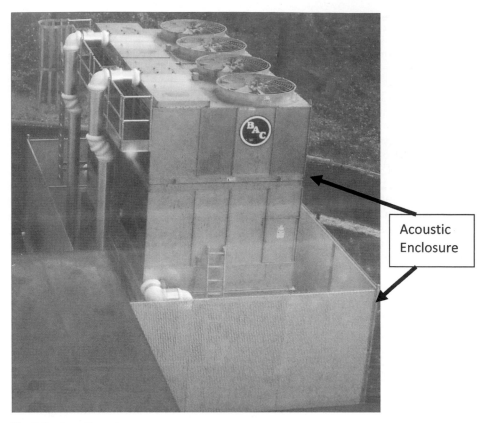

Fig. 3.5   Acoustic enclosures.

Table 3.4   Absorption Coefficients of Some Common Materials

Material	Sound absorption coefficient, α (describes the ability of the material to absorb sound energy)						Noise Reduction Coefficient
	Octave-band center frequencies (Hz)						
	125	250	500	1000	2000	4000	
Heavy carpet on concrete	0.02	0.06	0.14	0.37	0.60	0.65	0.29
Heavy carpet on felt	0.08	0.27	0.39	0.34	0.48	0.63	0.37
Heavy carpet on foam rubber	0.08	0.24	0.57	0.69	0.71	0.73	0.55
Polyester urethane foam (thickness: 0.5 inches, 2 lb/cu ft)	0.12	0.18	0.37	0.65	0.95	0.97	0.54
Polyester urethane foam (thickness: 1 inch, 2 lb/cu ft)	0.16	0.30	0.68	1.00	1.00	0.94	0.75
Polyester urethane foam (thickness 2 inches, 2 lb/cu ft)	0.32	0.68	0.92	0.96	1.00	1.00	0.90
Sprayed on (1 inch) cellulose fiber on timber lath	0.47	0.90	1.10	1.03	1.05	1.03	1.02

Use of Shields/Barriers between Noise Sources and Workers

Use of barriers is an option when any equipment cannot be fully enclosed. A barrier between the machine and other workers can reduce the noise reaching workers to some degree. A barrier's ability to block transmission of sound is indicated by its transmission loss (TL) rating. Measurement of TL at 16 different frequencies over a frequency range of 125 to 4000 Hz is required to determine a barrier's sound transmission class (STC). A higher STC rating indicates that more sound is blocked by the barrier. The STC depends on how the partition is constructed. Adding mass, increasing or adding air space, and adding absorptive materials to the partition can increase the STC rating. Doubling of the mass can increase STC rating by 5 dB. An airspace of 3 inches can improve the STC by 6 dB, and an airspace of 6 inches can improve the STC by approximately 8 dB. Installation of insulation within the barrier's airspace can further improve the STC by 4 to 6 dB. Any barriers should be built to be in the closest possible proximity to either the source or receiver and should have the largest possible width and height to allow extension well beyond the direct source-receiver path (Reeves, Randolph, Yantek, & Peterson, 2009).

In addition to the use of barriers, acoustic treatment of all nearby surfaces such as ceilings (acoustic ceilings) and walls (foam panels) can also reduce the noise levels. To be effective, all surfaces that reflect sound toward the worker's hearing zone should be treated with sound-absorbing materials.

Isolation of the Worker in an Insulated Booth or Room

Placement of workers in an insulated quiet booth or control rooms with windows from which equipment can be operated using remote controls can effectively reduce noise exposure. Office workers can also be isolated from noise in the same fashion. Soundproof glass or windows are a preferred solution to reduce the feeling of isolation that workers can feel in such areas. Call center operators can be isolated from each other as they often turn the volumes of their headsets high due to the background noise created by other operators, thus increasing the risk of exposure to loud sounds and acoustic shocks.

As an example, full enclosure of the environmental cab on a load haul dump can reduce the noise exposure of the cab operator by at least 20 dBA. In addition to reducing noise exposure, such an enclosure can create a comforting and protective environment for the cab operator and also reduce dust exposure. When enclosing an already existing cab, the original equipment manufacturer should be contacted to ensure continued integrity of the protection offered by the cab from falling objects. It is also necessary to ensure fresh air circulation in the cab at optimum temperatures without causing increase in noise. Inlets and outlets should not be placed opposite to each other, and the cab should be lined with sound-absorbing materials (Reeves, Randolph, Yantek, & Peterson, 2009).

Reorganize Workplaces and Workstations

It is important to evaluate the layout and design of workstations and workplaces. Workplaces can be reorganized to reduce noise exposure levels of several workers. If the primary work area of some workers is restricted, the primary workstation of such workers can be located in a relatively quiet area. For example, workers who inspect products for quality control are usually at their workstations in restricted areas. As mentioned previously, acoustical booths or barriers around such workstations can reduce noise exposure. Alternatively, wall, floor, and window constructions in such areas should allow maximum sound attenuation. Unused areas or rooms within workplaces should be examined to see if these can be converted into absorption chambers (**Fig. 3.6**) to reduce noise. Absorption chambers are created by covering walls of the space or a room with sound-absorbing materials. When the sound enters the chamber, the sound energy is absorbed by the walls. To prevent direct passage of high-frequency sounds, the inlets and outlets to the chamber should not be located opposite to each other. While planning new facilities or renovations, it is important to predict potential noise sources, including continuous or intermittent release of noise bursts that may startle workers (e.g., gaseous or high-pressure releases that may occur sporadically) and to preplan relevant noise controls.

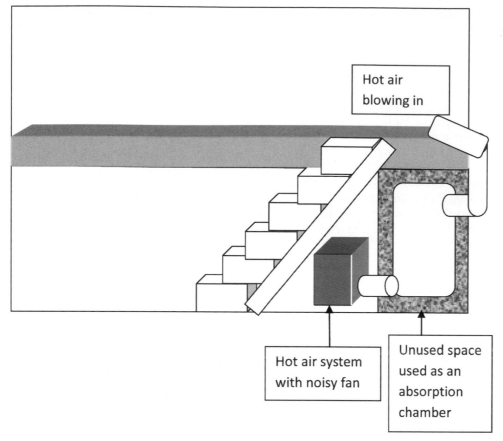

Fig. 3.6   Absorption chamber.

Maintaining and Servicing Equipment and Workplaces

Noise levels can increase to hazardous levels because of a lack of adequate maintenance. Inadequate lubrication of various parts of the machine or worn out mufflers can increase noise levels. Schedules should be developed carefully for maintenance and servicing of equipment and workplace systems and should be properly enforced. Any added controls or enclosures removed during maintenance should be carefully placed back. Any acoustic enclosures should be maintained carefully to avoid the following shortcomings:

◆ Acoustic enclosures can get damaged over time from contamination of internal surfaces from oil mist and other particles.
◆ Enclosures may be disassembled and reassembled inadequately by maintenance personnel, thus reducing their effectiveness.

Reduction of Noise Reaching the Receiver's Ears

All workers working in hazardous noise levels should be required to use hearing protection devices (see Chapter 6).

Mark Areas with High Levels of Noise and other Ototoxic Substances

Workplaces where workers are likely to be exposed to noise levels above 85 dBA or any other specified levels where implementation of hearing conservation programs is required should be clearly marked with highly visible signs at entrances or boundaries. Whenever possible, access to such areas should be restricted only for workers that work in these areas, and use of hearing protection devices should be required. When supervisors or managers enter such areas, they should use hearing protection devices. In addition, if any pieces of equipment produce noise levels greater than 85 dBA, including vehicles, these should be also marked as being potentially hazardous. The signs should include both words and symbols indicating hazardous noise and required use of hearing protection devices to accommodate multilingual workers.

Administrative Controls to Reduce Noise Exposure

For workers who are exposed to hazardous noise doses even after the use of engineering controls, one choice is to revise work schedules to limit the duration and intensity of noise exposure levels. For example, instead of one worker assigned to a duty that results in high noise exposure level during the entire day, two workers can be rotated through the task. The advantage is that both workers can perform relatively quiet duties for half a day. The disadvantage in such cases is that both workers are exposed to noise of concern.

Provide Adequate Rest Periods

The noise in the rest facilities should be reduced below 70 dBA to ensure that the rest periods will be effective in providing some recovery. Rest periods in proper rest facilities are important for at-risk workers.

◆ Medium-level Noise

Exposure to noise below the hazardous levels specified previously has the potential to cause the following nonauditory effects on health:

- ◆ Cardiovascular dysfunction (hypertension, changes to blood pressure and/or heart rate)
- ◆ Changes in breathing
- ◆ Annoyance
- ◆ Sleep disturbance and related physical and mental health effects

Other examples of negative effects of medium noise exposure are long-term interference with sleep and relaxation, interference with speech recognition and communication, and interference with tasks requiring a high degree of attention and concentration. Medium-level noise can negatively affect workers in the healthcare industry, academic professions, and production industries because of the increase in complexity of work and requirements for performing multiple tasks. In these types of environments, noise control measures should be employed. All the noise control measures discussed previously can be used to reduce medium-level noise. For example, in designing workplaces for production workers, noisy office equipment, such as noisy printers, should be avoided. The barriers should be of sufficient height and width and should have a high STC rating. In academic situations, use of acoustic ceilings in classrooms can reduce noise and reverberation. Another example of controlling noise in the academic setting is to encourage quiet social behaviors among students.

◆ Control of Exposure to Other Ototoxic Substances

In designing workplaces, proper and quiet ventilation systems must be considered to reduce exposure to toxic fumes. In addition, facemasks, protective clothing, and respirators should be provided to workers when necessary. To avoid skin contact with ototoxic chemicals, gloves should be worn; in case of accidental skin contact, the involved body part (e.g., hands) should be washed or cleaned immediately. In general, good personal hygiene practices, including washing hands before eating and taking a shower before leaving the worksite, can reduce exposure.

Review Questions

1. When is implementation of feasible engineering noise controls required by OSHA, MSHA, and DoD?
2. Review the factors that should be considered in determining the cost-effectiveness of engineering controls.
3. Outline the potential benefits of noise control measures.
4. Discuss the application of the source, path, and receiver model to noise control.
5. Outline some strategies for designing quiet machines.

6. Outline the two steps that should be taken before installing noise control measures on existing equipment.
7. Discuss the various types of silencers and their functions. What factors should be considered in purchasing silencers?
8. Review all possible ways of reducing the propagation of noise from a source toward workers.

9. In what type of work settings should attempts be made to reduce exposures to medium-level noise? Why?
10. Discuss potential measures for controlling the exposure to other ototoxic substances.

References

Aaberg D. (2008). Generator set noise solutions: Controlling unwanted noise from on-site power systems. *Pollution Engineering.* 40(3):47–54

Bolt RH, Ingard KU. (1957). System considerations in noise control problems. In: Harris CM, ed. *Handbook of Noise Control.* New York: McGraw-Hill: 22–31.

Bruce RD. (2006). It's time to buy quiet. *CAOHC Update.* 18(3):5.

European Agency for Safety and Health at Work. (2005). *Noise in Figures. Risk Observatory, Thematic Report.* Bilbao, Spain: European Agency for Safety and Health at Work.

European Parliament and Council Directive. (2006) *2006/42/EC of the European Parliament and of the council of 17 May, 2006 on Machinery and Amending Directive 95/16/EC.* http://eur-lex.europa.eu/LexUriServ/site/en/oj/2006/l_157/l_15720060609en00240086.pdf. Accessed June 26, 2011.

European Parliament and Council. (2003). *Directive 2003/10/EC on the Minimum Health and Safety Requirements Regarding the Exposure of Workers to the Risks Arising from Physical Agents (Noise).* (Seventeenth individual Directive within the meaning of Article 16(1) of Directive 89/391/EEC). *Off J Eur Union.* L42/38–L42/44.

Federal Railroad Administration. (2008). 71 FR 63123, Oct. 27, 2006, as amended at 73 FR 79702, Dec. 30, 2008. Part 227. *Occupational Noise Exposure.* Washington, DC: Federal Railroad Administration.

Franks JR, Stephenson MR, Merry CJ. (1996). *Preventing Occupational Hearing Loss. A Practical Guide.* DHHS (NIOSH) Publication No. 96–110. Washington, DC: U.S. Department of Health and Human Services, Public Health Service, Centers for Disease Control and Prevention, and National Institute for Occupational Safety and Health.

Gan WQ, Davies HW, Demers PA. (2011). Exposure to occupational noise and cardiovascular disease in the United States: the National Health and Nutrition Examination Survey 1999-2004. *Occup Environ Med.* 68(3):183–190.

Kovalchik PG, Matetic RJ, Smith AK, Bealko SB. (2008). Application of prevention through design for hearing loss in the mining industry. *J Safety Res.* 39(2):251–254.

Lyon RH, Bowen DL. (2007). Designing quiet products. *The Bridge.* 27(3):11–17.

Melamed S, Luz J, Green MS. (1992). Noise exposure, noise annoyance and their relation to psychological distress, accident and sickness absence among blue-collar workers—the Cordis Study. *Isr J Med Sci.* 28(8-9):629–635.

Mine Safety and Health Administration. (1999). *Health Standards for Occupational Noise Exposure: Final Rule* (30 CFR Part 62, 64 Fed. Reg. 49548–49634, 49636–49637). Arlington, VA: Mine Safety and Health Administration.

National Institute for Occupational Safety and Health. (1980). *Compendium of Materials for Noise Control,* NTIS Stock No. PB 298307. Pub. No. 80–116. Cincinnati, OH: National Institute for Occupational Safety and Health.

Occupational Health and Safety Administration. (1983). Occupational noise exposure; hearing conservation amendment, Occupational Safety and Health Administration, 29 CFR 1910.95. *Federal Register.* 48(46): 9738–9785.

Occupational Health and Safety Administration. (2010). 2010–0032; 29 CFR Parts 1910 and 1926 Interpretation of OSHA's Provisions for Feasible Administrative or Engineering Controls of Occupational Noise. http://edocket.access.gpo.gov/2010/pdf2010-26135.pdf. Accessed June 26, 2011.

Ping CW. (1986). Forensic audiology: Enforcement of safety regulations. *J Laryngol Otol Suppl.* 11:51–52.

Reeves ER, Randolph RF, Yantek DS, Peterson JS. (2009). *Noise Control in Underground Metal Mining. Information Circular 9518,* DHHS (NIOSH) Publication No. 2010–111. Washington, DC: U.S. Department of Health and Human Services, Centers for Disease Control and Prevention, and National Institute for Occupational Safety and Health.

Schmidt JW, Royster LH, Pearson KB. (1982). Impact of an industrial hearing conservation program on occupational injuries. *J Sound Vibration.* 16(1):16–20.

Soltani T, Hermann D, Cornu H, Sheikhzadeh H, Brennan RL. (2004). An Acoustic Shock Limiting Algorithm Using Time and Frequency Domain Speech Features. Proceedings of the 8th International Conference on Spoken Language, Jeju, Korea, October 4–8.

U.S. Department of Defense. (2004). *Instruction 6055.12. DoD Hearing Conservation Program.* Washington, DC: Department of Defense.

U.S. Department of Labor. (1980). *Noise Control. A Guide for Workers and Employees.* Washington, DC: U.S. Department of Labor.

Chapter 4

Monitoring of Auditory Sensitivity and Follow-up Procedures

A critical component of an effective hearing conservation program (HCP) is annual audiological monitoring of workers who are exposed to hazardous noise. Significant changes in auditory sensitivity of a group of workers can occur in the presence of an ineffective HCP. The key component of audiological monitoring is determination of air conduction audiometric thresholds for a series of tones at various frequencies. The threshold is the softest hearing level (HL) that the examinee responds to on at least 50% of the test trials during which tones are presented at decreasing HLs.

◆ Individuals Qualified to Monitor Auditory Sensitivity

The accuracy of both the baseline and annual audiometric thresholds is critical for a variety of purposes, including early detection of temporary or permanent hearing loss and evaluation of the efficacy of an HCP. Thus, only one of the qualified individuals listed here can conduct the testing (Occupational Safety and Health Administration [OSHA], 1983):

◆ A licensed or certified audiologist
◆ An otolaryngologist
◆ A physician
◆ A technician, if the following criteria are met:
  ◇ The technician is responsible to an audiologist, otolaryngologist, or physician.
  ◇ The technician is certified by the Council for Accreditation in Occupational Hearing Conservation (CAOHC) or has satisfactorily demonstrated competence in maintaining and checking proper calibration of the

audiometer, administering audiometric examinations, and obtaining valid audiograms. The Occupational Safety and Health Administration (OSHA) does not require certification for technicians who are using microprocessor audiometers to perform audiometry. However, in some cases valid audiograms are possible with only manual audiometric testing. Thus, the best approach is to train all individuals conducting auditory monitoring to establish thresholds manually even in the presence of microprocessor audiometers.

◆ Applicable Standards/ Recommendations for Monitoring

The standards or recommendations that apply to the monitoring of auditory sensitivity are shown in **Table 4.1**. In addition, annual audiometric tests are recommended for construction and demolition workers who have more than 30 days of exposure to noise above 85 dBA during the year (American National Standards Institute [ANSI]/American Society of Safety Engineers, 2007). Annual audiograms are highly recommended for workers whose airborne or dermal exposures to ototoxins are 50% or more of the occupational permissible exposure limit for the specific substance, regardless of the noise exposure levels (U.S. Army Center for Health Promotion and Preventive Medicine, 2003).

◆ Audiograms

Auditory thresholds can be either plotted in a graphic format or recorded in a table.

Table 4.1   Audiometric Monitoring Requirements/Recommendations

Regulation/ Recommendation	Hearing of which workers should be monitored?	Time of initial or baseline testing	Periodic audiometric monitoring	Exit/ termination audiogram
OSHA (1983); MSHA (1999)	Workers exposed to 85 dBA or higher TWA; MSHA: The test is at miner's discretion	Within 6 months of noise exposure; if mobile testing services are used, additional 6 months of exposure is allowed with the use of HPDs	Required annually	
FRA (2006)	Same as OSHA	Same as previous	Required every 3 years; must be offered annually	
DoD (2004)	All military personnel receive a reference or baseline audiogram; personnel exposed to hazardous noise levels receive annual audiograms	Every effort is required to obtain a reference audiogram on civilian workers before they are exposed to hazardous noise, and the maximum period allowed to obtain the audiogram is 1 month from the date of the worker's initial hazardous noise exposure	Required annually for workers assigned to duties involving hazardous noise exposure	Required for each worker who is about to stop working in hazardous noise
NIOSH (1998)	Same as OSHA; offer hearing tests to workers who are not exposed to hazardous noise levels to provide a valuable internal group for comparison to noise-exposed employees and to stress the importance of HCP for management and workers	Prior to beginning the job or within 30 days of exposure	Annually for all workers; best practice is to test workers exposed to greater than 100 dBA TWA every 6 months	Should be conducted when a worker leaves employment or is permanently moved to a job that does not involve exposure at or above 85 dBA TWA

DoD, U.S. Department of Defense; FRA, Federal Railroad Administration; HCP, hearing conservation program; HPD, hearing protection device; MSHA, Mine Safety and Health Administration; NIOSH, National Institute for Occupational Safety and Health; OSHA, Occupational Safety and Health Administration; TWA, time weighted average.

Graphic Representation

The thresholds obtained during audiological monitoring can be recorded on a graph called an audiogram (**Fig. 4.1**). The horizontal axis represents the frequency (Hz) of sounds and the vertical axis represents the dB HL. As an example, in **Fig. 4.1**, the softest sounds that the worker responded to on at least 50% of the test trials at the frequency of 500 Hz was 45 dB HL, while the softest sound he responded to at the frequency of 4000 Hz was 50 dB HL.

When the graphic form is used, one octave on the frequency scale is linearly adjusted to be equal to 20 dB on the HL scale. Thresholds for the right ear are plotted on the audiogram using a circle and those for the left ear are plotted using a cross, as shown in **Fig. 4.1**. If there is no response at the maximum output of the audiometer, an arrow is attached to the lower outside corner of the symbol and drawn downward and at approximately 45 degrees outward from the vertical ruling—to the right for the left-ear symbols and to the left for right-ear symbols. Other symbols used during audiometry are shown in **Table 4.2**.

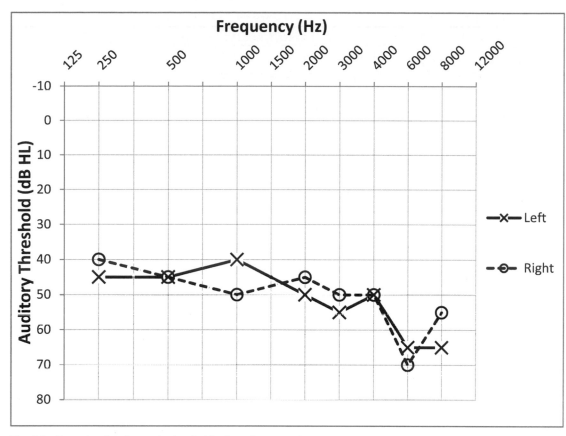

Fig. 4.1   Example of audiometric thresholds plotted on an audiogram.

Table 4.2   Audiogram Symbols Recommended by ASHA (1990)

		Right	Left	Both
Air conduction	Unmasked	○	X	
	Unmasked, no response at the intensity limit of the audiometer	○↙	X↘	
	Masked	△	□	
	Masked, no response at the intensity limit of the audiometer	△↙	□↘	
Bone conduction	Mastoid placement, unmasked	<	>	⌃
	Mastoid placement, unmasked, no response at the intensity limit of the audiometer	⟨↙	⟩↘	
	Mastoid placement, masked	[	]	
	Mastoid placement, masked, no response at the intensity limit of the audiometer	[↙	]↘	
	Forehead placement, unmasked			⋁
	Forehead placement, unmasked, no response at the intensity limit of the audiometer			⋁↓
	Forehead placement, masked	⌐	⌐	
	Forehead placement, masked, no response at the intensity limit of the audiometer	⌐↙	⌐↙	
Sound field				S

Table 4.3   Tabular Representation of Audiometric Thresholds Represented in Fig. 4.1

Ear	Frequency (Hz)							
	250	500	1000	2000	3000	4000	6000	8000
Left	45	45	40	50	55	50	65	65
Right	50	45	50	45	50	50	70	55

Tabular Representation

The thresholds obtained from audiological testing can also be recorded in a tabular format. **Table 4.3** shows the audiometric test results represented in **Fig. 4.1**.

◆ Hearing Level and Sound Pressure Level

Plotting of the audiograms in HLs versus sound pressure levels allows easier interpretation of normal versus impaired hearing (**Figs. 4.2** and **4.3**). In **Fig. 4.2**, it is easier to see how much of a hearing loss above the normal range is occurring at each frequency and that the hearing loss is worst at 4000 Hz compared with other frequencies, suggesting a notch that is typically apparent in individuals who are exposed to hazardous noise. In most cases, audiograms are plotted using HLs. During hearing aid fittings, audiograms are sometimes plotted using sound pressure levels.

◆ Air Conduction versus Bone Conduction Thresholds

Air conduction testing is conducted by using supra-aural earphones (**Fig. 4.4**) or insert earphones (**Fig. 4.5**). During air conduction testing, sounds travel through the outer ear, middle ear, and inner ear (**Fig. 4.6**). Thus abnormalities in any of the three parts can lead to elevated auditory thresholds or poor auditory sensitivity.

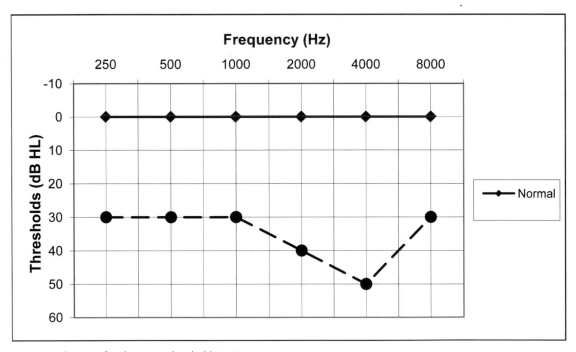

Fig. 4.2   Plotting of audiometric thresholds in HL.

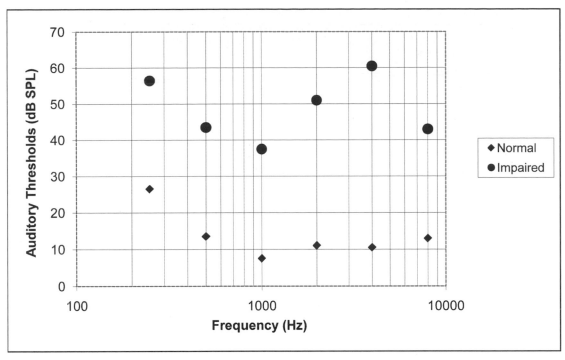

Fig. 4.3 Plotting of audiometric thresholds shown in Fig. 4.2 using sound pressure level.

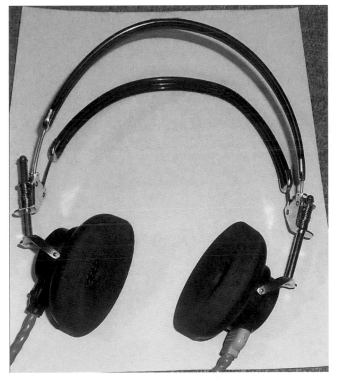

Fig. 4.4 Supra-aural earphones.

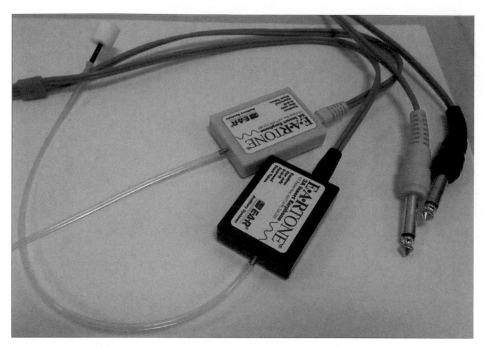

Fig. 4.5 Insert earphones.

In most cases, supra-aural earphones are used in occupational settings. However, supra-aural earphones can collapse the ear canals of some individuals, causing an artificial elevation of auditory thresholds. Use of insert earphones can prevent ear canal collapse, revealing true auditory sensitivity through air conduction. Through an interpretation letter, OSHA has stipulated establishment, if ER-3A insert earphones are used, of auditory thresholds using both supra-aural and insert earphones if baseline thresholds were previously obtained with supra-aural earphones. In addition, the final audiogram established with supra-aural earphones should be compared with the baseline audiogram to determine any occurrence of standard threshold shift (STS) and any need for revising the baseline audiogram. In addition, a baseline audiogram for comparing future audiograms obtained with ER-3A insert earphones should be compiled by using the lowest thresholds obtained with the two sets of earphones.

For regular use of insert earphones, the audiologist, otolaryngologist, or other physician responsible for conducting the audiological monitoring is expected to identify ear canals that prevent achievement of an adequate fit with insert earphones, or assure that any technician under his or her supervision is taught to recognize such ear canals and to not use insert earphones in such cases. In addition, anyone conducting

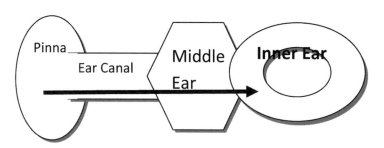

Fig. 4.6 Path of sound during air conduction testing.

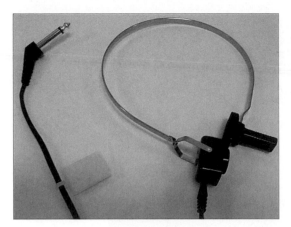

Fig. 4.7   Bone conduction vibrator.

the auditory monitoring should be trained in proper insertion of the insert earphones in the ear canals. If ear canals occluded with wax are excluded, occupational hearing conservationists who are certified by CAOHC appear to be able to obtain reliable thresholds using insert earphones (Bell-Lehmkuhler, Meinke, Sedey, & Tuell, 2009). Besides preventing ear canal collapse, insert earphones also provide greater interaural attenuation, better attenuation of background noise entering the ear canal, and better infection control. However, in the presence of excessive

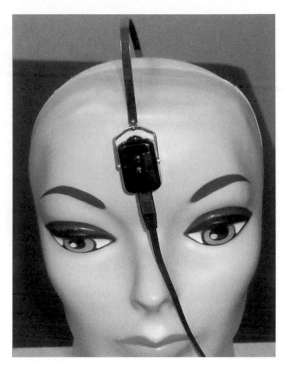

Fig. 4.9   Forehead placement for bone conduction testing.

wax, the wax can block the tubing and can cause artificial elevation of thresholds.

Bone conduction testing is conducted by placing a bone vibrator (**Fig. 4.7**) on the mastoid (**Fig. 4.8**) (behind the ears) or on the front of the forehead (**Fig. 4.9**). During bone conduction testing, an attempt is made to bypass the outer and the middle ear, and the inner ear is directly stimulated (**Fig. 4.10**). Thus, bone conduction testing allows evaluation of the integrity of the inner ear in the presence of outer and middle ear pathologies. Measurement of bone conduction thresholds is usually conducted by audiologists who take one or more courses on auditory assessment and have practicum in managing the complexity of bone conduction testing. Bone conduction thresholds are not required for audiological monitoring in occupational settings. We hear most external sounds through air conduction, and thus air conduction thresholds reflect the disability that can result from elevation of auditory thresholds. An individual who has abnormal air conduction thresholds will have difficulty hearing external sounds even if that person has normal bone conduction thresholds.

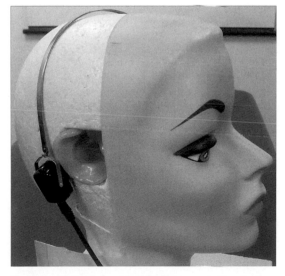

Fig. 4.8   Mastoid placement for bone conduction testing.

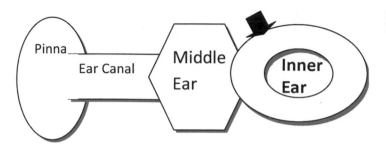

Fig. 4.10   Major path of sound during bone conduction testing.

◆ Audiogram Classifications

Audiograms can be classified using a variety of factors, including severity of hearing loss, location of the underlying pathology responsible for the hearing loss (type of hearing loss), audiometric configuration, modality of hearing loss (unilateral versus bilateral), and symmetry of hearing loss (**Fig. 4.11**)

Severity of Hearing Loss

Different criteria have been used to describe the severity of hearing loss. Most frequently, average thresholds at 0.5, 1, and 2 kHz are used in determining severity of hearing loss. The degrees of hearing loss can also be described using a variety of criteria. The criteria that are generally used in describing the severity of hearing loss in adults are presented in **Table 4.4**. Sometimes, severity of hearing loss is expressed in terms of percentage of hearing loss. Procedures for calculating percentage of hearing loss are shown in Chapter 11.

Type of Hearing Loss

Based on the approximate location of dysfunction in the ear, audiograms or hearing loss can be classified as conductive, sensorineural, or mixed.

Conductive Hearing Loss

In this case, when stimuli are delivered directly to the inner ear through the bone conduction vibrator, thresholds are within normal limits, suggesting normal inner ear function. However, when stimuli are delivered through headphones or the air-conduction path, the thresholds are elevated or are outside the normal limits, suggesting abnormality within the conductive pathway or the outer and middle ear. Conductive hearing loss can result from several causes including excessive cerumen in the outer ear canal, fluid in the middle ear, fixation of one of the bones in the middle ear (otosclerosis), disarticulation of the ossicular chain, and cholesteotoma. **Figure 4.12** shows the audiogram of a 33-year-old man with conductive hearing loss caused by fixation of the stapes. His bone conduction thresholds are within 15 dB HL, showing normal inner ear sensitivity, but his air conduction thresholds are outside the normal sensitivity, showing hearing loss.

Sensorineural Hearing Loss

In this case, both air and bone conduction thresholds are outside the normal limits and are similar, suggesting that the abnormality is in the inner ear or beyond. Sensorineural hearing loss can be further classified as sensory or neural. If the damage can be diagnosed as being located within the inner ear, the hearing loss is considered sensory. Hearing loss induced by noise or ototoxins usually tends to be at least initially sensory in nature. Other causes for sensory hearing loss include Meniere disease, viral infections, genetic hearing loss, and autoimmune conditions. If the hearing loss is due to abnormality beyond the inner ear, the hearing loss is considered neural. As an example, hearing loss caused by an auditory nerve tumor can be considered neural hearing loss.

Mixed Hearing Loss

In this case, both air and bone conduction thresholds are outside the normal limits, but

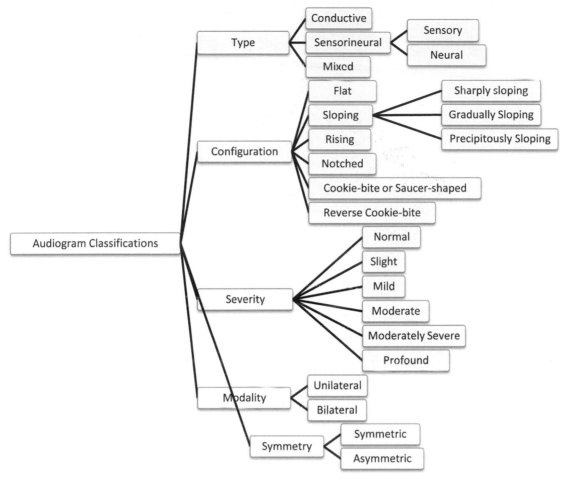

Fig. 4.11 Audiogram classifications.

bone conduction thresholds are better than air conduction thresholds. Stated differently, when an attempt is made to present stimuli directly to the inner ear by bypassing the outer and middle ears, the person is able to hear better than when stimuli are presented through the

outer ear. Mixed hearing loss can result from the presence of pathologies in both the conductive (outer and middle ear) and sensorineural (inner ear) mechanisms.

Audiometric Configurations

Flat

When auditory thresholds are similar across the test frequency range, the audiometric configuration is described as being flat (**Fig. 4.1**).

Sloping

When auditory thresholds are better in the lower frequencies and continue to get worse

Table 4.4 Severity of Hearing Loss Based on Audiometric Thresholds

Description of severity of hearing loss	Average of thresholds at 0.5, 1, and 2 kHz
Mild	26 to 40 dB HL
Moderate	41 to 55 dB HL
Moderately severe	56 to 70 dB HL
Severe	71 to 90 dB HL
Profound	Above 90 dB HL

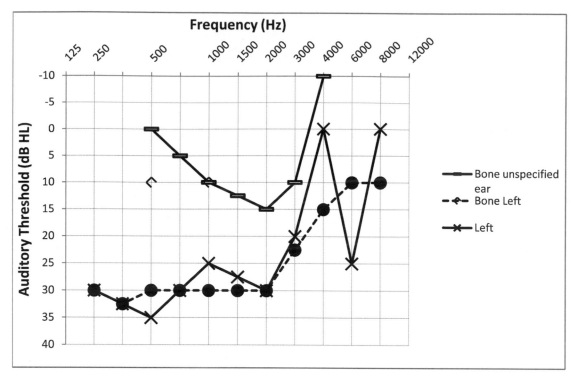

Fig. 4.12   Conductive hearing loss due to otosclerosis.

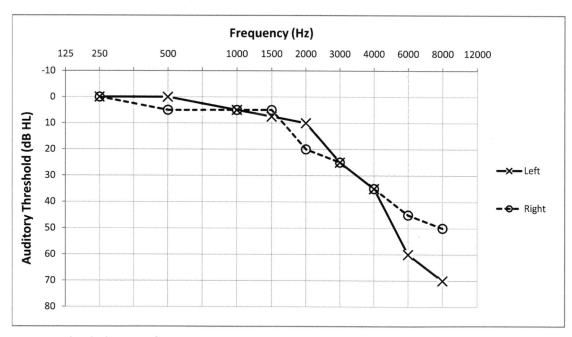

Fig. 4.13   Sharply sloping configuration in right ear and precipitous sloping in the left ear.

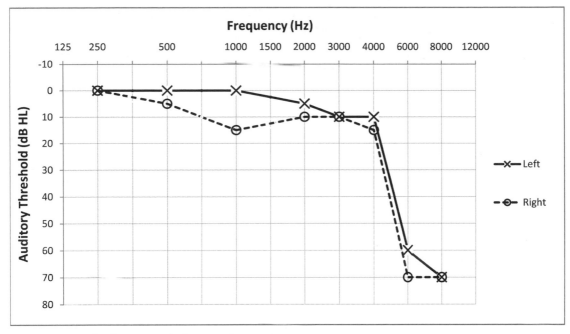

Fig. 4.14 Example of precipitously sloping audiogram.

with higher frequencies, the audiogram is referred to as having a sloping configuration. When the thresholds become worse by approximately 6 to 10 dB with each octave, the hearing loss is described as gradually sloping. When the thresholds become worse by 11 to 15 dB with each octave, the hearing loss is described as sharply sloping. When the thresholds become worse by more than 16 dB with each octave, the hearing loss is described as being precipitously sloping. **Figure 4.13** shows an audiogram from a 52-year-old woman with sharply sloping hearing loss in the right ear and precipitously sloping hearing loss in the left ear. **Figure 4.14** shows the audiogram of a 69-year old previous military pilot who is currently working as a dentist. In this case, a precipitous slope is apparent between 4 and 8 kHz. Some audiograms can display a mixture of different slopes between different octave frequencies, as shown in **Fig. 4.15**.

Rising

When thresholds are worse at lower frequencies but get better with increasing frequencies, the audiogram is considered to have a rising configuration (**Fig. 4.16**).

Notched

In this case, the thresholds are worse at 3, 4, or 6 kHz but are better at lower and higher frequencies. **Figure 4.17** shows a notched audiogram of a 47-year-old man with a history of noise exposure during service in the army. The exact definition for identification of the presence of an audiometric notch varies among investigators (**Table 4.5**). A high-frequency notch along with a history of hazardous noise exposure is suggestive of a noise-induced hearing loss (McBride & Williams, 2001). However, in 11% of cases, a notch can occur without any history of noise exposure (Nondahl, Shi, Cruickshanks, et al., 2009).

Cookie-bite or Saucer-shaped

When auditory thresholds are worse in the middle frequencies compared with those in the lower and higher frequencies, the configuration

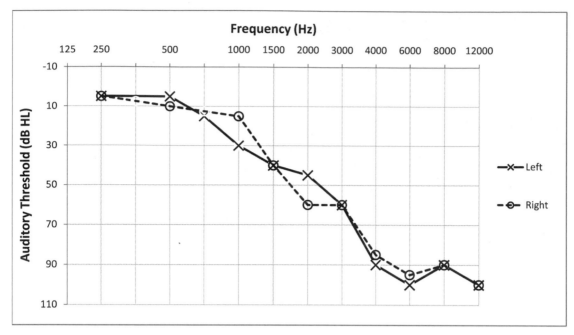

Fig. 4.15   Example of an audiogram with different sloping configurations.

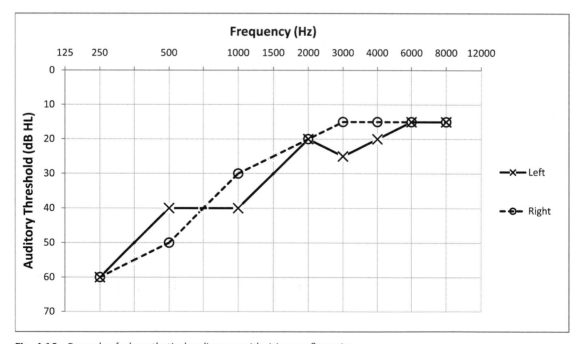

Fig. 4.16   Example of a hypothetical audiogram with rising configuration.

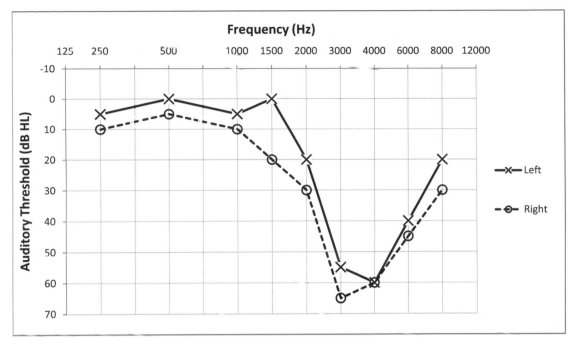

Fig. 4.17   Example of a notched audiogram.

is referred to as cookie-bite configuration. The audiogram of a woman with congenital hearing loss showing cookie-bite configuration is shown in **Fig. 4.18**.

Reverse Cookie-bite

In this case, the auditory thresholds are normal or near normal in the middle frequencies and worse in the lower and higher frequencies, as represented in **Fig. 4.19**.

Modality

Unilateral Hearing Loss

When hearing is normal in one ear in the presence of hearing loss in the other ear, the hearing loss can be considered unilateral. Medical referrals should be initiated in the presence of unilateral hearing loss to determine the cause and appropriate treatment unless the cause and treatment options are already known to the patient. **Figure 4.20**

Table 4.5   Criteria Used for Detecting a Notched Audiogram

Investigators	Criteria used for detecting audiometric notch
Coles, Lutman, and Buffin (2000)	Thresholds worse by at least 10 dB at 3, 4, or 6 kHz than those at 1 or 2 kHz and 6 or 8 kHz.
McBride and Williams (2001)	Narrow or V-shaped notch: Only one frequency in the depth of the notch and the depth is at least 15 dB.
	Wide or U-shaped notch: More than one frequency in the depth of the notch, depth of 20 dB, thresholds better by at least 10 dB at the high frequency end.
Dobie and Rabinowitz (2002)	NI is obtained by subtracting the average thresholds at 1 and 8 kHz from the average thresholds at 2, 3, and 4 kHz. Noise index greater than 0 dB may indicate the presence of a bulge or a notch.
Hoffman, Ko, Themann, Dillon, and Franks (2006)	Thresholds worse by at least 15 dB at 3, 4, or 6 kHz than the average thresholds at 0.5 and 1 kHz and the thresholds at 8 kHz better by at least 5 dB than the worst threshold at 3, 4, or 6 kHz.

NI, notch index.

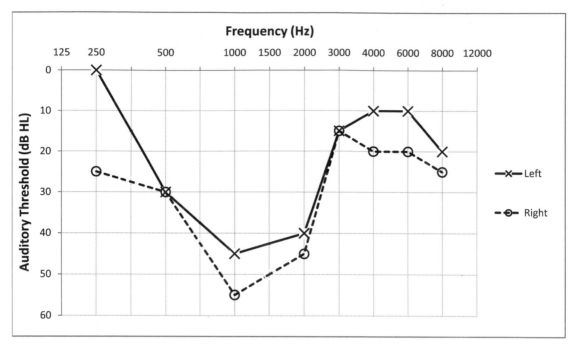

Fig. 4.18   Example of an audiogram with cookie-bite configuration.

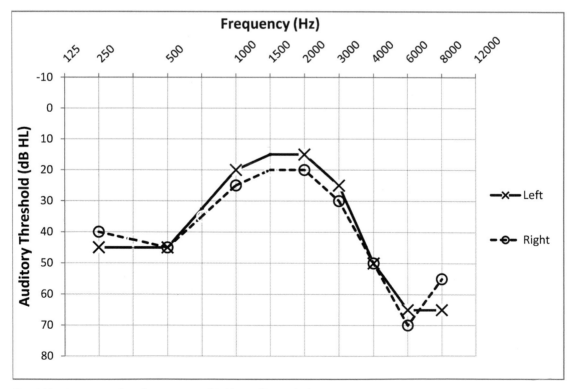

Fig. 4.19   Representation of a reverse cookie-bite audiometric shape.

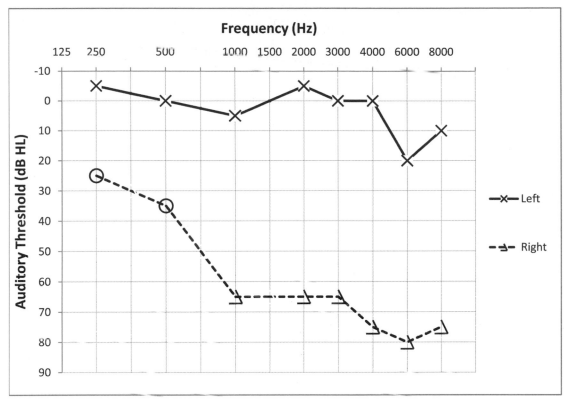

Fig. 4.20   Unilateral hearing loss.

shows the audiogram of a woman who suffered from a sudden sensorineural hearing loss in the right ear but suffers from continuous tinnitus in both ears.

Bilateral Hearing Loss

When hearing loss is apparent in both ears, the hearing loss is considered bilateral (**Fig. 4.1**)

Symmetry

Symmetric Hearing Loss

When hearing loss in both ears is similar, the hearing loss is considered symmetric (**Fig. 4.1**)

Asymmetric Hearing Loss

When hearing loss in the two ears is different, the hearing loss can be described as asymmetric. Medical referral should be initiated in the presence of asymmetrical hearing loss. In the United Kingdom, a difference of 20 dB at 0.5, 1, 2, or 4 kHz is used as a criterion for asymmetry; in the United States, a difference of 15 dB in the average thresholds of 0.5, 1, 2, and 3 kHz is used as a criterion for asymmetry to determine the need for medical referral. Using a criterion of 15 dB or more difference in the average thresholds at 0.5, 1, 2, and 4 kHz, approximately 1% of the general non-noise–exposed U.K. population between the ages of 18 to 80 years have asymmetric audiometric configurations (Lutman & Coles, 2009). Thus a few individuals can be expected to have asymmetric hearing of unknown origin. **Figure 4.21** shows an asymmetric audiogram of a 34-year-old man with no reported history of noise exposure or ototoxicity. **Figure 4.22** shows an asymmetric audiogram of a 54-year-old worker with history of occupational noise exposure and a history of ear infections and mastoidectomy on the right side. His postmedical referral magnetic resonance imaging on the right side revealed a tumor in the right mastoid space area, which was surgically removed and found to be benign.

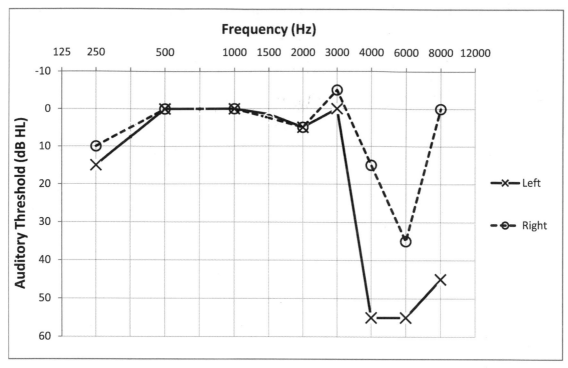

Fig. 4.21   No noise exposure in a 34-year-old with asymmetric narrow and broad notch.

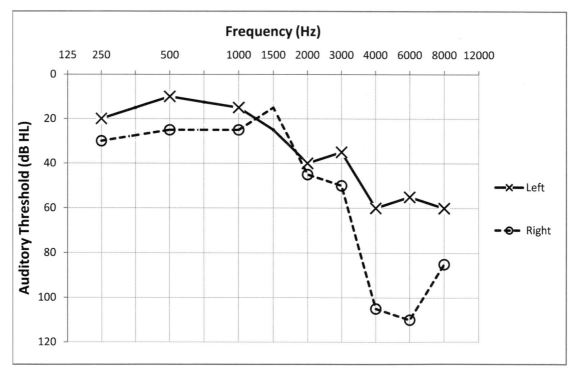

Fig. 4.22   Example of an asymmetric audiogram of a 54-year-old individual.

Classifications Based on More than One Audiogram

Depending on the onset and progression of hearing loss, the hearing loss can be described as progressive, sudden, or fluctuating. If the hearing continues to deteriorate over longer periods, the hearing loss can be described as a progressive hearing loss. Hearing loss caused by occupational noise exposure is usually progressive in nature. If a significant hearing loss occurs suddenly, it is described as a sudden hearing loss. Such a hearing loss can occur following exposures to sudden loud noises such as bomb blasts or firecrackers. In some cases, the hearing can appear to become better and then become worse again over time. In such cases, the hearing loss can be described as fluctuating. Examples of diseases or conditions in which fluctuations in auditory sensitivity are apparent are Meniere disease or middle ear infections.

◆ Preparations Prior to Testing

Scheduling for Baseline or Periodic Audiograms

Full cooperation from management, union leaders, and employees before establishing schedules for audiometric testing can reduce absenteeism and lead to more efficient audiometric monitoring. If all involved personnel fully understand the importance of audiometric testing and employees do not feel threatened about potential negative outcomes such as demotion, job reassignment, or termination due to temporary or permanent threshold shifts, most employees can be expected to fully cooperate with audiometric testing. Existence of motivating reasons such as civil penalties for employees who willfully do not report for audiometric testing (Federal Railroad Administration [FRA], 2006) is likely to improve the attendance rates for monitoring audiometry.

Ensuring a Sufficiently Quiet Test Environment

The test environment needs to be sufficiently noise-free to allow accurate threshold measurements. High ambient noise levels can cause artificial elevation of auditory thresholds. In practice, it is difficult to have an environment that is completely free of noise. Therefore, OSHA and other agencies have specified maximum permissible noise levels for audiometric monitoring of workers, as shown in **Table 4.6**. To ensure a quiet test environment, OSHA (1983) requires the measurement of sound pressure levels in the test environment using at least a sound level meter that meets the requirements of ANSI for

Table 4.6 Maximum Acceptable/Permissible Sound Pressure Levels for Audiometric Test Rooms Assuming a Test Frequency Range of 500 to 8000 Hz

Octave band center frequency (Hz)	Supra-aural and insert OSHA, (1983)	Supra-aural earphones ANSI S3.1–1999 (reaffirmed by ANSI, October 2008). If 250 Hz is included in the test frequency range, noise levels at 125 and 250 Hz should be 10 dB lower.		FRA, (2006)	Insert earphones ANSI S3.1–1999 (reaffirmed by ANSI, October 2008). If 250 Hz is included in the test frequency range, noise levels at 125 and 250 Hz should be 11 dB lower.	
		For 0 dB HL testing	For −10 dB HL testing		For 0 dB HL testing	For −10 dB HL testing
125		49	39		78	68
250		35	25		64	54
500	40	21	11	50	50	40
1000	40	26	16	47	47	37
2000	47	34	24	49	49	39
4000	57	37	27	50	50	40
6000						
8000	62	37	27	56	56	46

ANSI, American National Standards Institute; FRA, Federal Railroad Administration; OSHA, Occupational Safety and Health Administration.

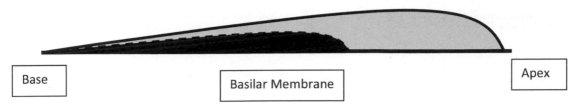

Base

Basilar Membrane

Apex

Fig. 4.23 Illustration of excitation of upward spread of masking.

octave, half octave, and third octave band filter sets as specified in the ANSI specifications for sound level meters, S1.4–1971 (ANSI, 1971).

Ideally, testing should be conducted in a quiet environment that does not exceed the maximum sound pressure levels specified in ANSI S3.1–1999 (ANSI/Acoustical Society of America [ASA], 1999) shown in **Table 4.6**. The maximum noise levels permitted by OSHA (1983) for supra-aural earphones are higher and can interfere in establishing very low thresholds such as −10 dB HL in young adults with very good hearing who are just beginning their careers. It is also important to monitor the noise levels at 125 and 250 Hz, even though these frequencies are not included in testing. High noise levels at these frequencies can elevate thresholds at higher frequencies because of upward spread of masking. Upward spread of masking occurs due to the fact that the traveling wave in the cochlea always travels from base

to apex, and the maximum excitation for low frequencies occurs at the apex. Thus, when the ear is stimulated with low frequency noise, the related traveling wave, while moving toward the apex, can cause masking of high-frequency tones whose excitation patterns are located toward the base. In **Fig. 4.23**, the excitation pattern created by a soft, near-threshold high-frequency tone is represented by a dotted line, and the excitation pattern created by low frequency noise is shown by a solid line. To be audible above the low-frequency noise, the level of the high-frequency tone will have to be increased. ANSI/ASA (1999) derived the maximum permissible ambient noise levels at 125 and 250 Hz by assuming a slope of 14 dB/octave for the upward spread of masking function below the lowest test frequency. Therefore, the permissible maximum noise level for 250 Hz is 14 dB higher than that permitted at 500 Hz (e.g., for supra-aural earphones, 21 + 14 = 35)

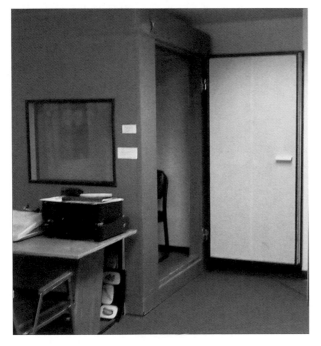

Fig. 4.24 A double wall booth for hearing evaluations.

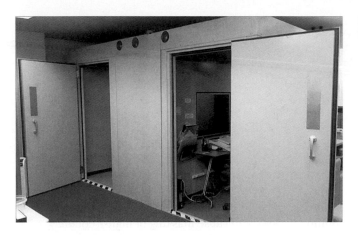

Fig. 4.25 A double wall booth set up for both patient and examiner rooms.

and that at 125 Hz is 14 dB higher than that permitted at 250 Hz.

A sound-treated double-wall booth (**Fig. 4.24**) is ideal for testing because it allows attenuation of even transient bursts of loud sounds such as jet airplanes flying by. When speech audiometric testing is being conducted, the best practice is to have both the patient and examiner areas sound treated (**Fig. 4.25**). Sound booth manufacturers often provide sound absorption and noise reduction data for their booths that can be used in determining if the noise levels in the booth will be within the maximum permissible noise levels specified by the ANSI/ASA (1999) standards. However, in evaluating the data provided by manufacturers, whether or not the data was obtained using standard testing procedures and with the air ventilation system on should be considered. Adequate ventilation and temperature control in the booth is necessary to minimize fatigue and discomfort during testing, which can affect thresholds. It should also be noted that the booths need to be properly installed to achieve the attenuation characteristics provided by the manufacturers. Examples of the determination of expected noise levels in the booths using the attenuation characteristics of the booth are provided in **Table 4.7** for a single-wall booth and in **Table 4.8** for a double-wall booth.

Continuous Monitoring of the Test Environment

When testing is being conducted in non-ideal environments, such as within a manufacturing plant, use of a continuous noise monitor can ensure compliance with the standard. The monitor can alert the examiner when the noise exceeds the OSHA (1983) standard through a light indicator so that the testing can be discontinued until the noise levels are within acceptable limits.

◆ Audiometric Functional Checks and Calibration

Audiometric testing should not begin until the audiometer (**Fig. 4.26**) is properly calibrated and

Table 4.7 Predicting the Noise Levels in the Booth Based on Noise Levels Where the Booth Will be Located and Manufacturer Specifications about Attenuation Provided by a Single-Wall Booth

Center frequency (Hz)	125	250	500	1000	2000	3000	4000	8000
Hypothetical noise levels in the manufacturing plant where the booth will be located	81	93	94	87	89	82	79	73
Hypothetical attenuation characteristics of a single wall booth	28	36	43	50	55	56	55	61
Expected noise levels in the booth	53	57	51	37	34	26	24	12
Are expected noise levels within OSHA (1983) permissible limits?			40 (No)	40 (Yes)	47 (Yes)	57 (Yes)		62 (Yes)

OSHA, Occupational Safety and Health Administration.

Table 4.8   Predicting the Noise Levels in the Booth Based on Noise Levels Where the Booth Will be Located and Manufacturer Specifications about Attenuation Provided by a Double-Wall Booth

Center frequency (Hz)	125	250	500	1000	2000	3000	4000	8000
Hypothetical noise levels in the manufacturing plant where the booth will be located	81	93	94	87	89	82	79	73
Hypothetical attenuation characteristics of a double wall booth	43	68	83	81	83	83	84	90
Expected noise levels in the booth	38	25	11	6	6	−1	−5	−17
S3.1-1999 (ANSI/ASA, 1999; R2008) maximum permissible noise levels for testing under supra-aural headphones for −10 dB HL testing	39	25	11	16	24	25	27	27
Are expected noise levels within permissible limits?	Yes	Yes	Yes	Yes	Yes	Yes	Yes	Yes

ANSI, American National Standards Institute; ASA, Acoustical Society of America.

is in a good working condition. Failure to ensure a calibrated audiometer can lead to inaccurate auditory thresholds. Three types of audiometric calibration procedures are specified in the OSHA (1983) standard: daily functional checks, annual acoustic calibrations, and an exhaustive calibration every two years. The functional check and calibration sequence is shown in **Fig. 4.27**.

Daily Functional Checks

The functional operation of the audiometer should be checked at the beginning of each day of testing and at each facility where the testing is being conducted. The daily check should have the components described as follows.

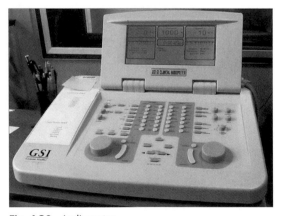

Fig. 4.26   Audiometer.

Visual Check

◆ Earphone cushions: Check the earphone cushions for any cracks or stiffness. The cushions should be cleaned periodically and replaced when cracks appear or when they are stiff.
◆ Cords: Check the cords for any discontinuities and make sure that the right and left earphones are plugged in correctly.

Listening Check

◆ Check for distortions: Listen to the output of the audiometer at both soft and moderately loud levels to ensure that there are no distortions or unwanted sounds mixed with the presented pure tones.
◆ Check for acoustic crosstalk: Press one earphone on one ear and present tones through the other earphone. Check to see if the tones are audible in the earphone placed on the ear. If the tone is audible, recheck to see if the right and the left earphones are plugged into the corresponding jacks. Sometimes crosstalk can occur even after accurate plugging of headphones, although this is less likely to occur with new audiometers.

Threshold or Biological Check

During the threshold check, the examiner makes sure that the output of the audiometer at each test frequency has not changed on the day of

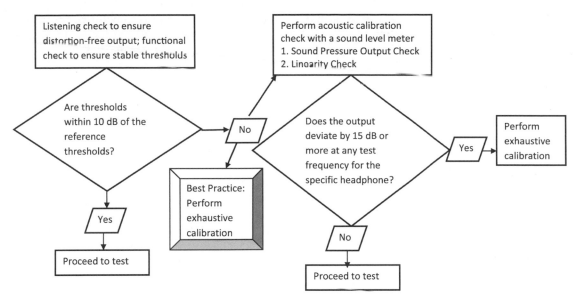

Fig. 4.27 Audiometric calibration sequence.

testing. This can be accomplished by using the following procedures:

- Test a person with known stable hearing and compare his thresholds with his previously established thresholds. It is better to have the reference audiograms of at least two individuals available for comparison in case one person is absent or experiences elevated thresholds because of illness or other factors.
- Use an instrument that simulates a human subject or ear. The instrument (**Fig. 4.28**) is referred to as a bioacoustic simulator or an electroacoustic ear. The earphones are placed on the simulator, and the thresholds are determined as they would be determined for an individual.

If the threshold check yields deviations equal to or above 10 dB, acoustic calibration is required by OSHA. The best practice is to temporarily remove and/or recalibrate (exhaustive calibration) the audiometer if the daily biological test results differ from the baseline audiogram by more than 5 dB at 500 to 4000 Hz, or more than 10 dB at 6000 Hz as required by the U.S. Navy (Navy and Marine Corps Public Health Center [NMCPHC], 2008). Such recalibrations will allow fairly accurate documentation of test results on an ongoing basis and are easier with modern digital audiometers and calibration equipment.

Modern calibration equipment can automatically correct the reference equivalent threshold sound pressure levels (RETSPLs) and test supraaural and insert earphones, extended frequency earphones, bone vibrators, and speakers based on limits in the ANSI standard specifications for audiometers. Examples of such equipment include the ACS 100 software from Audiological Service and Supply Company (Chicago, IL) and the AUDit™ with System 824 from Larson Davis (Depew, NY). Spare audiometers should be available in cases when an audiometer cannot

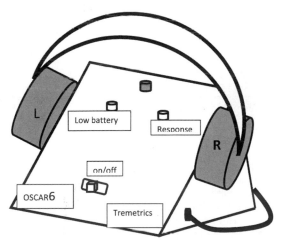

Fig. 4.28 Example of equipment for biological check.

be immediately recalibrated because of lack of calibration equipment or expertise.

Record Results

A record of the daily functional checks should be maintained using a checklist. The best practice is to keep biologic calibrations available for review (upon request) for up to 5 years.

Annual Acoustic Calibration Checks

A sound level meter, octave band filter set, and a National Bureau of Standards 9A coupler is necessary to perform the acoustic calibration checks. The calibrating equipment itself needs to be adequately calibrated on an annual basis.

The acoustic calibration has two components, including a sound pressure output check and a linearity check.

Sound Pressure Output Check

During this check, the earphone is coupled to the microphone of the sound level meter through a coupler. The audiometer is then set to provide 70 dB HL at each of the test frequencies. The sound pressure levels shown by the sound level meter should be within the tolerance range shown in **Table 4.9** for TDH-39 earphones and in **Table 4.10** for TDH-49 earphones. The RETSPLs (dB re 20 μPa) for insert earphones are shown in **Table 4.11**. OSHA (1983) requires the acoustic calibration at least annually, but outputs at test frequencies below 500 Hz and above 6000 Hz need not be evaluated. If the outputs during acoustic calibration show deviations equal to or greater than 15 dB, exhaustive calibrations are required. Best practice is to perform exhaustive calibrations when the output levels are outside the range specified in row 4. Waiting until the values are outside the range specified in row 5 will make it difficult to interpret and explain their audiometric thresholds to workers in the context of normal hearing thresholds.

Linearity Check

The purpose of this check is to ensure that the attenuator of the audiometer is functioning properly. With the earphone still coupled to the microphone of the sound level meter through the coupler, a tone of 1000 Hz is presented at 70 dB HL. The sound levels are then noted for each 10-dB decrement from 70 to 10 dB. For each 10-dB decrement in the HL dial, a dB decrement in the sound level is expected. A linear check can also be performed using a voltmeter connected to the earphone terminals and viewing a linear decrease in voltage with each 10-dB decrease in HL.

Record Results

A record of the results of acoustic calibration can be maintained in tabular formats.

Exhaustive Calibration

Exhaustive calibrations involve resetting the output of the audiometer to meet ANSI standards. Exhaustive calibrations of the audiometer as specified in 4.1.2, 4.1.3., 4.1.1.4.3, 4.2, 4.4.3, and 4.5 of the S3.6-1969 (ANSI, 1969) is required every 2 years. The 1969 standard has been revised and appears as the S3.6–1989 (ANSI/ASA, 1989) standard. The

Table 4.9   Levels for Checking Sound Pressure Output of the Audiometer for TDH-39 Earphones (OSHA, 1983) Using the NBS 9A Coupler

Frequency	500 Hz	1000 Hz	2000 Hz	3000 Hz	4000 Hz	6000 Hz
Reference dB SPL for 0 dB HL (reference equivalent threshold sound pressure levels)	11.5	7	9	10	9.5	15.5
Audiometric dial setting	70	70	70	70	70	70
Expected dB SPL output with the audiometeric dial set at 70 dB HL	81.5	77	79	80	79.5	85.5
Tolerance range for recommending exhaustive calibration	78.5–84.5	74–80	76–82	77–83	75.5–83.5	80.5–90.5
Tolerance ranges for requiring exhaustive calibration	66.5–96.5	62–92	64–94	65–95	64.5–94.5	70.5–100.5

Table 4.10   Levels for Checking Sound Pressure Output of the Audiometer for TDH-49 Earphones (OSHA, 1983) Using the NBS 9A Coupler

Frequency	500 Hz	1000 Hz	2000 Hz	3000 Hz	4000 Hz	6000 Hz
Reference dB SPL for 0 dB HL (reference equivalent threshold sound pressure levels)	13.5	7.5	11	9.5	10.5	13.5
Audiometric dial setting	70	70	70	70	70	70
Expected dB SPL output with the audiometeric dial set at 70 dB HL	83.5	77.5	81	79.5	80.5	83.5
Tolerance range for recommending exhaustive calibration	80.5–86.5	74.5–80.5	78–84	76.5–82.5	76.5–84.5	78.5–88.5
Tolerance ranges for requiring exhaustive calibration	68.5–98.5	62.5–92.5	66–96	64.5–94.5	65.5–95.5	68.5–98.5

record of the date on which each exhaustive calibration was performed should be carefully noted.

Calibration Record Retention

The best practice is to maintain calibration records for at least 5 years (National Institute for Occupational Safety and Health [NIOSH], 1998) including the results of the daily functional checks.

Case History

A detailed case history is presented in Appendix A of this chapter. A detailed history is important for the following reasons:

1. To meet the recordkeeping requirements of regulatory organizations such as OSHA

2. To monitor any changes in noise levels, hearing protection devices (HPDs), etc.
3. As a tool for health surveillance
4. To determine any contributing factors other than workplace noise that might be contributing to hearing loss
5. To provide insights into the factors that increase the risk of hearing loss and to indicate closer surveillance for workers who are at higher risk

◆ Otoscopic Examination

An otoscopic examination should be performed before proceeding with the test procedures using an otoscope (**Fig. 4.29**). During the otoscopic examination, both the eardrum and ear canal should be observed for any signs of drainage

Table 4.11   Reference Equivalent Threshold Sound Pressure Levels (dB re 20 μPa) for Insert Earphones

Frequency (Hz)	Occluded ear simulator		HA-1		HA-2 with rigid tube
125	ANSI S3.6–1989 Appendix G, Interim levels; OSHA (1993) interpretation letter	ANSI S3.6–2004; ISO 389–2	ANSI S3.6–1989 Appendix G, Interim levels; OSHA (1993) interpretation letter	ANSI S3.6–2004	ANSI S3.6–2004; ISO 389–2
125	30.0	28.0	27.5	26.5	26.0
250	19.0	17.5	15.5	14.5	14.0
500	12.0	9.5	8.5	6.0	5.5
1000	9.0	5.5	3.5	0.0	0.0
2000	15.0	11.5	6.5	2.5	3.0
3000	15.5	13.0	5.5	2.5	3.5
4000	13.0	15.0	1.5	0.0	5.5
6000	13.0	16.0	−1.5	−2.5	2.0
8000	14.0	15.5	−4.0	−3.5	0.0

ANSI, American National Standards Institute; OSHA, Occupational Safety and Health Administration.

and occluding cerumen. In the presence of drainage or occluding cerumen, the best practice is to postpone the evaluation until medical management is complete, as these conditions can elevate thresholds. In addition, the pinna should be pressed gently to mimic the positioning of supra-aural earphones to visualize any possibility of ear canal collapse, which can lead to poor test-retest reliability and artificial elevation of thresholds (Mahoney & Luxon, 1996). If ear canal collapse is apparent, best practice is to use insert earphones following the OSHA recommendations discussed previously. Another possibility is to retest with supra-aural earphones while the worker is holding his jaw open (Reiter & Silman, 1993), provided that there is no discomfort involved in holding the jaw open through the duration of the test. When possible, a video-otoscope (**Fig. 4.30**) should be used, which can allow individuals to visualize the conditions of their ear canals and eardrums. Such visualization can motivate them to follow any recommendations for medical management.

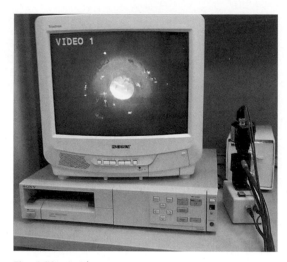

Fig. 4.30   A videotoscope.

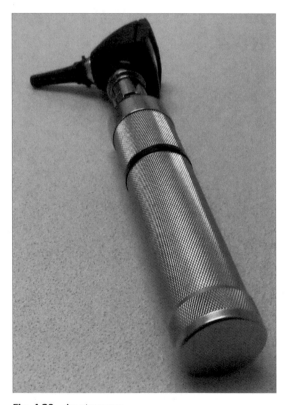

Fig. 4.29   An otoscope.

◆ Test Procedures

The most current standard for manual procedures for determination of auditory thresholds is the American National Standard S3.21–2004 (ANSI, 2004), which was reaffirmed by ANSI in April 2009. This standard is a revision of the American National Standard ANSI S3.21–1978.

Instructions

The individual should be asked to remove any jewelry or eyeglasses, as such items can make accurate placement of headphones difficult and cause discomfort to the patient. In addition, request that the individual remove gum or tobacco, as chewing can make it difficult to hear sounds near thresholds. The individual should also be asked to turn off or put away items such as cell phones or pagers, as these can interfere with the testing and prolong it.

Instructions for the Test Procedure

Proper instructions are extremely important for establishing accurate thresholds and completing the test in an efficient manner without the need for retest. If the person uses hearing aids, these should be left on while giving instructions. Detailed instructions are given in **Table 4.12**.

Table 4.12   Instructions for Audiometric Testing and Related Goals

Goal	Instruction
Describe the purpose of the test.	We need to determine the softest sounds you can hear in each ear.
Inform the individual what to expect to reduce anxiety.	You will be hearing tones/beeps; some are going to be easy to hear, and some are going to be really soft. Some sounds will be high pitched, and some will be lower in pitch. We will test one ear at a time.
Tell the individual how to respond.	Please press this button (or raise your hand) as soon as you hear the tones/beeps and let the button go (or lower your hand) as soon as the tones/beeps stop.
Emphasize the need for paying attention and responding to sounds near thresholds.	Please pay close attention and respond to any tones/beeps you hear, regardless of how soft they are.
Give an opportunity to ask questions.	Do you have any questions?
Make the individual feel comfortable in the booth (some individuals feel claustrophobic in the booth; others may feel fatigued during the test).	If you have any questions/concerns during testing or need a break, please feel free to speak. I can hear you from outside the booth.
For individuals with severe to profound hearing loss, confirm the comprehension of instructions.	Please tell me what you are supposed to do during the test procedures.

Earphone Placement

The earphone should be centered over the ear; the examinee should be asked to adjust the position of the earphones to achieve loudest perception of an audible tone presented at 250 Hz.

Characteristics of Tones

The presented tones should be 1 to 2 seconds in duration, and the interval between successive presentations should be longer than the duration of tones and should be varied so that the timing of the tonal presentation cannot be predicted by the subject. During tonal presentations, the examiner should make sure that the examinee cannot see or receive any cues about when each tone is being presented. Some agencies such as the FRA require the use of pulsed tones during testing with on-off time of 225 ± 35 milliseconds, which approximates the critical duration for temporal summation.

Familiarization to the Listening and Response Task

The frequency of 1000 Hz is generally used during the familiarization phase. Two approaches have been suggested for familiarizing the subject with the task:

◆ Present the tone at a HL of 30 dB. If a clear or quick response occurs, threshold search

can begin. If there is no response, present the tone at 50 dB HL and at increments of 10 dB above 50 dB HL until a clear and quick response is apparent. A clear response indicates that the individual knows what to listen for and how to respond.

◆ Set the intensity dial at the softest level (−10 or 0 dB HL) and turn it continuously on. Slowly increase the sound pressure level until a clear response is apparent. Turn off the tone for a minimum period of 2 seconds and then present it again at the same level. If a clear response is apparent, familiarization is complete. If there is no response, repeat the procedure.

◆ Frequencies to be Tested

OSHA (1983) requires auditory monitoring at the following frequencies: 500, 1000, 2000, 3000, 4000, and 6000 Hz. In addition to these frequencies, some agencies such as the FRA require threshold determination at 8000 Hz.

Order

If information is available, it is advantageous to test the better ear first, as the task is easier when the tones are easily audible. To maintain consistency in the testing approach, testing should begin with the frequency of 1000 Hz and should proceed to higher frequencies. After thresholds at all higher frequencies are determined, the threshold should be reestablished at 1000 Hz to determine the reliability of thresholds. If the re-established thresholds at 1000 Hz differ by more than 5 dB, then the lower of the two thresholds may be accepted, but thresholds should be re-established for at least one more frequency. If thresholds continue to differ by more than 5 dB, it may be better to reinstruct the individual before proceeding. Finally, thresholds are established at 500 Hz and during complete evaluation at 250 Hz.

Level of Tonal Presentations

The level of the first presentation of tone should be 10 dB below the level at which the subject responded during the familiarization procedure. After each response, the level is decreased by 10 dB; after each failure to respond, the tone is increased by 5 dB. This procedure is illustrated in **Fig. 4.31**.

Manual Determination of Threshold

The lowest HL at which a response is apparent on at least 50% of ascending trials with at least two responses out of three tonal presentations

at the same level is considered the threshold. In **Fig. 4.31**, the subject provided a clear response at 30 dB HL during the familiarization procedure. Thus the level of the first presentation was 10 dB below 30 dB or 20 dB. The subject did not respond at 20 dB. Therefore, the second presentation of the tone occurred at a 5 dB higher or 25 dB level. The subject responded to 25 dB HL. Thus during the third trial, the level was lowered by 10 dB and the tone was presented at 15 dB HL. There was no response to the 15 dB tone. Thus, the level was raised to 20 dB on the fourth trial and the subject responded. On the fifth trial, the level was lowered by 10 dB and there was no response to 10 dB HL. On the sixth trial, the level was raised by 5 dB and the subject did not respond to 15 dB HL. On the seventh trial, the level was raised by another 5 dB and the subject still did not respond to 20 dB HL. On the eighth trial, the level was raised by another 5 dB and the subject responded to 25 dB HL. On the ninth trial, the level was dropped by 10 dB to 15 dB HL and there was no response. On the tenth trial, the level was increased by 5 dB and the subject responded. Because the lowest level at which the subject responded on two out of three ascending trials (trials where the tone level was increased) was 20 dB, the threshold of the subject is 20 dB HL.

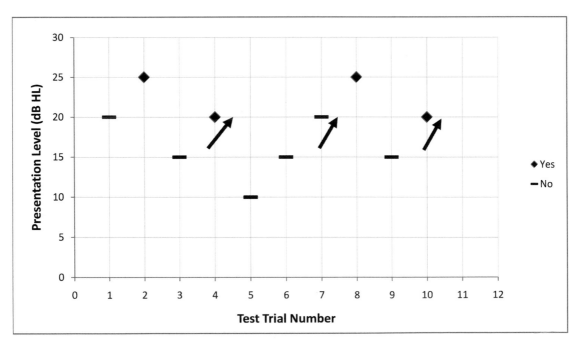

Fig. 4.31   Illustration of determination of thresholds.

Automatic Determination of Thresholds Using Microprocessor-based or Computerized Audiometers

Computerized audiometers are programmed to follow the same procedures that are used during manual audiometry. Thus, after each response the level is decreased by 10 dB, and after each failure to respond by the subject, the tone is increased by 5 dB. All individuals cannot perform well with automatic audiometry. In such cases, it is necessary to use manual override to obtain valid thresholds. The advantage of computerized audiometry is that several individuals can be tested simultaneously. Some agencies require the use of microprocessor audiometers (e.g., the U.S. Navy for all active duty personnel) except in evaluating difficult-to-test patients (NMCPHC, 2008).

Potential Sources of Unreliable Thresholds

1. The examiner: Variations in content and delivery of instruction, placement of earphones, and variation in testing techniques including masking procedures can result in poor inter- and intratest reliability.
2. Calibration of test equipment: Failure to regularly and properly calibrate test equipment can increase test-retest threshold variability.
3. Test environment: Excessive noise in the test environment or uncomfortable test environment due to poor temperature control causing excessive heat or cold can lead to unreliable thresholds.
4. Characteristics of the examinee:
   - The dynamic nature of auditory sensitivity: Minor fluctuations in physiological activity can lead to minor fluctuations in thresholds. Presence of tinnitus can add to these fluctuations.
   - Motivation: If the claimant is motivated to make the hearing loss more severe, he or she may wait for the tones to become clearly loud before responding.
   - Possible presence of a temporary threshold shift due to noise exposure before testing.
   - Psychological and emotional state: Fatigue, anxiety, and physical sickness can interact with the examiner's experience and demeanor. If the audiologist is viewed as either an impersonal authority figure or as an adversary, the worker may become antagonized and may not fully cooperate.

Postponing Examination and Rescheduling Employees

In some cases, to achieve valid results, it is necessary to postpone testing and reschedule employees. Examples of when rescheduling is necessary include the presence of excessive occluding cerumen in the ear canals, discharging ears, and signs of excessive fatigue or drug/alcohol abuse.

Hygiene and Infection Control

It is important to maintain proper hygiene around the test area and to control for the spread of any infections. After testing, each set of employee headphones, including earphone cushions, should be cleaned carefully with disinfection wipes. It is important to wipe surfaces that are touched by patients such as chair arm rests, response buttons, and any other surfaces.

Nondisposable otoscopic specula that are contaminated by ear drainage or blood can be first cleaned and then sterilized by soaking them in 2% glutaraldehyde or in 7.5% hydrogen peroxide solutions for 10 hours. Another option is to use an autoclave, which can sterilize the specula by high-pressure steam at 121°C for 10 to 20 minutes. It may not be easy to determine the presence of ear drainage or blood in the presence of cerumen. Thus sterilization of nondisposable specula is preferred (American Academy of Audiology Infection Control Task Force, 2003).

When there is a clear indication of clear ear canal and lack of blood or fluid drainage, specula can be first cleaned off for any visible organic matter such as cerumen with cotton swabs, washed with soap and water and dried, and then soaked in 70% alcohol for 10 to 20 minutes. In case of lack of time to soak the pieces between patients, after washing with soap and water the pieces can be wiped thoroughly with an alcohol-soaked cotton ball, rinsed with water, and then dried. If this is done, at the end of each day the pieces should be soaked in 70% alcohol for 10 minutes (Texas Department of State Health Services, 2009).

◆ Baseline or Reference Air Conduction Audiogram

Baseline audiogram is a valid initial audiogram of the employee and serves as a reference for subsequent audiograms to track any changes in hearing and thus to indicate any problems with the efficacy of the HCP.

Timeline for Establishing the Baseline Audiogram

As shown in **Table 4.1**, OSHA (1983) and some other agencies allow the baseline audiogram to occur within 6 months of the worker's first exposure at or above 85 dBA time weighted average (TWA). OSHA also allows an additional 6-month period to perform the baseline audiogram where mobile test vans are used, provided that the employee has been wearing HPDs for any period beyond the initial 6 months after first hazardous noise exposure until the baseline audiometry is complete.

The Mine Safety and Health Administration (MSHA; 1999) allows the mine operator to use an existing audiogram as a baseline audiogram if the audiogram meets the specified audiometric testing requirements.

The best time for establishing a baseline audiogram is before the employee begins work in the noisy place or before he or she is exposed to any hazardous noise levels. However, if this is not possible, it should occur within 30 days of exposure (NIOSH, 1998) because of the possibility of a permanent hearing loss occurring within months or even days in susceptible workers, especially when noise exposure levels are high (International Organization for Standardization [ISO,] 1990). This recommendation is adopted by the U.S. Department of Defense.

Noise-free Period before the Baseline Test

If the employee is exposed to hazardous noise levels before the baseline audiogram is established, the baseline thresholds can be contaminated by a temporary hearing loss. To minimize this possibility, the employee is required to be free from all hazardous noise exposures including occupational and nonoccupational noise exposure for at least 14 hours before the baseline testing can occur. However, if the employee cannot be away from work for 14 hours preceding the baseline audiometry test session, testing can still occur provided that the employee has been using HPDs (OSHA, 1983). Although the best day to perform baseline audiometry may appear to be Monday, after the employee has been away from work, recreational noise exposure may be greater during this period for some workers. Thus, the employers are required to inform the employees about the need to avoid hazardous levels of nonoccupational noise exposures during the 14-hour noise-free period (OSHA, 1983).

NIOSH (1998) recommends a minimum of 12 hours of unprotected quiet. Thus, to the best extent possible, use of hearing protectors should not be substituted for an actual quiet period because of the uncertainties involved in the attenuation provided by HPDs (see Chapter 6).

Review of Baseline Audiogram

The occupational hearing conservationist should perform a preliminary review of the baseline audiogram to determine the need for any referrals to the audiometric supervisor. Some characteristics of patients or baseline audiograms that will need a referral or further review by the supervising professional are as follows:

1. Recent or chronic history of pain and drainage in one or both ears (American Academy of Otolaryngology-Head and Neck Surgery [AAO-HNS], 1997), as this suggests the possibility of current or chronic middle ear pathology that needs to be treated or managed, especially before fitting and use of HPDs.
2. History of dizziness; severe, persistent tinnitus; sudden, fluctuating, or rapidly progressive hearing loss; or a feeling of fullness or discomfort in one or both ears within the preceding 12 months (AAO-HNS, 1997). These symptoms are associated with ear pathologies and need to be treated or managed.
3. Presence of excessive cerumen in the ear canal (AAO-HNS, 1997) that completely obstructs the flow of sound to the eardrum. This may elevate thresholds and can cause discomfort with the use of earplugs or insert earphones.
4. Inability to obtain a valid audiogram using standard manual test procedures, as demonstrated by one or more of the following characteristics:
   ◆ Too much test-retest variability: Test-retest difference at 1000 Hz is 10 dB or more.
   ◆ Inconsistent response patterns: Thresholds vary greatly on ascending and descending trials of tonal presentation.
   ◆ False responses: These can consist of either the patient responding in the absence of tonal presentation (false-positive) or not responding to a tone to which a clear and immediate response was apparent during previous trials (false-negative).

5. Asymmetric or unilateral hearing loss: In the presence of an asymmetric or unilateral hearing loss, a full evaluation is necessary to determine type and degree of hearing loss and to treat or manage any underlying pathology such as an acoustic nerve tumor. The following air conduction threshold characteristics suggest an asymmetric or unilateral hearing loss:

- Difference of 40 dB or more between ears at any frequency on baseline (NM-CPHC, 2008). This suggests a significant asymmetric hearing loss and needs to be investigated further to rule out any significant pathology in one ear.
- Difference in average HL between ears of more than 15 dB at 500, 1000, and 2000 Hz or more than 30 dB at 3000, 4000, and 6000 Hz (AAO-HNS-1997).

6. A significant hearing loss: In the presence of a significant hearing loss, the loss needs to be fully evaluated to determine the type of hearing loss, possible treatment, and accurate recordkeeping in case the hearing loss progresses further during the course of employment and the employee seeks compensation. The following characteristics suggest the presence of a significant hearing loss:

- Average HL greater than 25 dB at 500, 1000, and 2000 Hz. Expected speech reception thresholds will be 25 dB HL suggesting hearing loss.
- Average HL at 500, 1000, 2000, and 3000 Hz greater than 25 dB in either ear (AAO-HNS, 1997).
- Average HL at 2000, 3000, and 4000 Hz of 25 dB or greater (OSHA, 2002, Federal Register [67 FR 77165–77170]).

◆ Periodic Monitoring of Auditory Sensitivity

OSHA and other agencies require additional audiometric tests after the baseline tests and most require annual monitoring. However, MSHA allows miners to decide if they wish to undergo audiometric tests. FRA requires that annual testing be offered; workers are required to undergo audiometric evaluation every 3 years. For workers who are exposed to greater than 100 dBA TWA, NIOSH (1998) recommends auditory threshold monitoring every 6 months, which will allow early detection of hearing loss in the most susceptible population. The ISO (1990) data suggest that the most susceptible 10% of the population could develop a hearing loss with noise exposures of 100 dBA TWA prior to the end of 1 year without the use of effective hearing protection.

Best Time to Perform Periodic Monitoring Tests

The best practice for obtaining annual or periodic audiograms is at the end of the work shift to catch any temporary hearing losses before the hearing recovers after a night of rest (NIOSH, 1998). Temporary hearing losses can serve as an alert for the presence of deficiencies in the HCPs.

Audiogram Review to Determine Validity of Findings

OSHA (1983) requires comparison of the monitoring or current audiogram to the baseline audiogram to determine if the audiogram is valid; this comparison can be done by a technician. The occupational hearing conservationist should perform a preliminary review of the monitoring audiogram to determine the need for any referrals to the audiometric supervisor. All of the criteria that are listed under the section for the review of the baseline audiogram can be used for referral unless referrals and adequate follow-up procedures were already followed at the time of the baseline audiogram for the presence of significant sensorineural hearing loss. In addition, the following criterion can be used for the review of the periodic or annual audiogram:

A worsening of average thresholds in either ear on the periodic audiogram compared with the baseline audiogram of more than 15 dB at 500, 1000, and 2000 Hz or more than 20 dB at 3000, 4000, and 6000 Hz. (AAO-HNS, 1997)

Too much discrepancy in the current audiogram compared with the baseline audiogram in the absence of any relevant medical history can point to the possibility of an invalid current audiogram. If the audiogram is valid, it should be reviewed to rule out the presence of an STS and to determine the need for reporting the hearing loss to any regulatory agency.

Standard Threshold Shift

If the average thresholds at 2000, 3000, and 4000 Hz show a worsening of 10 dB or more, the

Table 4.13   Example of Calculation of a Standard Threshold Shift Using Left Ear Air Conduction Thresholds (dB HL) of a Hypothetical Male Worker

	Age (Years)	Frequency (kHz)						
		500	1000	2000	3000	4000	6000	8000
Current confirmed thresholds	49	10	10	10	15	20	30	15
Baseline	21	0	0	5	5	5	10	10
Step 1	Calculate the average threshold shift at 2000, 3000, and 4000 Hz for the current audiogram.	$10 + 15 + 20 = 45/3 = 15$						
Step 2	Calculate the average threshold shift at 2000, 3000, and 4000 Hz for the baseline audiogram.	$5 + 5 + 5 = 15/3 = 5$						
Step 3	Examine if the current average thresholds at 2000, 3000, and 4000 Hz are 10 dB or worse than the baseline thresholds.	$15 - 5 = 10$. The current average thresholds are worse by 10 dB; thus there appears to be a standard threshold shift.						

employee is considered to have an STS (OSHA, 1983). Most agencies use this criterion to determine if the worker has lost hearing ability since the baseline. An example of determination of an STS using hypothetical auditory thresholds is shown in **Table 4.13**.

Significant Threshold Shift

NIOSH (1998) recommends a criterion of a change of 15 dB or more at any of the test frequencies between 500 and 6000 Hz for determining worsening of auditory thresholds. If this criterion is applied for the audiogram in **Table 4.13**, a significant threshold shift is apparent at 4000 Hz (15 dB) and 6000 Hz (20 dB).

Use of Age Corrections in Determining Standard Threshold Shift

Age correction refers to a procedure for compensating for age-related hearing loss assuming that all individuals will suffer from hearing loss due to aging. In reality, this assumption is not true. Approximately one-third of the population over the age of 60 years does not have a significant hearing loss. Nonetheless, OSHA and MSHA allow the use of age correction in determining STSs. Appendix F of the OSHA (1983) regulations provides tables that include expected thresholds

for men and women at ages ranging from 20 to 60 years. Example of how these tables can be used in applying age correction is presented in **Table 4.14**.

Periodic Monitoring Retest

Although an immediate retest is not required (OSHA, 1983), the best practice is to repeat the test immediately after reinstructing the patient in the presence of a STS. The immediate retest strategy can lead to a reduction in the number of workers that need to be rescheduled for confirming the threshold shift or ruling out a temporary threshold shift (NIOSH, 1998). MSHA (1999) allows only one retest. Thus, for miners it may be best to reschedule the patient after a 14-hour noise-free period if an STS is apparent.

Periodic Monitoring Confirmation Test

If the temporary threshold shift persists following an immediate retest, hearing should be retested after 14 hours away from occupational or other hazardous noise exposure within 30 days. If the STS is confirmed on the retest, the results of the retest can be recorded as the annual audiometric test results (OSHA, 1983). Note that a confirmation retest is not required by OSHA (1983).

Table 4.14   Example of Application on Age Correction for Determination of a Standard Threshold Shift

	Age (Years)	Frequency (kHz)						
		500	1000	2000	3000	4000	6000	8000
Current	49	10	10	10	15	20	30	15
Baseline	21	0	0	5	5	5	10	10
Step 1	Locate expected thresholds at the age of 49 years for men from Table F-1 of OSHA (1983) Appendix F.			9	15	21		
Step 2	Locate expected thresholds at the age of 21 years for men from Table F-1 of OSHA (1983) Appendix F.			3	4	5		
Step 3	Calculate the difference between the values in steps 1 and 2. This difference reveals the expected deterioration in thresholds due to the effect of aging from the age of 21 to 49 years.			6	11	16		
Step 4	Correct the current audiogram by subtracting the assumed age-related threshold shift obtained in step 3.			10 6 4	15 11 4	20 16 4	Current Age correction from step 3 Age corrected current	
Step 1	Calculate the average threshold shift at 2000, 3000, and 4000 Hz for the age-corrected current audiogram.			$4 + 4 + 4 = 12/3 = 4$				
Step 2	Calculate the average threshold shift at 2000, 3000, and 4000 Hz for the baseline audiogram.			$5 + 5 + 5 = 15/3 = 5$				
Step 3	Examine if the current average thresholds at 2000, 3000, and 4000 Hz are 10 dB or worse than the baseline thresholds.			The current age-corrected thresholds are better than the baseline thresholds. Thus, there is no age-corrected standard threshold shift.				

OSHA, Occupational Safety and Health Administration.

Determination of the Need for Reporting the Hearing Loss

In the presence of a confirmed STS, calculate the average thresholds at 2, 3, and 4 kHz in the ear with STS to determine if the average is 25 dB or worse. In the example in **Table 4.14**, the average threshold at these frequencies is 15 dB HL. Thus, the hearing loss need not be reported. If the current average thresholds are 25 dB or worse in the presence of an STS, it is necessary to determine if the hearing loss is related to noise exposure at work. If the hearing loss is determined to be work-related, it should be reported on the OSHA 300 Form (log of work-related injuries and illnesses) in the "Hearing Loss" column within 37 days or within 7 days of retest. This process is shown in **Fig. 4.32**.

In this process, it is necessary to determine if the hearing loss is work-related. Such determination is not straightforward, but a detailed case history as presented in the Appendix along with the following guidelines can help:

◆ Are there any health factors that can cause hearing loss? If there are more than two contributing factors, then the hearing loss is less likely to be work-related.
◆ Is there any use of ototoxic medications? (See Chapter 10.)
◆ Is there unprotected recreational or other (e.g., wood workshop at home) noise exposure?
◆ What are the noise levels that the worker is exposed to? If the noise level exposures are

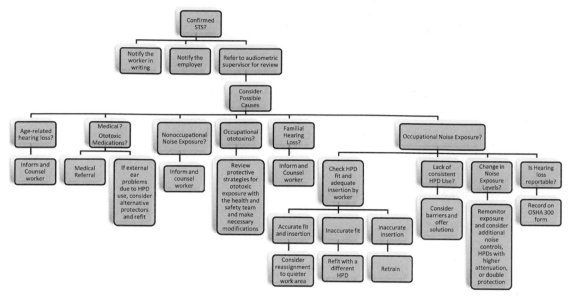

Fig. 4.32   Follow-up procedures after confirmed STS.

less than 90 dBA, the chance of work-related noise-induced hearing loss is less.

- HPD use: Does the worker use HPDs? If yes, are they used all of the time or some of the time when exposed to loud noises? Are the HPDs used correctly? What is the estimated attenuation provided by the HPDs? What is the estimated protected noise exposure with the use of HPDs? If the protected noise exposure is less than 85 dBA, then the hearing loss is less likely to be work-related.
- Is the STS age-related?
- Is there a family history of hearing loss without noise exposure?
- Does there appear to be a noise-induced notch? If the STS appears to be caused by similar threshold shifts at 2, 3, and 4 kHz, suggesting a flat configuration, the shift is less likely to be caused by occupational noise exposure. As a cautionary note, the presence of notch can occur in approximately 11% of the population without any history of noise exposure (Nondahl, Shi, Cruickshanks, et al., 2009). Some ototoxic medications also lead to notches on the audiogram.

Revision of the Baseline Audiogram

In the presence of STS in one or both ears, the baseline or reference audiogram should be revised in both ears; the new periodic audiogram becomes the baseline audiogram. When the reference or baseline audiogram of a worker is revised on three different occasions because of deterioration in hearing, the probability that the employee is at a greater risk for hearing loss should be considered and all attempts to reduce the employee's hazardous noise exposure should be made. Baseline audiograms should also be revised in the presence of significant improvement in thresholds, because significant improvements suggest that the original baseline audiogram may not have been a valid record of the employee's hearing. More specifically, if the average of thresholds at 2, 3, and 4 kHz for either ear show a 5 dB or more improvement, and the improvements persists on two annual tests, the record should be identified for review by the professional supervisor (National Hearing Conservation Association, 1996).

Other Follow-up Procedures in the Presence of Standard Threshold Shift

OSHA (1983) requires notification of employees about STS within 21 days, although the best practice would be to inform the employee immediately (NIOSH, 1998). In addition, employees that have not been wearing HPDs because of exposures below 90 dBA TWA should be fitted with HPDs,

Table 4.15   Classifications of Individuals with Hearing Loss into Four Profiles Required by the U.S. Department of Defense

Profile		Follow-up
H1	Unaided hearing loss in either ear but no single threshold greater than 25 dB HL at 500, 1000, and 2000 Hz, 35 ṣ IL at 3000 Hz, and 45 dB HL at 4000 and 6000 Hz.	No follow-up is required unless there is a specific problem of complaint.
H-2	Unaided hearing loss is either ear with no single threshold greater than 35 dB HL at 500, 1000, and 2000 Hz, 45 dB HL at 3000 Hz, and 55 dB HL at 4000 Hz.	Referral to a medical officer is required who will whenever possible refer workers to an audiologist or otolaryngologist when H-2 levels are met or exceeded.
H-3	Any hearing loss that exceeds the values noted in the definition of an H-2 profile.	Consider disqualifying. Evaluation and waiver is required. An auditory fitness for duty evaluation is also required to determine eligibility for continued employment in hazardous noise.
H-4	Hearing loss sufficient to preclude safe and effective performance of duty, regardless of degree of pure tone hearing loss, or unknown thresholds.	This indicates an incomplete follow-up or a medical evaluation board referral.
Other	Hearing loss in both ears in which the sum of thresholds at the frequencies of 3000, 4000, and 6000 Hz exceeds 270.	Will not be assigned to duties in hazardous noise without a fitness for duty evaluation and clearance.

trained in their use, and required to use them. Employees that have been using HPDs should be refitted (if necessary with a different type of HPD) and retrained in proper and consistent use. In addition, when necessary, employees should be referred for a complete audiological evaluation. Employees who have non-work–related ear problems should be informed about the need for an otological evaluation. Unless an audiologist or a physician determines that the STS is neither work-related nor aggravated by occupational noise, MSHA (1999) has requirements similar to OSHA (1983) with an additional requirement of the appraisal of the effectiveness of engineering and administrative controls to spot and correct any deficiencies. Some agencies require additional follow-up procedures in the presence of a hearing loss. For example, the U.S. Department of Defense (2004) requires classification of individuals into the four profiles shown in **Table 4.15** to help in making follow-up recommendations.

The need for follow-up procedures and recordkeeping can be made accurate and efficient by using a database software. Such software can perform calculations for the determination of STS and percent binaural impairment and generate letters informing workers about the test results. It can also flag workers who may have OSHA-recordable shifts, although the work-relatedness

of such shifts needs to be determined by the supervising professional.

◆ Audiometric Recordkeeping Requirements

In relation to each audiogram, the following information should be recorded and kept for the duration of employment or duration of the employee's enrollment in the hearing conservation program and 6 months after the termination of employment (MSHA, 1999; OSHA, 1983). The records should be transferred to the successor if the employer/mine operator goes out of business (OSHA, 1983). NIOSH has recommended maintenance of hearing tests for 30 years beyond duration of employment. As mentioned previously, the use of database software can improve the efficiency of the process of recordkeeping. The audiometric test records should include:

◆ Name and job classification
◆ A copy of all audiograms with dates
◆ Examiner's name
◆ Evidence that the audiograms were conducted in accordance with audiometric test requirements

- Audiometer model and serial number
- Date of last acoustic and exhaustive calibration at the time of each evaluation
- A record of biological checks performed on the equipment
- Background noise levels in test rooms
- The number of hours the employee was away from noise prior to the test
- Any personal noise exposure data obtained closest in time to the date of each evaluation
- Audiogram classification code (e.g., military personnel)
- The results of follow-up examinations/recommendations

◆ Audiological Monitoring of Patients with Ototoxic Drug Exposure

Early detection of ototoxic hearing loss is important, as such detection can allow a reduction in drug dose or a change in prescribed medication. When this is not possible, early detection can provide an opportunity for early aural rehabilitation and early counseling related to coping strategies for the progressive nature of such loss.

The auditory thresholds of patients who are scheduled to receive drugs with a high incidence of ototoxicity should be monitored. Such patients can be identified by medical personnel who are prescribing the drugs and/or monitoring the patient's pathology or by the pharmacists dispensing the medications.

Baseline/Reference Audiometry

Ideally, the baseline audiogram should be obtained before initiation of any ototoxic drug intake. In cases when this is not possible, the baseline audiogram can be obtained within 72 hours following initiation of aminoglycosides. However, chemotherapeutic drugs such as cisplatin can damage hearing after a single dose. Thus, baseline audiometry should be performed before the administration of the first dose. A complete audiometric test battery can allow the documentation of thresholds, word recognition scores, otoacoustic emissions, and the type of hearing loss if present before administration of the drugs. Test reliability should

be assessed by repeating some parts of the tests (e.g., word recognition score in one ear, threshold determination at some frequencies). History of tinnitus should also be noted. If tinnitus is present during baseline testing, it should be carefully investigated and documented (see Chapter 5). If patient illness and related fatigue is a major factor, the key information that should be recorded is the audiometric thresholds in the range of 0.25 to 8 kHz. When possible, thresholds should be documented for up to 20 kHz (American Speech-Language-Hearing Association [ASHA], 1994).

Monitoring Audiometry

These evaluations can mainly comprise the pure tone thresholds. For chemotherapeutic drugs, the periodic evaluations can occur before each dose; for aminoglycosides, these can occur once or twice per week depending on the dose schedule. In the presence of significant changes, a retest should be performed to confirm the changes and to reduce false-positive rates (ASHA, 1994). Transient evoked otoacoustic emissions may reveal cochlear damage before it is seen on the audiogram. A complete tinnitus evaluation (see Chapter 5) is important for those who complain of increase in the severity of preexisting tinnitus and those who complain of onset of tinnitus during treatment because tinnitus onset is associated with chemotherapy and certain ototoxic antibiotic treatments (Dille, Konrad-Martin, Gallun, et al., 2010).

Post-treatment Completion Audiometry

The monitoring test schedule should continue for as long as threshold changes are apparent on the audiogram. The recommended schedule is every week for chemotherapeutic drugs and every 2 days for aminoglycosides.

Long-term Follow-up Audiometry

Long-term follow-up testing at around 3 and 6 months is recommended to confirm that hearing is stable (ASHA, 1994), because the related deterioration in hearing can occur 6 months or some years following drug exposure (Al-Khatib, Cohen, Carret, & Daniel, 2010; Kolinsky, Hayashi, Karzon,

Mao, & Hayashi, 2010). Patients who receive radiation to the posterior fossa and are fitted with hearing aids are at higher risk for late-onset deterioration of hearing (Kolinsky, Hayashi, Karzon, Mao, & Hayashi, 2010). If threshold deterioration is apparent during follow-up tests, weekly tests are recommended until the hearing becomes stable (ASHA, 1994).

Significant Threshold Shifts

There is a critical need for international consensus on ototoxicity assessment criteria (Neuwelt & Brock, 2010). In the interim, the following criteria can be used for determining significant changes in auditory sensitivity, provided that the changes are confirmed by retest (ASHA, 1994):

- Worsening of thresholds by more than 20 dB at any single frequency
- Worsening of thresholds by more than 10 dB at any two consecutive test frequencies
- Previous response obtained close to the limits of the audiometer changing to "no response" status at three consecutive test frequencies, specifically at high frequencies

Extended High-frequency Testing

For frequencies between 9 and 14 kHz, test-retest variability can be within 10 dB. In addition, false-positive rates indicating a change in ultra-high–frequency thresholds in patients that were not exposed to ototoxic drugs is reportedly low in young and older adults, when testing is conducted in the hospital ward under controlled conditions. However, test-retest variability is generally greater in young children (Konrad-Martin, Helt, Reavis, et al., 2005).

Some investigators have recommended determination of a sensitive range of ototoxicity (SRO)

for each individual. The SRO is defined as the highest frequency in the 0.25 to 20 kHz range at which the threshold is 100 dB SPL or less and the six consecutive lower frequencies in one-sixth octave steps (Fausti, Henry, Helt, et al., 1999) or three consecutive lower frequencies in one-third octave steps. Best overall test performance for detecting ototoxicity has been noted by using a criterion of a 10 dB or greater shift at two or more adjacent frequencies tested in one-sixth octave steps in the SRO (Konrad-Martin, James, Gordon, et al., 2010). Because these protocols have been mainly tested using drug-induced ototoxicity, further research is necessary to see if they might be applicable to audiometric threshold shifts caused by other ototoxins.

Follow-up Procedures

In the presence of significant threshold shifts and/or complaints of aural fullness, tinnitus, and/or dizziness, a complete test battery including the following tests should be administered:

- Tympanometry and bone conduction testing to rule out threshold shifts because of middle ear dysfunction.
- Speech audiometry to evaluate the impact of the hearing loss on speech recognition.
- Otoacoustic emissions and auditory brainstem response testing to confirm the results of behavioral tests in children. In the presence of normal middle ear function and good baseline hearing, otoacoustic emissions can provide early indication of ototoxicity.
- Hearing aid fittings and aural rehabilitation in the presence of a stable confirmed sensorineural hearing loss.
- Tinnitus evaluation and management in the presence of tinnitus.
- Vestibular assessment and appropriate treatment when possible.

Review Questions

1. Discuss the various schemes used in classifying audiograms.
2. Describe all the steps involved in conducting baseline or periodic audiometry of individuals enrolled in an HCP, including preparations prior to testing.
3. Which factors should be controlled to avoid unreliable audiometric thresholds?
4. Why is it necessary to have a noise-free period before the baseline audiogram? How long should the person be free from noise exposure before the baseline test?

Test year/no	Right ear thresholds (dB) at each frequency (kHz)						Left ear thresholds (dB) at each frequency (kHz)					
	0.5	1	2	3	4	6	0.5	1	2	3	4	6
1993 Revised baseline	25	45	55	55	45	60	10	40	25	35	45	50
1994/6	30	50	55	55	55	55	15	35	40	40	40	40
1995/7	30	50	55	55	50	55	15	45	45	45	50	45
1996/8	30	50	45	45	45	60	10	40	40	45	50	45
1997/9	30	50	55	45	45	60	15	50	55	50	50	40

5. Review the characteristics of patients or baseline audiograms that will need a referral or further review by the supervising professional.

6. Examine the following audiometric results of a hypothetical female who is 45 years old in 1997. Is there an STS? Is there an age-corrected STS? Is there any NIOSH-significant threshold shift?

7. When is it necessary to report a hearing loss on the OSHA 300 Form? How will you determine that the hearing loss is work-related?

8. Outline the follow-up procedures that should be performed in the presence of an STS.

9. Review the recordkeeping requirements for audiometric monitoring of individuals enrolled in an HCP.

10. Discuss audiological monitoring test procedures for patients who are on ototoxic medications.

References

Al-Khatib T, Cohen N, Carret A-S, Daniel S. (2010). Cisplatinum ototoxicity in children, long-term follow up. *Int J Pediatr Otorhinolaryngol.* 74(8):913–919.

American Academy of Audiology Infection Control Task Force. (2003). Infection control in audiological practice. *Audiology Today.* 15:12–19.

American Academy of Otolaryngology-Head Neck Surgery. (1997). *Otologic Referral Criteria for Occupational Hearing Conservation Programs.* Alexandria, VA: AAO-HNS Foundation Inc.

American National Standards Institute.(1969). ANSI S3.6–1969 (R1989). *American Standard Specifications for Audiometers.* New York: American National Standards Institute.

American National Standards Institute. (1971). *American National Standard Specifications for Sound Level Meters, S1.4–1971 (R1976).* New York: American National Standards Institute

American National Standards Institute. (2004). *ANSI S3.6–2004 (Revision of ANSI S3.6–1996). Specification for Audiometers.* New York: American National Standards Institute.

American National Standards Institute, Acoustical Society of America. (1989). *ANSI S3.6–1989 (ASA 81–1989) Revision of ANSI S3.6–1969. Specification for Audiometers.* New York: American National Standards Institute.

American National Standards Institute, Acoustical Society of America. (1999). *ANSI/ASA S31–1999. (R 2008) Maximum Permissible Ambient Noise Levels for Audiometric Test Rooms.* New York: American National Standards Institute.

American National Standards Institute, American Society of Safety Engineers. (2007). *ANSI/ASSE A10.46–2007. Hearing Loss Prevention in Construction and Demolition Work.* New York: American National Standards Institute.

American Speech-Language-Hearing Association. (1990). Committee on Audiologic Evaluation. (1990, Apr). Guidelines for audiometric symbols. *ASHA Supplement.* 32(2):25–30.

American Speech-Language-Hearing Association. (1994). Guidelines for the audiologic management of individuals receiving cochleotoxic drug therapy. *ASHA.* 36:11–19.

Bell-Lehmkuhler B, Meinke DK, Sedey A, Tuell C. (2009). Reliability of audiometric thresholds obtained with insert earphones when used by certified audiometric technicians. *Noise Health.* 11(42):59–68.

Coles RR, Lutman ME, Buffin JT. (2000). Guidelines on the diagnosis of noise-induced hearing loss for medicolegal purposes. *Clin Otolaryngol Allied Sci.* 25(4):264–273.

Dille MF, Konrad-Martin D, Gallun F, et al. (2010). Tinnitus onset rates from chemotherapeutic agents and ototoxic antibiotics: results of a large prospective study. *J Am Acad Audiol.* 21(6):409–417.

Dobie RA, Rabinowitz PM. (2002). Change in audiometric configuration helps to determine whether a standard threshold shift is work-related. *Spectrum (Lexington, Ky.).* 19(Suppl 1):17.

Fausti SA, Henry JA, Helt WJ, et al. (1999). An individualized, sensitive frequency range for early detection of ototoxicity. *Ear Hear.* 20(6):497–505.

Federal Railroad Administration. (2006). *71 FR 63123, (Oct. 27, 2006). As amended at 73 FR 79702, Dec. 30, 2008. Part 227. Occupational Noise Exposure.* Washington, DC: Federal Railroad Administration.

Hoffman HJ, Ko C-W, Themann CL, Dillon CF, Franks JR. (2006). Reducing noise-induced hearing loss (NIHL) to achieve U.S. Healthy People 2010 goals. *Am J Epidemiol.* 163(Suppl):487.

International Organization for Standardization. (1990). *Acoustics: Determination of Occupational Noise Exposure and Estimation of Noise-Induced Hearing Impairment,* 2nd ed. Geneva, Switzerland: International Organization for Standardization.

Kolinsky DC, Hayashi SS, Karzon R, Mao J, Hayashi RJ. (2010). Late onset hearing loss: a significant complication of cancer survivors treated with Cisplatin containing chemotherapy regimens. *J Pediatr Hematol Oncol.* 32(2):119–123.

Konrad-Martin D, Helt WJ, Reavis KM, et al. (2005). Ototoxicity: Early detection and monitoring. *The ASHA Leader.* www.asha.org/Publications/leader/2005/050524/ 050524b.htm. Accessed June 28, 2011.

Konrad-Martin D, James KE, Gordon JS, et al. (2010). Evaluation of audiometric threshold shift criteria for ototoxicity monitoring. *J Am Acad Audiol.* 21(5):301–314, quiz 357.

Lutman ME, Coles RRA. (2009). Asymmetric sensorineural hearing thresholds in the non-noise-exposed UK population: a retrospective analysis. *Clin Otolaryngol.* 34(4):316–321.

Mahoney CFO, Luxon LM. (1996). Misdiagnosis of hearing loss due to ear canal collapse: a report of two cases. *J Laryngol Otol.* 110(6):561–566.

McBride DI, WilliamsS. (2001). Characteristics of the audiometric notch as a clinical sign of noise exposure. *Scand Audiol.* 30(2):106–111.

Mine Safety and Health Administration. (1999). *Health Standards for Occupational Noise Exposure: Final Rule* (30 CFR Part 62, 64 Fed. Reg. 49548–49634, 49636–49637). Arlington, VA: Mine Safety and Health Administration.

National Hearing Conservation Association. (1996). Guidelines for audiometric baseline revision recommended by the National Hearing Conservation Association. *Spectrum (Lexington, Ky.).* 13(2):5.

National Institute for Occupational Safety and Health. (1998). *Criteria for a Recommended Standard: Occupational Noise Exposure—Revised Criteria 1998. Publication No, 98–126.* Cincinnati: National Institute for Occupational Safety and Health.

Neuwelt FA, Brock P. (2010). Critical need for international consensus on ototoxicity assessment criteria. *J Clin Oncol.* 28(10):1630–1632.

Nondahl DM, Shi X, Cruickshanks KJ, et al. (2009). Notched audiograms and noise exposure history in older adults. *Ear Hear.* 30(6):696–703.

Occupational Safety and Health Administration. (1983). 29 CFR 1910.95 OSHA. Occupational Noise Exposure; Hearing Conservation Amendment; Final Rule, effective 8 March 1983. *Federal Register.* 48:9738–9785.

Occupational Safety and Health Administration. (1993). Use of Insert Earphones for Audiometric Testing Letter of Interpretation. www.osha.gov/pls/oshaweb/owadisp .show_document?p_table=INTERPRETATIONS&p_ id=21245. Accessed June 28, 2011.

Occupational Safety and Health Administration. (2002). Occupational injury and illness recording and reporting requirements; final rule. *Federal Register.* 47:44037–44048.

Reiter LA, Silman S. (1993). Detecting and remediating external meatal collapse during audiologic assessment. *J Am Acad Audiol.* 4(4):264–268.

Texas Department of State Health Services. (2009). *Infection Control Manual for Ambulatory Care Clinics.* Austin, TX: Texas Department of State Health Services.

U.S. Army Center for Health Promotion and Preventive Medicine. (2003). *Just the Facts. . . Occupational Ototoxins (Ear Poisons) and Hearing Loss* (Pub No. 51-002-0903). Aberdeen Proving Ground, MD: U.S. Army Center for Health Promotion and Preventive Medicine.

U.S. Department of Defense. (2004). Department of Defense Instruction Number 6055.12. DoD Hearing Conservation program. Washington, DC: U.S. Department of Defense.

U.S. Navy and Marine Corps Public Health Center. (2008). *Navy Medical Department Hearing Conservation Program Procedures.* (Technical Manual. NMCPHC – TM 6260.51.99-2). Portsmouth, VA: U.S. Navy and Marine Corps Public Health Center

◆ Appendix A

Identification

Name: _____

Age: _____ Date of birth: _____ Gender: _____

Employee number: _____ Job code: _____ Dept: _____

Occupation title: _____ Duration of current occupation: _____

Second current job with noise or other ototoxic substance exposure: _____

Test date: _____ Test time: _____ Hours since last noise exposure: _____

Test type: Baseline/Periodic/Exit

Education: Highest level attained: _____

Ethnicity: _____

Native language: _____ Handedness: Left _____ Right _____

If your native language is other than English, are you fluent in English? Yes _____ No _____

Noise Exposure Information

Noise monitoring results: _____ dBA TWA _____ % dose peak exposure levels: _____

Do you feel that you have temporary hearing loss at the end of the workday? (Frequently, Sometimes, No)

During the last week were you exposed to

- A noise level over 85 dBA (Not sure/yes/no/duration)
- Noise with shocks or impulses (yes/no/duration)
- Other disturbing noise (yes/no/duration)
- Ultrasounds (yes/no/duration)
- Does noise interfere with your ability to work?

Do you have any hobbies that expose you to loud noises (loud music/bands/concerts, hunting/shooting, motorcycles, car racing, other loud vehicles, using power tools, other)?

_____

Have you ever been previously exposed to hazardous noise or other ototoxins in an occupational setting?

Yes _____ No _____

If yes, where: Military service: _____

State any other occupation _____

Hearing Protection Device Use

Do you wear HPDs during current job?

Yes _____ No _____ Sometimes _____ % of the time

Type of hearing protection worn: _____

Have you worn HPDs during previous jobs with hazardous noise exposure: Yes _____ No _____

Sometimes _____ %

Type of hearing protection worn:

Do you wear HPDs during any recreational noise exposure:

Not applicable _____ Yes _____ No _____ Sometimes _____ % of the time

Type of hearing protection worn: _____

Occupational Ototoxin Exposure

Are you exposed to or have been exposed to the following substances during work?

Potential ototoxin	Yes	No	Current job	Current second job	Previous job
Asphyxiant (carbon monoxide)					
Metals					
Arsenic					
Organic tin					
Mercury and derivatives					
Manganese					
Solvents					
Carbon disulfide					
Ethylbenzane					
n-propylbenzene					
n-hexane					
p-xylene					
Styrene or methylstyrenes					
Toluene					
Trichloroethylene					
Other chemicals					
Hydrogen cyanide					
Diesel fuel					
Kerosene fuel					
Jet fuel					
JP-8 fuel					
Organophosphate pesticides					
Chemical warfare nerve agents					

Are you exposed to excessive heat during work? Yes _____ No _____
If yes, approximate % of time: _____
Are you exposed to vibrations during work? Yes _____ No _____ Frequency _____
If yes, approximate % of time: _____

Medical History

Have you ever consulted an ear, nose, and throat specialist before? Yes: _____ No: _____
Have you ever had ear surgery? Yes _____ No _____
If yes, please list the date, the ear and procedures, if known:

_____

Did you ever experience any of the following? If so, please state the duration and severity:
1. Earaches: Yes _____ No _____ Which ear/s _____ Frequency _____ Severity _____
2. Draining in ears: _____
3. Noises, ringing, or buzzing in your ear(s): _____
   – Do you hear ringing or experience tinnitus at the end of the workday? (frequently, sometimes, no)
   – How bothersome is your tinnitus? (highly, somewhat, minimally, not at all)
4. Dizziness (vertigo): _____
5. Nausea: _____
6. Chronic headaches: _____
   – Do you get headaches at the end of each workday? Yes _____ No _____
7. Concussion or severe blows on the head: _____
8. Mastoiditis: _____
9. Meningitis: _____
10. Pneumonia: _____
11. Frequent colds or respiratory infections: _____
12. Allergies: _____
13. Diabetes: _____
14. Heart disease: _____
15. High cholesterol: _____
16. Cerebrovascular disease: _____
17. Kidney problems: _____
18. Liver problems: _____
19. Hypothyroidism: _____
20. Hyperlipidemia: _____
21. Hypertension: _____
22. Stroke: _____
23. Arthritis: _____
24. Chronic lung disease: _____
25. Viral/bacterial infections: _____
26. Cancer: _____
26. Seizures: _____
27. White fingers: _____
Did you ever use any of the following or any other medications over a prolonged period of time?
Aspirin: Yes _____ No _____
Diuretics: Yes _____ No _____
Chemotherapeutic agents: Yes _____ No _____
Aminoglycosides: Yes _____ No _____
Warfarin or other blood thinners: Yes _____ No _____
Did you ever use any other medications over a prolonged period of time?
If yes, please list the medications and their purposes: _____

_____

Are you currently taking any medications regularly? Yes _____ No _____
If yes, please list the medications and their purposes:
Do you smoke? Yes _____ No _____ If yes, how frequently? _____
Do you use any other recreational drugs? Yes _____ No _____ If yes, how frequently? _____
How is your general health now? Good _____ Fair _____ Poor _____

Hearing History: (Fill in this section only if you think you have a hearing impairment.)

When did you first notice your problem? _____

In which ear? Right _____ Left _____ Both _____

Did the problem appear: Suddenly _____ Gradually with progression _____

How do you think your hearing problem started? _____ _____

Is there any history of hearing problems in your family? Yes _____ No _____

If yes, please describe who and the age of onset of hearing difficulties.

How do you hear in the following situations?

Quiet: Good _____ Fair _____ Poor

Noisy: Good _____ Fair _____ Poor

How well do you understand conversation when someone is speaking at a fast or slow rate?

Fast rate: Good _____ Fair _____ Poor

Slow rate: Good _____ Fair _____ Poor

Hearing Aid/Assistive Device Use History (Fill in this section only if you have worn or currently wear hearing aids.)

Do you wear an aid now? Yes _____ No _____

Is your hearing aid satisfactory? Yes _____ No _____

How frequently do you wear your current aids? _____

Have you worn another hearing aid in the past? Yes _____ No _____

How long have you been wearing hearing aids? _____

Do you use any other assistive listening devices? Yes _____ No _____

If yes, specify each and the satisfaction with each.

Rehabilitation History

Have you ever had speechreading training? Yes _____ No _____

Have you ever had auditory training? Yes _____ No _____

If you have had any other type of training to improve your communication, please describe: _____

_____

Chapter 5

Comprehensive Audiological, Tinnitus, and Auditory Processing Evaluations

Some workers who are exposed to hazardous noise will have to undergo comprehensive audiological evaluations, as stated in Chapter 4. In addition, some workers might need a comprehensive evaluation for the purpose of workers' compensation claims. Most audiology students are required to take one or two courses in conducting a comprehensive audiological evaluation, including instruction in the use of masking to obtain accurate thresholds in cases with conductive or unilateral hearing loss. A detailed discussion of the comprehensive test battery is out of the scope of the current textbook. Thus, only the aspects that are most relevant to noise-induced or ototoxic hearing loss are discussed in this chapter.

◆ Standard Requirements

Many standards require a complete audiological evaluation depending on the outcomes of the baseline or annual monitoring. As an example, the U.S. Navy requires a standard audiological evaluation of personnel exceeding an H-2 profile (see Chapter 4) inclusive of the following components:

- Pure tone air conduction (AC) under phones
- Pure tone bone conduction (BC)
- Speech reception threshold (SRT) under phones using prerecorded standardized word list(s)
- Ipsilateral and contralateral reflexes and reflex decay
- Word recognition abilities under phones using prerecorded standardized speech list(s)

- Word recognition abilities in noise under earphones using the speech recognition in noise test without hearing aids
- Phonetically balance rollover or other VIIIth cranial or vestibulocochlear nerve screening to assist in determining if the hearing loss is due to noise exposure or a medical condition
- Otoacoustic emissions (OAEs)
- Auditory brainstem response (ABR) evaluations at the discretion of the clinical audiologist and the availability of these services

To avoid any effects of fatigue, speech recognition abilities in noise are assessed in a separate evaluation session.

◆ Medicolegal Audiological Evaluations

When comprehensive audiological evaluations are being conducted on noise-exposed employees, there is potential for medicolegal involvement because of issues such as workers' compensation (Miller, Crane, Fox, & Linstrom, 1998) or fitness for duty (see Chapter 12). When audiological evaluations are conducted in current or potentially future medicolegal contexts, it is important to follow systematic protocols so that the results cannot be questioned during any legal proceedings (see Chapter 11).

◆ Case History/Intake Interview

A sample case history form was presented in the Appendix of Chapter 4. It is important to obtain any additional information about the onset and descriptions of different conditions/complaints, including tinnitus, diplacusis, hyperacusis, and/or auditory processing difficulties.

◆ Nonorganic Hearing Loss

The audiometric findings of some noise-exposed employees may suggest a nonorganic hearing loss, indicating a deficit that is greater than can be explained based on expected organic pathology (Austen & Lynch, 2004). In other cases, nonorganic components can be superimposed on existing organic hearing loss (Gelfand & Silman, 1985, 1993; Johnson, Work, & McCoy, 1956; Wolf, Birger, Ben Shoshan, & Kronenberg, 1993). In such cases, the audiologist has the responsibility for determining accurate thresholds.

The prevalence of nonorganic hearing loss in the general population may be as low as 2% (Rintelmann & Schwan, 1999), but in individuals with histories of noise exposure, the prevalence is higher. Based on the cortical slow vertex response, Alberti, Hyde, and Riko (1987) found that 8% of compensation claimants had excessively high behavioral thresholds. In another study of 246 workers' compensation claimants, 9% were found to be malingering (Barrs, Althoff, Krueger, & Olsson, 1994), but as many as 34% of medicolegal cases of industrial workers may exaggerate hearing loss (Gosztonyi, Vassallo, & Sataloff, 1971). An Australian study of 333 workers identified 17.7% of claimants with exaggerated hearing loss (Rickards & De Vidi, 1995). Among military personnel, the estimated prevalence of nonorganic hearing loss can range from 10 to 50% (Johnson, Work, & McCoy, 1956). Among patients who are suspected to be malingering based on the basic audiometric test battery findings, exaggerated thresholds can be found in 71.25% of ears (Balatsouras, Kaberos, Korres, Kandiloros, Ferekidis, & Economou, 2003).

Underlying Causes of Nonorganic Hearing Loss in Employees

Among military personnel, older workers may malinger to increase benefits before retirement. In younger individuals, especially recruits, unconscious malingering may occur as a result of the shock of being thrust in the disciplined military regimen away from family and home (Gold, Hunsaker,

& Haseman, 1991), along with some conscious malingering as a means to avoid obligations or to hide failures. Thus, the underlying motivations among noise-exposed individuals for nonorganic hearing loss can be conscious and/or unconscious. It is important to consider the possibility of unconscious motivations in completing a diagnostic test battery to determine accurate thresholds.

Referral Sources/Reasons

Under the following circumstances, a nonorganic component or nonorganic hearing loss should be considered a possibility:

- ◆ Failure to establish reliable AC thresholds during annual audiological monitoring
- ◆ Referral for evaluation from lawyers, insurance companies, worker compensation boards, or other related agencies
- ◆ Referral due to other related legal issues such as accidents, pensions, compensations, etc.

Case History Considerations

Illiterate individuals (43.5% of illiterate individuals) are more likely to present with pseudohypacusis than individuals with higher education levels (17.5% of individuals with higher education). Closer attention to the education levels can be helpful in cases of workers seeking compensation (Mahdavi, Mokari, & Amiri, 2011). When patients report that they have completely normal hearing in one ear but total deafness in the other ear due to noise exposure, possible nonorganic components or hearing loss should be considered.

◆ Test Battery and Sequence

The recommended test battery and sequence for audiological evaluations in medicolegal contexts or in cases with potential for nonorganic hearing loss or a nonorganic component added to an organic component is presented in **Fig. 5.1**.

Otoscopic Evaluation

Otoscopic evaluations are performed using a handheld or videotoscope to serve the following purposes:

- ◆ To examine the condition of the ear canal and eardrum.

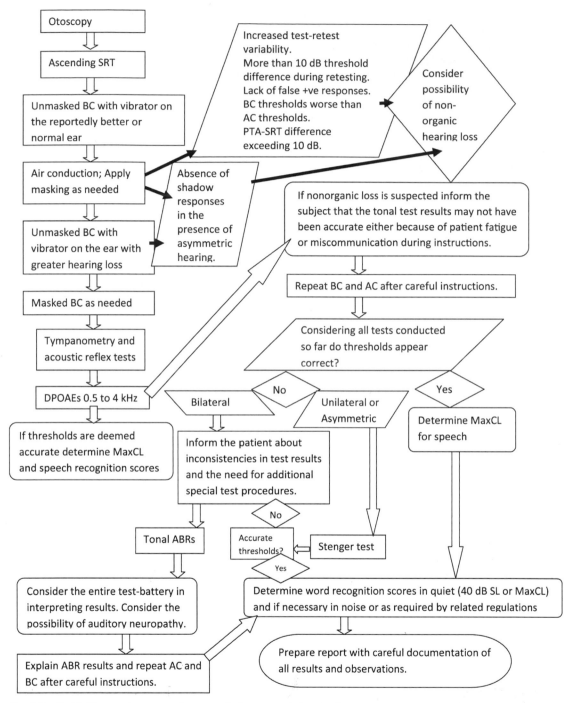

Fig. 5.1 Test battery and sequence for suspected nonorganic hearing loss.

◆ To ensure that the ear canal is free from impacted cerumen that can elevate thresholds. In the presence of impacted cerumen, the cerumen should be removed before proceeding with the remaining test battery.

◆ To examine the possibility of ear canal collapse with the use of supra-aural earphones and the need to use insert earphones.

Speech Reception Thresholds

The SRT is the softest level at which the examinee can repeat half of spondee words (bisyllabic words with equal emphasis on both syllables) accurately through insert or supra-aural earphones. This level is usually within 8 to 10 dB of the average tonal thresholds at 500, 1000, and 2000 Hz (Chaiklin & Ventry, 1965a) or at 0.5 kHz and 1.0 kHz (Chaiklin & Ventry, 1965a; Jahner, Schlauch, & Doyle, 1994). If the audiogram has a steep slope, the SRT can be similar to the average thresholds at 500 and 1000 Hz. Thus, the test is useful in confirming the accuracy of pure tone thresholds at these frequencies.

In patients with nonorganic hearing loss, the pure tone average (PTA)-SRT difference often exceeds 12 dB (Ventry & Chaiklin, 1961). Thus, the PTA-SRT difference can be used to determine the possible presence of a nonorganic component. SRTs obtained with the ascending procedure provide the largest difference in SRT and PTA in the presence of pseudohypacusis (Conn, Ventry, & Woods, 1972). Thus, an ascending approach with an initial level of -10 dB hearing level (HL) is recommended in determining SRTs (Schlauch, Arnce, Olson, Sanchez, & Doyle, 1996).

Establishing SRTs using an ascending approach at the beginning of the audiological test battery minimizes opportunities for the patient to establish a loudness reference based on tonal stimuli that are used during air or BC testing. In cases of unilateral hearing loss, no responses from one ear in the presence of normal SRTs in the other ear is suggestive of nonorganic pathology. In the presence of a true hearing asymmetry, the need for masking should be evaluated after establishing ear-specific BC thresholds; if necessary, masked SRTs should be obtained.

Tonal Thresholds

Unmasked Bone Conduction Thresholds

Following SRTs, unmasked BC testing is recommended by placing the bone vibrator on the mastoid process behind the reportedly normal or better ear. The procedure for obtaining thresholds is similar to that described in Chapter 4. BC thresholds are usually determined at 500, 1000, 2000, and 4000 Hz.

In most cases of noise-exposed individuals, BC thresholds match the AC sensitivity of the better ear unless there is a conductive component. Thus, BC thresholds can be used to judge test-retest reliability during AC testing. In addition, knowledge of BC thresholds before AC testing allows the determination of need for masking and the amount of masking for establishing ear-specific AC thresholds.

Air Conduction Thresholds

These thresholds are similar to those described in Chapter 4 with the following exceptions:

◆ Test frequencies of 250 and 8000 Hz are always included.
◆ When the thresholds at two adjacent test frequencies differ by 20 dB or more, thresholds are also determined at midoctave frequencies.
◆ Masking is used when the participation of the non-test ear is suspected.

Consideration of Possible Errors at 6 kHz

◆ The TDH-39 and TDH-39P earphones have some problems at 6000 Hz because their resonance frequency is close to 6000 Hz. The thresholds at 6 kHz can be worse by 6 dB when obtained with TDH-39 earphones calibrated on the IEC 303 reference coupler, compared with those obtained with TDH-39P earphones calibrated on the IEC 318 coupler (Lutman & Qusem, 1997).
◆ When testing is conducted using headphones, the test-retest reliability at this frequency can be poor because of the presence of standing waves.

Age-Related Versus Noise-Induced Hearing Loss

These two types of losses tend to occur at higher frequencies and thus are not always easy to separate. One proposed approach to this problem is to compare the PTA thresholds at 1 and 8 kHz (PTA18) with the PTA thresholds at 2, 3, and 4 kHz (PTA234). If the PTA234 exceeds PTA18, there is a positive notch index suggesting a noise component. If PTA234 minus PTA18 is negative, the chance of noise-induced damage is less (Rabinowitz & Dobie, 2003).

Bone Conduction Thresholds of the Worse Ear

Unmasked Bone Conduction Thresholds

BC thresholds should be re-established by placing the bone vibrator on the mastoid process of the reportedly worse ear. These thresholds should be similar to those obtained from the better ear because the interaural attenuation for bone conducted stimuli is minimal. If these thresholds are worse by more than 15 dB than those obtained from the reportedly better ear, nonorganic hearing loss is suspected.

Masked Bone Conduction Thresholds

Obtain ear-specific thresholds by using masking as necessary. Ear-specific BC thresholds allow determination of the type (conductive, sensorineural, or mixed) of hearing loss, as explained in Chapter 4.

Questionable Tonal Threshold Test Findings

The following indicators suggest the possibility of a nonorganic hearing loss component.

♦ Increased variability in response patterns during ascending and descending trials.
♦ Threshold differences of greater than 10 dB during repeat testing: It is a standard practice to retest the thresholds at 1000 Hz. If the difference on retest is 15 dB or higher, retesting should be performed at least at one more frequency. If both retested thresholds are not within 10 dB, nonorganic hearing loss should be considered.
♦ Absence of false-positive responses with an apparently higher number of false-negative responses: Most patients with organic hearing losses respond a few times in the absence of any tones, showing an attempt to respond to the softest sounds they can hear. Patients with nonorganic hearing losses are less likely to respond in the absence of tones even in the presence of extended-duration (1 minute) silent trials (Chaiklin & Ventry, 1965b).

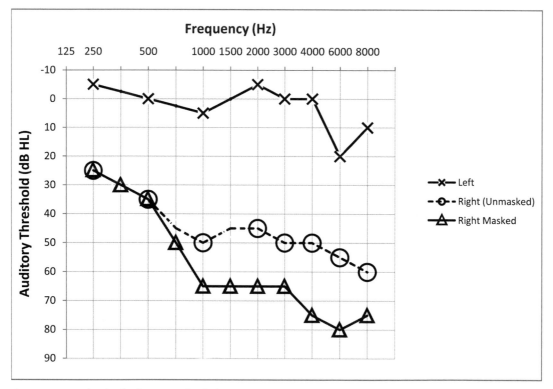

Fig. 5.2 Example of a shadow curve (circles).

◆ BC thresholds worse than AC thresholds in the presence of accurate placement of the bone conduction vibrator: In most cases of organic hearing loss, BC thresholds are usually similar to or better than AC thresholds.

◆ Absence of the shadow responses for unmasked thresholds in the impaired ear in cases of unilateral hearing losses: When one ear has normal BC thresholds, it is not possible to have no responses to unmasked tones in the other ear. Usually, shadow responses are apparent in the other ear. Example of a shadow curve is apparent in **Fig. 5.2** in a case with true unilateral hearing loss. As can be seen, the unmasked AC thresholds shadow the AC thresholds of the better ear. The maximum possible interaural attenuation for the particular earphones (insert or supra-aural) should be considered in making a determination of absence of shadow responses. The interaural attenuation is higher for insert earphones. Hypothetical responses such as those shown in **Fig. 5.3** are not possible for stimuli presented through AC or BC and are

indicative of nonorganic hearing loss in one ear.

Disagreement Between Pure Tone Average and Speech Reception Threshold

The PTA is usually much worse than the SRT in most individuals who are asked to feign hearing loss (Aplin & Kane, 1985; Martin, Champlin, & McCreery, 2001). A difference in the two values of 12 dB or greater is suggestive of nonorganic hearing loss (Ventry & Chaiklin, 1965).

Tympanometry

Tympanometry is performed using a tympanometer or middle ear analyzer (**Fig. 5.4**) to evaluate the function of the middle ear and to confirm or rule out any conductive component to any hearing loss. A normal tympanogram is shown in **Fig. 5.5**. In the presence of some abnormal findings suggesting reduced mobility of the middle ear system or eardrum rupture, acoustic reflex tests cannot be conducted. Also, results of OAE testing should be interpreted with caution in the presence of middle ear dysfunction.

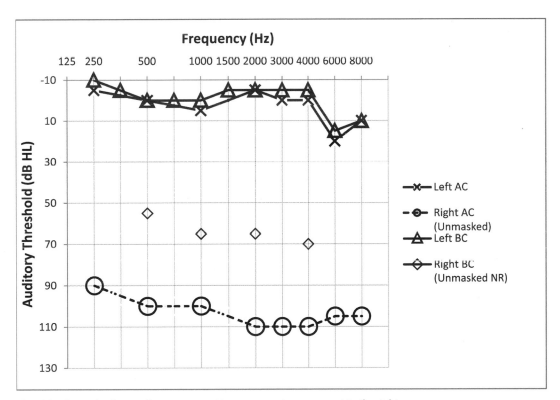

Fig. 5.3 Example of an audiogram suggesting nonorganic component in the right ear.

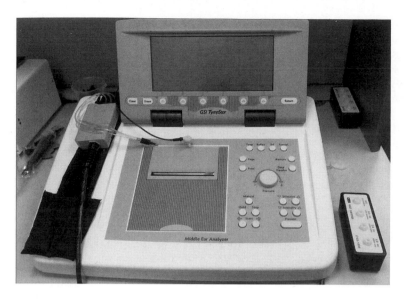

Fig. 5.4 Tympanometer or middle ear analyzer.

Acoustic Reflex Testing

Acoustic reflex tests are performed using the middle ear analyzer. The acoustic reflex occurs when relatively loud stimuli are presented to the ear.

Acoustic Reflex Thresholds

The softest stimulus level that causes a minimal recordable (specified) change in middle ear admittance is referred to as acoustic reflex threshold (ART). **Figure 5.6** shows establishment of ARTs using a criterion of a minimum

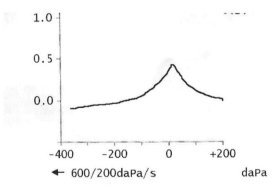

EARCANAL VOLUME: 1.1

	daPa	ml
TYMP 1:	15	0.4

Fig. 5.5 Example of a normal tympanogram.

change of 0.02 mL in admittance. At 80 dB HL, no change in admittance is apparent. Thus using a 5 dB step size, the lowest level at which a recordable change is apparent is 85 dB HL. Therefore, the ART is 85 dB HL in this case. ARTs should be established at 500, 1000, and 2000 Hz using a 226 Hz probe tone in adults, though reflex thresholds can also be established using high-frequency probe tones (Rawool, 1998a) and broadband stimuli such as clicks (Rawool, 1995). In normal individuals, ARTs can be recorded at levels between 85 and 100 dB sound pressure level (SPL) for pure tones and approximately 20 dB lower for broadband stimuli (Gelfand, 1984).

Acoustic Reflex Decay

During the reflex decay test, a tone is presented continuously for 10 seconds at a level 10 dB above the reflex thresholds. The magnitude of the reflex response either stays the same or decreases over the 10-second period. Reflex decay or positive reflex decay is noted when the magnitude of the response decreases by 50% or more during the 10-second period, as shown in **Fig. 5.7**. In the presence of elevated ARTs, it is not always possible to conduct threshold decay testing because of the upper limit of presentation levels or loudness tolerance difficulties.

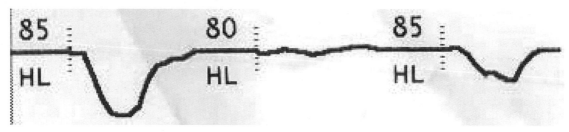

Fig. 5.6 Example of ARTs at 85 dB HL.

Applications of Acoustic Reflex Test Results

Retrocochlear Pathologies

Acoustic reflex abnormalities, including reflex thresholds at elevated levels, absent reflexes, and/or positive reflex decay, are associated with retrocochlear pathologies in the ear receiving the stimulus tone. In the presence of hearing loss, ARTs that fall above the 90% range established for individuals without known retrocochlear pathologies should be considered elevated. The normative data for various AC thresholds is provided by Gelfand (2001a). Consideration of positive findings on either or both reflex threshold or reflex decay tests has a hit rate of approximately 85% for retrocochlear pathologies and a relatively low false-positive rate of 11% (Silman & Silverman, 1991).

Auditory Neuropathy

In cases with auditory neuropathy, acoustic reflexes are often absent in the presence of normal OAEs.

Nonorganic Hearing Loss

Because of the wide variability of ARTs in individuals with AC thresholds below 60 dB HL,

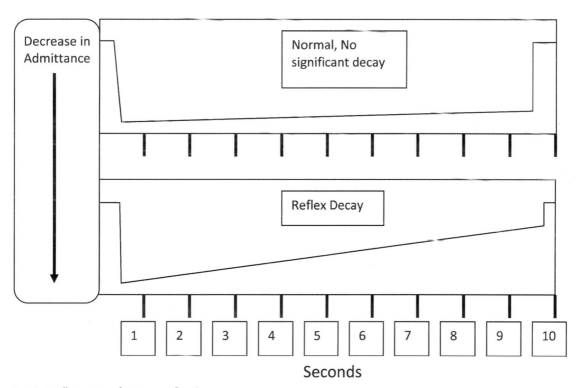

Fig. 5.7 Illustration of acoustic reflex decay.

it is difficult to differentiate between organic or nonorganic hearing loss. For 60 dB HL or higher AC thresholds, nonorganic hearing loss is suspected when the patient's ARTs are below the admitted pure tone AC thresholds or below the ARTs specified in **Fig. 5.8** (Gelfand, 2001b). For example, if the patient's audiogram shows an AC threshold of 75 dB HL, but the ARTs are established at 85 dB HL at 500, 1000, or 2000 Hz, presence of nonorganic hearing loss should be considered.

Otoacoustic Emission Testing

OAEs are sounds generated in the cochlea and are recorded by presenting clicks or tonal stimuli to the ear. The equipment for measuring OAEs comprises a probe tip assembly that is placed in the ear canal. The probe tip assembly has receivers for presenting stimuli to the ear and a microphone to pick up sounds elicited by the cochlea. The sounds picked up by the microphone are amplified and filtered to detect the emissions of interest. Background noise is also minimized by applying signal averaging.

From a clinical standpoint, OAE testing is very useful because it allows quick evaluation at more discrete frequencies in an objective manner that is unaffected by fatigue factors.

In addition, the only requirement from subjects is to sit still and not speak during the testing.

Transient evoked OAEs (TEOAEs) are elicited in response to stimuli of very brief duration (transients) such as clicks. Distortion product (DP) OAEs (DPOAEs) are elicited by simultaneous presentation of two tones with different but relatively close frequencies that are referred to as primaries. The tone with lower frequency is referred to as *f1* and the tone with higher frequency is referred to as *f2*. The ear generates different DPs in response to the two tones, including *2f1-f2*, *2f2-f1*, *f2-f1*, etc. The *2f1-f2* DP has the largest amplitude (Gaskill & Brown, 1990), allowing easier detection, and is thus the most commonly measured DPOAE for clinical applications.

For clinical applications, DPOAEs are usually elicited for several different primary frequencies by holding the primary levels and frequency ratio constant. The amplitudes of the recorded DPOAEs are then plotted as a function of *f2* (Gorga, Neely, Ohlrich, Hoover, Redner, & Peters, 1997) or the geometric mean of the primaries (Lonsbury-Martin & Martin, 1990). The assumption underlying plotting DPOAEs as a function of *f2* is that the level of the DPOAE reflects cochlear function near the *f2* place (generator component) on the basilar membrane, where there is maximum overlap of excitation patterns generated

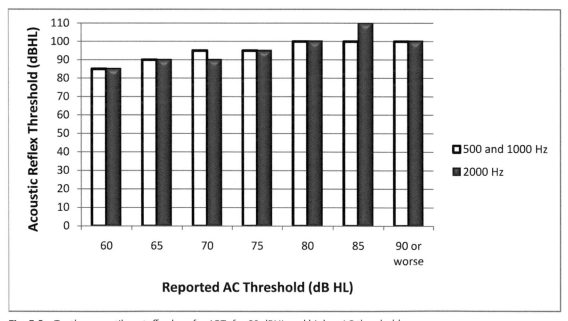

Fig. 5.8 Tenth percentile cutoff values for ARTs for 60 dBHL and higher AC thresholds.

by $f1$ and $f2$. However, when the DP frequency is lower than the $f2$ frequency, a proportion of the DP energy appears to travel to the characteristic place for that DP frequency and is reflected from there (Shaffer, Withnell, Dhar, Lilly, Goodman, & Harmon, 2003). This component of DPOAE is referred to as the reflection component, and it can be larger than the generator component because energy traveling from the base to the DP characteristic place is amplified (Talmadge, Long, Tubis, & Dhar, 1999). The DPOAE fine structure (relatively large changes in DPOAE amplitudes with small changes in frequency) may be a result of the interaction of the generator and reflection components. When the frequencies of the primaries are changed, the phase of both the generator and reflection components is expected to change. However, the phase change is slower for the generator component compared with that for the reflection component. When the generator and the reflection components are in phase, DPOAE amplitudes can be expected to be larger; when they are out of phase, the magnitude is expected to be smaller, leading to the DPOAE fine structure. The DPOAE fine structure is indicative of a healthy cochlea and has been used for differential diagnosis of outer hair cell damage (Mauermann, Uppenkamp, van Hengel, & Kollmeier, 1999). Use of rapidly sweeping tones has been proposed to obtain quicker estimates of DPOAE fine structure or to obtain estimates of DOPAE from the generator component uncontaminated by the reflection component (Long, Talmadge, & Lee, 2008).

Otoacoustic Emissions for Early Indication of Noise-Induced Deterioration of the Cochlea

OAEs are useful in monitoring noise-induced deterioration of the cochlea if they can be measured initially or if there is enough room for recordable deterioration of OAEs (no floor effect). Significant reduction in DPOAEs obtained in half-octave bands centered at 1.4 to 6 kHz has been demonstrated following a 30-minute 85 dBC exposure to music in young adults in the absence of audiometric threshold shifts (Bhagat & Davis, 2008). OAEs show reduction at more frequencies than audiometric thresholds, suggesting better sensitivity for detecting noise-induced damage (Helleman, Jansen, & Dreschler, 2010). Following impulse noise exposure, significant reduction in DPOAE amplitudes can occur in some ears with no

changes in audiometric thresholds (Balatsouras, Tsimpiris, Korres, Karapantzos, Papadimitriou, & Danielidis, 2005).

The main shifts in DPOAEs in a noise-exposed population are apparent in the 4 to 8 kHz range, but all workers may not have reliable OAEs at the baseline in this range. OAEs may also be useful in screening for susceptibility to noise-induced hearing loss, as individuals with low-level OAEs appear to be at a greater risk of noise-induced hearing loss (Job, Raynal, Kossowski, et al., 2009; Lapsley-Miller, Marshall, Heller, & Hughes, 2006; Marshall, Lapsley Miller, Heller, et al., 2009).

Otoacoustic Emissions in Nonorganic Hearing Loss

If an individual suspected of nonorganic hearing loss has thresholds that are within normal limits, OAE testing can quickly rule out hearing loss. **Figure 5.9** shows two test runs of DPOAEs from a 55-year-old woman using tones presented with a $f1/f2$ ratio of 1.22 at 65 and 55 dB SPL. The same data are shown in **Fig. 5.10** for midoctave frequencies. At 2000 and 4000 Hz, a 9 dB DPOAE/noise ratio is suggested as a criterion for assuming normal auditory sensitivity in older adults (Torre, Cruickshanks, Nondahl, & Wiley, 2003). Using this criterion, DPOAEs in **Fig. 5.10** indicate normal sensitivity at 2000 and 4000 Hz. Application of the same strict criterion of +9 dB DPOAE/noise ratio (Dorn, Piskorski, Gorga, Neely, & Keefe, 1999; Gorga, Neely, & Dorn, 1999) to 1000, 3000, and 6000 Hz, frequencies that are relevant to noise-induced hearing loss, also indicate normal sensitivity, ruling out the presence of a hearing loss.

DPOAEs are present in almost all normal ears and are absent in the presence of a sensory hearing loss of approximately 50 to 60 dB HL. Recording of OAEs in the presence of AC thresholds above 50 to 60 dB HL strongly suggests the presence of a nonorganic hearing loss, although in some cases with retrocochlear pathology, OAEs can be normal.

In some noise-exposed workers, TEOAEs can be absent in the presence of normal audiometric thresholds because of subclinical cochlear damage (Attias, Furst, Furman, Reshef, Horowitz, & Bresloff, 1995; Prasher & Sułkowski, 1999). Even if OAEs may be present in a relatively small percentage of cases with noise exposure because of subclinical pathology, the objectivity of the test can encourage some patients to yield more accurate

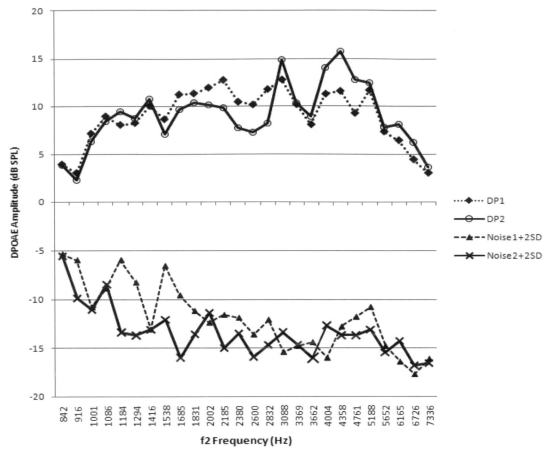

Fig. 5.9 Two recordings of DPOAEs from a 55-year-old woman with normal auditory sensitivity.

Repetition of Tonal Threshold Measures

AC thresholds following acoustic immittance and OAE tests (Balatsouras, Kaberos, Korres, Kandiloros, Ferekidis, & Economou, 2003; Kvaerner, Engdahl, Aursnes, Arnesen, & Mair, 1996).

Repetition of Tonal Threshold Measures

It is not necessary to repeat tonal threshold measures if the initial tonal thresholds are deemed accurate and reliable. However, in cases of suspected nonorganic hearing loss, the tonal thresholds should be re-established after having some objective data from acoustic reflex and OAE measures. In the presence of a suspected nonorganic component, the patient should be informed that the initial measurements performed by presenting tones may be inaccurate probably because of miscommunications during instructions or patient fatigue. It is important to

not accuse the patient of malingering to ensure continued cooperation and to minimize negative behaviors or lack of cooperation during the remaining test procedures. It is also possible that the patient may not be consciously malingering.

Although repetition of the test following reinstruction can often improve the ability to obtain accurate thresholds, it is important to minimize a learning effect. With practice, the patient's ability to consistently produce false thresholds at similar stimulus levels can improve (Monro & Martin, 1977) perhaps because of the opportunity to think about additional strategies for feigning hearing loss. Thus initially, the employee may use the loudness judgment strategy, which involves responding to sounds to reach some predetermined amount of reference loudness level. After this, the employee may use a counting strategy. For example, the employee

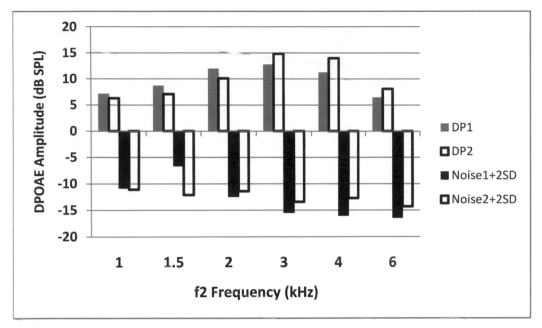

Fig. 5.10   DPOAE data from Fig. 5.8 plotted in half-octave bands.

may respond to every third presentation following the predetermined loudness reference (Martin, Champlin, & McCreery, 2001).

Thus, repetition of the tonal threshold measures immediately following the initial measures should be avoided. Instead, it is ideal to repeat tonal threshold measures after acoustic immittance and OAE measures (Balatsouras, Kaberos, Korres, Kandiloros, Ferekidis, & Economou, 2003). These tests do not require active participation from the patient, thus allowing the patient to recover from any fatigue. It also allows the patient to realize that objective tests of hearing are available, which can motivate some patients to yield more accurate thresholds during retesting.

In most cases, repetition of tonal threshold tests will yield accurate thresholds (Qiu, Yin, Stucker, & Welsh, 1998). In the presence of accurate thresholds, maximum comfortable levels and speech recognition testing should be conducted. If accurate thresholds are still not obtained after repeating the tonal thresholds tests and the hearing loss is unilateral, a Stenger test should be conducted immediately following the tonal tests. If the loss is bilateral, frequency-specific ABR or auditory steady state response (ASSR) testing should be conducted to obtain thresholds at least at 500, 1000, 2000, 3000, and

4000 Hz, which are the most relevant frequencies in the majority of workers' compensation cases (see Chapter 11).

Stenger Test

As indicated previously, absence of shadow responses on tonal and/or speech threshold measures indicates the presence of a nonorganic hearing loss in one ear or a nonorganic component in one ear. Workers with unilateral profound or total hearing loss may be considered unfit for performing military duty (Durmaz, Karahatay, Satar, Birkent, & Hidir, 2009). Thus, it is important to determine the true frequency-specific thresholds in the poor ear. Careful administration of the Stenger test can allow estimation of true thresholds in the worse ear. The test has a sensitivity of 99.4% and specificity of 70% in military personnel with unilateral, profound hearing loss (Durmaz, Karahatay, Satar, Birkent, & Hidir, 2009).

Stenger Effect or Principle

When two tones of the same frequency are presented simultaneously to the right and left ears, only the tone with higher sensation level is perceived. More specifically, the two sounds are fused in a single image that is perceived only in the ear that is receiving the tone at a higher sensation level. This is illustrated in **Fig. 5.11**.

Necessary Asymmetry for Performing the Stenger Test

A difference of at least 20 dB should be apparent in the thresholds between the ears to be able to perform the tonal or speech Stenger test.

Test Instructions

Because the patient is already in the booth for repetition of thresholds and has already been instructed to respond to all tones including the softest tones, the examiner can proceed to perform the Stenger test without any instructions. However, if a different test sequence is used, the same instructions used for tonal threshold measures should be used. From the patient's perspective, the Stenger test need not be different than the tonal threshold tests.

Test Procedure

The procedure for determining true thresholds is illustrated in **Fig. 5.12**. In the illustration, it is assumed that the normal ear has a 0 dB HL threshold at the test frequency. Thus, 10 dB sound level (SL) is equal to 10 dB HL in the right ear. The sensation levels for the left or reportedly poor ear are shown inside the boxes, representing the amplitude of the tone on the left side. As shown in the figure, initially a tone of 10 dB SL is presented to the normal or better ear, to which a clear and quick response is expected because the level is 10 dB above the threshold. This response is important because during each test trial, except for the control trial, the right ear will be presented with the same 10 dB SL tone during the remaining procedure, ensuring an audible tone even if the patient has a true hearing loss in the poor ear.

Following this step, two tones are simultaneously presented to the right and left ear. The presentation level of the tone in the right ear is always 10 dB SL. The presentation level in the left ear is initially 0 dB HL. With each test trial, the level is increased in 5-dB steps until the patient's admitted thresholds. If the patient has a true hearing loss, the patient will respond for each trial

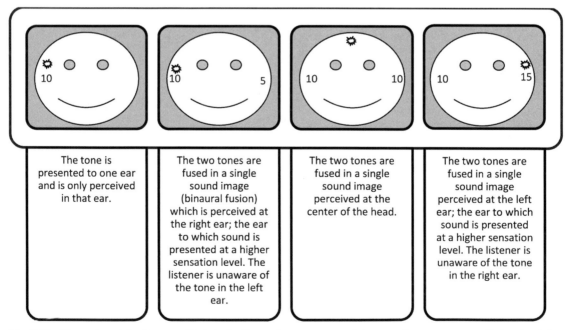

| The tone is presented to one ear and is only perceived in that ear. | The two tones are fused in a single sound image (binaural fusion) which is perceived at the right ear; the ear to which sound is presented at a higher sensation level. The listener is unaware of the tone in the left ear. | The two tones are fused in a single sound image perceived at the center of the head. | The two tones are fused in a single sound image perceived at the left ear; the ear to which sound is presented at a higher sensation level. The listener is unaware of the tone in the right ear. |

Fig. 5.11   Illustration of the Stenger effect. In the illustration, two tones of the same frequency are applied to the right and left ears. The presentation levels at each ear are indicated in dB SL.

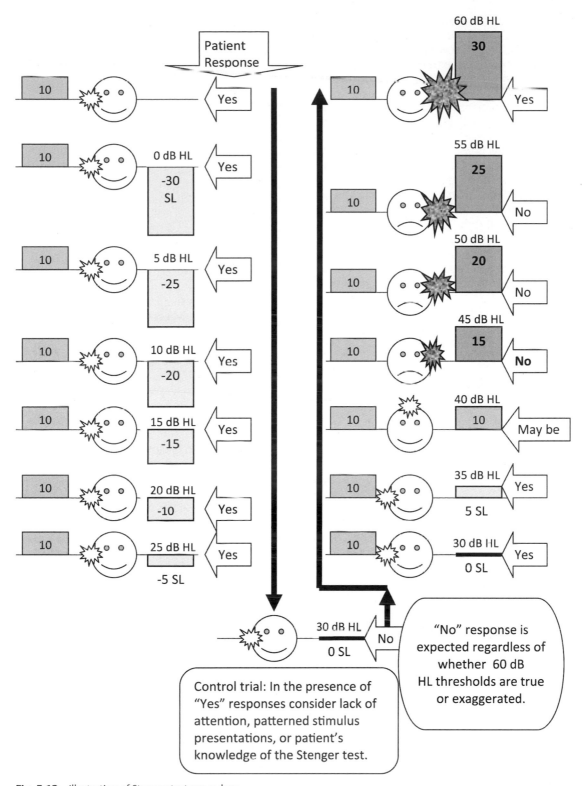

Fig. 5.12   Illustration of Stenger test procedure.

because of the presence of a clearly audible tone in the right ear. If the patient has a nonorganic component, he or she is expected to not respond at 15 dB above the true thresholds or 15 dB SL. In **Fig. 5.12**, the patient does not respond at 45 dB HL. This level is 15 dB above the true threshold (15 dB SL); thus, the patient's true threshold is very likely to be (45 − 15) 30 dB HL. The patient with nonorganic hearing loss does not respond at 15 dB SL, because at this point the fused image of the two tones is on the left side. The left ear has the louder 15 dB SL tone, and the right ear has the softer 10 dB SL tone. Thus, provided that the tones are presented simultaneously, the patient is unaware of the tone in the right ear. The level at which the patient stops responding is also referred to as the minimum contralateral interference level (MCIL). If the hypothetical patient in **Fig. 5.12** would have stopped responding at 50 dB HL, the patient's true threshold would be at (50 − 15) 35 dB HL. With increasing presentation levels, the patient is expected to begin to respond when the level approximates the previously admitted thresholds.

Precautions in Conducting the Stenger Threshold Test

It is important to vary the pattern of tonal presentations during any tonal tests. The onset of the tones to the right and left ear should be simultaneous. If the tone in the right ear begins sooner than the tone in the left ear, some patients will become aware of the presence of the tone in the right ear and will respond to it. This is especially critical at the MCIL, where the difference in the tones in the two ears differs only by 5 dB SL. As the patient gets more practice with the Stenger test through testing at different frequencies, the patient may become aware of the tone in the right ear and is less likely to be confused by MCILs (Martin & Shipp, 1982).

When a patient continues to respond to several tones, it is important to mix the test sequence with a few trials with the tone only in the left ear below the patient's admitted threshold to elicit a "no" response (see bottom of **Fig. 5.12**). If a patient is aware of the test and thus continues to respond, the trials with no tone in the right ear can serve as "catch" trials. Practice in performing the Stenger test by asking several normal subjects to feign hearing loss in one ear is highly recommended before performing the test on patients with suspected nonorganic hearing loss. When

administered correctly, the Stenger test is expected to be efficient in identifying nonorganic hearing loss (Kinstler, Phelan, & Lavender, 1972).

Auditory Brainstem and Steady State Response

In response to sounds presented to ear(s), the auditory nervous system produces electrical signals or auditory-evoked potentials that can be picked up by surface electrodes that are placed on the head.

The response occurring within 7 to 8 seconds following the stimulus onset is referred to as the ABR if conventional averaging is used and the averaged waveform is displayed in the time domain. ABR relies on peak detection in a time-versus-amplitude plot. ABR amplitudes are measured in microvolts, and ABR is usually elicited using clicks or tone bursts, though more complex stimuli can be used. The threshold is estimated by using the softest stimulus level at which wave V of the ABR can be detected. The tonal ABR threshold in normal individual is usually at 10 to 20 dB nHL or normalized hearing level (nHL). The nHL is established by averaging the behavioral thresholds of several normal individuals for the specific stimuli such as tonal bursts or clicks used in eliciting the ABR. This average threshold is referred to as 0 dB nHL. Responses within 20 dB above this level or at 20 dB nHL are usually considered normal although stricter criteria for normalcy such as 15 dB nHL can be used when children are involved. In adults with sensorineural hearing loss, tone-evoked ABR thresholds are detected at 5 to 15 dB above behavioral thresholds (Stapells, 2000). The click-evoked ABR waveforms in **Fig. 5.13** from a 29-year-old man suggests that he has hearing within normal limits because wave V of the ABR is detectable at 10 dB nHL. In this case, auditory neuropathy and other retrocochlear pathologies can also be ruled out from the presence of clear ABR waveforms from I to V and normal peak and interpeak latencies (I to III, III to V) at 70 dB nHL.

If a statistical analysis of the probability of responses is conducted, the technique is referred to as ASSR. ASSR relies on peak detection from amplitude and phases of the response. It is usually measured in nanovolts and is elicited by using amplitude or frequency-modulated sounds. A technique called multiple hertz ASSR allows evaluation of multiple frequencies simultaneously in both ears (Lins & Picton, 1995). In this technique, the ASSR is elicited by presenting a

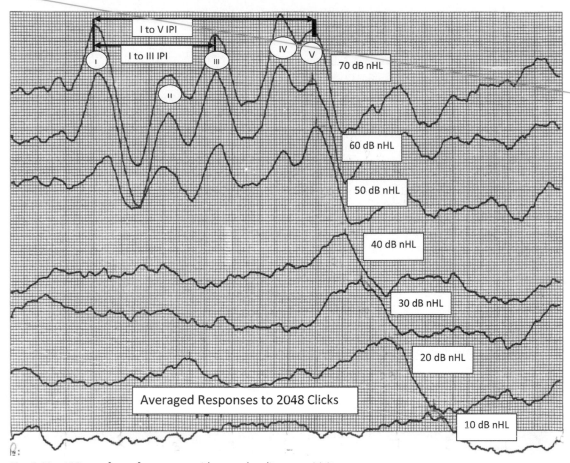

Fig. 5.13 ABR waveforms from a man with normal auditory sensitivity.

complex stimulus comprising multiple amplitude modified (AM) tones, which are at least one octave apart in frequency and are modulated at different rates. Actual data for correcting ASSR thresholds to predict behavioral thresholds depends on many variables, including the equipment used to obtain ASSR resulting from variations in response detection algorithms, age and sleep state of the subject, and specific stimulus parameters. Using the 40 Hz multiple ASSR technique, thresholds at 500, 1000, 2000, and 4000 Hz in each ear can be recorded within 45 minutes with an average recording time of 21 minutes. The mean difference in ASSR thresholds and behavioral thresholds with this technique can vary from 1 to 14 dB (Van Maanen & Stapells, 2005). A meta-analysis of studies using 70 to 110 Hz multiple ASSRs indicated mean difference of 15 dB at 0.5 and 1 kHz, 12 dB at 2 kHz, and 8 dB at 4 kHz between the ASSR and behavioral thresholds (Herdman & Stapells, 2003). In general, ASSR is good at predicting behavioral thresholds at the frequencies of 500, 1000, 2000, and 4000 Hz and may be more reliable than ABR (Lin, Ho, & Wu, 2009).

In some cases, statutory regulations require ABR testing to confirm behavioral tonal thresholds (Durmaz, Karahatay, Satar, Birkent, & Hidir, 2009). In other cases, discrepancies in test results may continue after completion of the previous test battery. In these cases, ABR or ASSR testing is necessary. Before conducting the test, it is important to inform the patient that the test allows direct and objective evaluation of the function of parts of the auditory system. This may promote admission of true thresholds following the objective evaluation. In conducting these tests, it is important to use frequency-specific stimuli and stimulus and response parameters that are known to yield accurate thresholds, as well as well-established norms for estimating audiometric frequency-specific thresholds based on ABR or ASSR thresholds. It is important to keep the patient alert and quiet during ASSR. During ABR, the patient needs to be quiet (preferably asleep) and thus does not need to be alert. The difference in evoked potential thresholds and behavioral thresholds is minimal at 4 kHz, which is where hearing loss is most prevalent in populations exposed to noise and many ototoxins.

Consideration of the Presence of Auditory Neuropathy/Auditory Dyssynchrony

If the patient yields abnormal ABRs or no responses to ABR, the possibility of auditory neuropathy (AN)/auditory dyssynchrony (AD) should be considered. In cases of AN, the response can be absent even in the presence of perception of the sound (Lin & Staecker, 2006). Auditory thresholds in patients with AN can vary from normal findings to severe hearing loss. **Table 5.1** shows the different results for patients with sensory hearing loss, AN/AD, and auditory processing disorders.

Repeat Behavioral Tonal Threshold Measures

Although ABRs allow evaluation of the functional and anatomical integrity of the auditory pathways, they do not truly test hearing. Therefore, it is important to establish reliable behavioral thresholds to the best extent possible.

Maximum Comfort Level

This is the maximum level of words or tones that the patient can listen to without perceiving them as being uncomfortably loud. Although the maximum comfort level (MaxCL) can be very close to tonal or speech thresholds in patients with severe hearing losses and recruitment, it should not be within 10 dB SL. Testing with reinstructions can be helpful in establishing accurate MaxCL. If MaxCLs occur at 0 dB SL, possibility of a nonorganic component to AC thresholds should be considered, unless other reported symptoms suggest the presence of hyperacusis.

Word Recognition Scores

This is the percentage of words that the individual can repeat correctly when presented at the MaxCL. Some regulations specify the particular speech materials that are to be used in evaluating the ability to recognize speech in quiet and noise. Word recognition scores can vary depending on the presentation level. Thus, it is important to accurately determine the MaxCL and to present the words at the MaxCL or 40 dB above the SRT or the PTA. Information about word recognition ability can serve the following purposes:

◆ These scores are sometimes considered in awarding workers' compensation. Poorer scores can lead to a greater award (see Chapter 11).

Table 5.1   Test Battery Results for Patients with Sensory Hearing Loss, AN/AD, and Auditory Processing Disorders

Test	Sensory	AN/AD	Auditory processing disorder
Auditory thresholds	Abnormal	Normal or abnormal	Usually normal; auditory processing disorder can be present in cases with sensory hearing loss
OAEs	Abnormal in most cases	Normal	Normal unless accompanied by sensory loss
Acoustic reflex	Depending on the degree of hearing loss; normal, elevated, or absent	Absent	Normal or abnormal
ABR	Level at which wave V of the ABR can be detected depends on the degree of hearing loss	Absent	Normal or abnormal
Word recognition score	Proportional to the degree of hearing loss	Disproportionately poor compared with AC thresholds	Usually normal on conventional word recognition tests in quiet

ABR, auditory brainstem response; AC, air conduction; AN/AD, auditory neuropathy/auditory dyssynchrony; OAE, otoacoustic emission.

- The scores allow prediction of the potential benefit from hearing aids or indicate candidacy for cochlear implants.
- Poorer word recognition than expected from AC thresholds can be suggestive of auditory neuropathy.

◆ Tinnitus Evaluation

When the patient reports disabling or bothersome tinnitus, it is important to perform a comprehensive evaluation that should begin with a detailed case history. Based on the case history, a test battery can be developed and administered. Some test procedures included in a comprehensive tinnitus evaluation are shown in **Table 5.2**. Note that when the patient has hearing loss, results for many of the tests included in **Table 5.2** should already be available and need not be repeated. For example, AC thresholds at most frequencies should already be available.

Detailed Case History/Intake Interview

In medicolegal cases, the case history can help in determining if the tinnitus is work-related or if other causes may have contributed to the tinnitus. In this context, it is important to note that approximately one-third of the general population reports tinnitus. It is also important to note whether or not the patient spontaneously

Table 5.2   Possible Tests for Inclusion of Comprehensive Tinnitus Evaluations

Test	Purpose
Self-report instrument	To assess the impact of tinnitus. To assess the coping strategies used by the patient. To assist in determining the severity of the tinnitus.
Pure tone audiometry at octave and interoctave frequencies from 250 to 12,000 Hz	To record any associated hearing loss and the frequency of maximum hearing loss which often matches the frequency of tinnitus. To determine the types of hearing loss.
Extended high-frequency audiometry	This can be useful in selecting high-frequency masking if hearing is within normal limits at frequencies between 250 and 12,000 Hz.
Speech audiometry	To confirm the pure tone audiometric findings and to determine work recognition skills.
ABR	When the reliability of pure tone findings is in question, degree of hearing loss can be determined using the ABR. Although expensive, ABR can in some cases reduce the amount of worker compensation significantly (Miller, Crane, Fox, & Linstrom, 1998).
Tinnitus pitch match Tinnitus loudness match	To determine the loudness and pitch of tinnitus. Credibility of the tinnitus report can be assessed using these measures, which produce similar findings on repeated evaluations. Pitch matching information can also be useful in providing a tinnitus masker. Loudness matching can be useful in determining the efficacy of treatment. Louder sounds tend to be more annoying than softer sounds, and any treatment or management strategy that reduces the loudness of tinnitus can be considered beneficial.
MML of tinnitus	To determine if masking noise can be helpful in reducing the annoyance of tinnitus. To determine the minimum level that will be necessary if a masker is used as treatment. To document the credibility of the tinnitus report; repeated evaluations should result in similar outcomes.
Residual inhibition	This measurement is useful if tinnitus maskers are used. The greater the amount of residual inhibition, the less the levels required to mask the tinnitus. Patients can be informed about their residual inhibition to maintain as low a masking level as possible. The acceptability of tinnitus masker is better with lower masking levels. Residual inhibition can also provide insight into how the patients may continue to find relief at night from tinnitus after a full day use of hearing aids.
ULLs at all test frequencies including the frequency that matches with the tinnitus	To gain insight into any accompanying hyperacusis. To determine the maximum output limits for hearing aids and any tinnitus maskers used for alleviation of the tinnitus. The maximum output limits should be below the ULL.

ABR, auditory brainstem response; MML, minimum masking level; ULL, uncomfortable loudness level.

reported the tinnitus before the detailed tinnitus-related history is noted. Spontaneous reports of tinnitus can improve the credibility and integrity of the tinnitus claims in worker compensation cases (see Chapter 11). The patient should also be asked if the tinnitus is continuous or intermittent, if it is inside the head or outside the head, and if it is in one specified ear or both ears.

Assessment of Impact of Tinnitus and Coping Strategies

Self-report instruments can allow the assessment of the impact of tinnitus on the patient and the coping strategies used by the patient. Several self-report instruments have been developed. For example, the Tinnitus Questionnaire (TQ) (Hallam, 1996) can be administered in a longer or a shorter version. The full version has 52 items covering sleep, emotional disturbances, audiological and perceptual difficulties, and intrusiveness. The shorter version has 33 items that assess helplessness, capacity for rest and relaxation, acceptability of change, emotional effects and related beliefs, hearing speech and sounds, and ability to ignore (Hiller & Goebel, 2004). Administration of a Chinese (Cantonese) version of the TQ (TQ-CH) has also identified five factors including auditory perceptual difficulties, cognitive and emotional distress, somatic complaints, sleep disturbances, and intrusiveness. In addition, significant correlations were apparent between the TQ-CH and psychological distress, tinnitus-related problem ratings, and severity ratings. High construct validity and high test-retest reliability was also apparent (Kam, Cheung, Chan, et al., 2009). Other examples of self-report instruments include the Tinnitus Handicap Questionnaire (Kuk, Tyler, Russell, & Jordan, 1990) and the Tinnitus Handicap Inventory (Newman, Jacobson, & Spitzer, 1996). In addition, a new questionnaire titled Tinnitus Functional Index has been specifically developed to measure tinnitus treatment outcomes (Snow, 2006).

Determination of Tinnitus Severity

Determination of severity is important for deciding treatment options, for estimating prognosis, and for determining the award of compensation in jurisdictions where tinnitus is compensable with the amount of award depending on the severity of the tinnitus. Determination of severity is also important for documenting the effect of treatments. Several different procedures have been suggested for determining the severity of the tinnitus. **Table 5.3** shows one of the two severity rating systems used in Sweden (Axelsson, 1996).

Tinnitus questionnaires often provide an index score to quantify the impact of tinnitus on the patient's everyday life. For example, a patient's score on the Tinnitus Handicap Inventory (Newman, Sandridge, & Jacobson, 1998) determines the patient handicap severity as either none, mild, moderate, or severe. Patients with tinnitus who hear multiple types of sounds tend to have higher scores on the Tinnitus Handicap Inventory (Lim, Lu, Koh, & Eng, 2010). Information generated from tinnitus questionnaires should be combined with that gained from the case history/intake interview to determine overall severity of the tinnitus (Schechter & Henry, 2002).

Pitch Matching

The goal of the test is to determine the frequency of an external tone or narrowband noise that closely matches the pitch of the perceived tinnitus (tinnitus frequency of F_T). Test-retest reliability in the matched pitch can be helpful in documenting the authenticity of the reported tinnitus in workers' compensation cases.

If the tinnitus is described as noise and the noise is described as being high-pitched or low-pitched, narrowband noises can be used. In some cases, the pitch can be higher than those that can be presented through conventional audiometers, and audiometers with extended high-frequency range can be useful. If pitch of the noise

Table 5.3   Example of One of the Severity Ratings

Rating	Description
Mild	Intermittent, noticeable in quiet environments, easy to suppress
Moderate	Continuous, more noticeable in quiet environments, sometimes irritating especially during activities that require concentration, can affect sleep, can be suppressed by different activities, patient unaware of tinnitus for several hours each day
Severe	Continuously annoying, disturbing concentration and sleep, constant awareness of tinnitus, marked effect on quality of life

cannot be described, white noise can be used for matching the loudness. Typically, during pitch matching, a reference signal is presented to the patient, and the patient is asked to describe if the pitch of the reference tone is higher or lower than the pitch of his or her tinnitus. The frequency of the reference tone is then changed first in larger step sizes and then in smaller step sizes (1 Hz) to match the tinnitus pitch.

Loudness Matching

The goal of this test is to measure the intensity of an external sound that closely matches the loudness of the tinnitus. The intensity of the external tones should be varied first in 5 dB steps and then in 1 dB steps when it approaches the loudness of the perceived tinnitus. The matching should be performed at the tinnitus frequency and another frequency where the hearing is best.

Considerations in Determining the Loudness of Tinnitus

Coles and Baskill (1996) noted the following difficulties with the tinnitus matching procedure:

◆ Tinnitus matching is different than other loudness balancing techniques where the patient is asked to match the loudness of two tones, which are alternately switched on and off. During tinnitus loudness matching, the patient is asked to match the loudness of the continuous sound of tinnitus with an external sound when the tinnitus is still on. Some patients may have difficulty in attending to the loudness of the tinnitus and then listening to the loudness of the external tone when the tinnitus is still "on."
◆ Some patients have tinnitus that is characterized as "unpleasant" or "dysphonic." Such patients may have difficulty in matching the loudness of an external tone to the tinnitus because of the difference in the quality of the two sounds.
◆ Some patients may confuse tinnitus loudness and tinnitus masking. They might judge the loudness of the external tone as being as loud as the tinnitus only when the external tone completely masks the tinnitus.
◆ When tinnitus is measured at the approximate frequency that matches the pitch of the tinnitus, the tinnitus usually is only 5 to

15 dB SL regardless of the subjective loudness of the tinnitus. The correlation between loudness of the tinnitus and self-reported severity of tinnitus is poor. Workers with very low levels of tinnitus can be seriously disturbed by it, whereas others with high levels of tinnitus appear to cope quite well with it.

Minimum Masking Level

The lowest intensity of the external tone (F_T) or narrowband noise (F_{NB}) that masks the tinnitus or where the patient cannot perceive the tinnitus is recorded as the minimum masking level (MML). Using a narrowband of noise centered at F_T, masking is expected to be successful in providing relief from tinnitus if the MML is established at 0 to 3 dB SL. In the presence of MMLs that are greater than 11 dB SL, the prognosis for tinnitus masking is expected to be poor (Vernon & Fenwick, 1984).

Residual Inhibition

This is the temporary depression of tinnitus immediately following masking, and 91% of patients demonstrate some residual inhibition (Vernon & Fenwick, 1984). This measurement is useful if tinnitus maskers are used.

In this procedure, the masking stimulus is presented at 10 dB above the MML of the F_T or F_{NB} for 60 seconds. If the tinnitus disappears, it is referred to as complete residual inhibition. If the tinnitus does not disappear but is only suppressed, the amount of time for the tinnitus to return to the original severity is recorded. The patient can also be asked to indicate the degree of suppression using a visual analog device (Vernon & Fenwick, 1984).

◆ Hyperacusis and Uncomfortable Loudness Levels

The point prevalence rate of self-reported hyperacusis may be approximately 8 to 9% in the general population, including those with hearing loss. It is associated with use of hearing protection devices and sensitivity to light and colors (Andersson, Lindvall, Hursti, & Carlbring, 2002). Many patients with hyperacusis also suffer from tinnitus (86%) and headaches (49%). Patients with hyperacusis can be divided into those hypersensitive to the loudness of sounds with a decreased pure tone uncomfortable loudness level (ULL) and those hypersensitive to certain specific sounds showing relatively high pure tone ULLs. Forty percent of the individuals with hyperacusis report occupational noise exposure, including more frequent exposure to loud music. Spontaneous recovery can occur is some patients (Anari, Axelsson, Eliasson, & Magnusson, 1999). A disturbance in serotonin (5-hydroxytryptamine [5-HT]) function may be a mediating factor for hyperacusis because serotonin function is often disturbed in conditions that are accompanied by hyperacusis, including depression and post-traumatic stress (Marriage & Barnes, 1995).

The average ULL among patients with hyperacusis can range from less than 45 to above 110 dB HL, with an average ULL of 77 dB HL. Hyperacusis may have a serious impact on everyday life for patients who yield ULLs below 70 dBHL. Such patients are less likely to work full-time and are more likely to take full- or part-time sick leave (Anari, Axelsson, Eliasson, & Magnusson, 1999). This would be specifically true for workers who are exposed to occupational noise. Thus, it is important to establish the ULLs for patients who report hypersensitivity to sounds and provide necessary support. Because many patients with hyperacusis also suffer from tinnitus, treatment offered for tinnitus (see Chapter 12), including sound therapy or desensitization, may alleviate the hypersensitivity. Some patients who constantly use earplugs to cope with their extreme hypersensitivity may experience communication difficulties. Such patients may benefit from in-the-ear electronic devices that provide mild gain to low-level sounds but compress moderate- and high-level inputs to bring the sound levels within those that are tolerated by the patient (Sammeth, Preves, & Brandy, 2000).

Before obtaining ULLs, it is important to inform the patient that the goal is to establish the level that is so loud that it causes discomfort but not pain. The starting level should be around 40 dB HL because some patients have such low ULLs. The level should then be increased first in 5 dB steps and then in 1 dB steps around the ULL. Another approach is to use categorical loudness scaling, which can yield information about ULLs and the dynamic range at the same time, which is useful in hearing aid fittings.

◆ Diplacusis and Pitch Deviation

Some individuals perceive the same tone as being different in pitch in the two ears. Such differing perception is referred to as diplacusis, and it can interfere with music perception (see Chapter 9). Diplacusis can be evaluated and documented using an adaptive procedure by presenting tonal signals alternating to the right and left ears. First, the subject should be requested to match the loudness of a clearly audible tone (e.g., 40 dB SL) presented to one ear to that of the same frequency (e.g., 1000 Hz) tone presented to the other ear. The examiner can vary the loudness in the other ear around 40 dB SL in 1 dB steps to get loudness match. Using the same loudness levels in two ears, the pitch in one ear is kept constant by presenting the same frequency. The frequency in the other ear is then adjusted in 1 Hz steps around 1000 Hz to obtain a pitch match. In the presence of diplacusis, the pitch deviation between the ears can be expressed as a percentage of the reference frequency. For example, if a 1000 Hz tone presented to the right ear is matched to the pitch of a 1025 Hz tone, the pitch deviation is 2.5% (Jansen, Helleman, Dreschler, & de Laat, 2009).

◆ Evaluation of Auditory Processing Skills

Some studies indicate the effects of various metals and solvents on vision, hearing, olfactory function, touch, and taste. Different pathogenic mechanisms may be involved that may act on sensory receptors, nerve fibers, and the central nervous system (Gobba, 2003). More specifically, processing of auditory stimuli can be poor in workers exposed to solvents (Laukli & Hansen, 1995; Morata, Engel, Durão, et al., 1997; Niklasson, Arlinger, Ledin, et al., 1998; Odkvist, Arlinger, Edling, Larsby, & Bergholtz, 1987), even in the presence of auditory sensitivity within normal limits (Fuente & McPherson, 2007). Damage to the central auditory pathways is also possible following noise exposure, as discussed in Chapter 1. In cases where possibility of damage to the central auditory systems is suspected because of patient complaints or exposure to ototoxic substances, an auditory processing test battery is recommended. A matched control group of employees that is not exposed to solvents and/or noise should be included in evaluations. In evaluating individual patients, use of a normative database established in each clinic is recommended.

◆ WorkSafe Australia Guidelines

Employees who are exposed to ototoxins and complain of hearing difficulties but have normal audiometric test results should be referred for evaluation of the central parts of the auditory system (see www.commerce.wa.gov.au/Work-Safe/Content/Safety_Topics/Noise/Further_information/Ototoxin.html).

◆ Recommended Test Battery

Further research will be useful in identifying the type of auditory processing skills that are affected because of exposure to ototoxins including solvents and metals like mercury. In the interim, a recommended battery for evaluating auditory processing skills in the context of occupational exposure to ototoxins is shown in

Fig. 5.14. The test battery should be preceded by a complete audiological evaluation, as described previously, to document any peripheral hearing loss and word recognition difficulties in quiet and noise. The inclusion of tests within the auditory processing test battery in **Fig. 5.14** is based on the following considerations:

- ◆ Ease of administration and interpretation in clinical settings.
- ◆ Evaluation of brainstem and cortical auditory pathways.
- ◆ Evaluation of binaural (dichotic) and temporal auditory processing skills.
- ◆ Minimal effect of hearing loss.
- ◆ Minimal effect of linguistic competency: Individuals with poor linguistic competency may do poorly on tasks involving words or sentences, making it difficult to distinguish auditory processing from linguistic deficits.
- ◆ Minimal effect of cognitive variables including attention: Solvent-exposed workers may have some difficulty in modulating their attentional resources according to task demands, as apparent in similar P300 amplitudes for rare and oddball stimuli (Massioui,

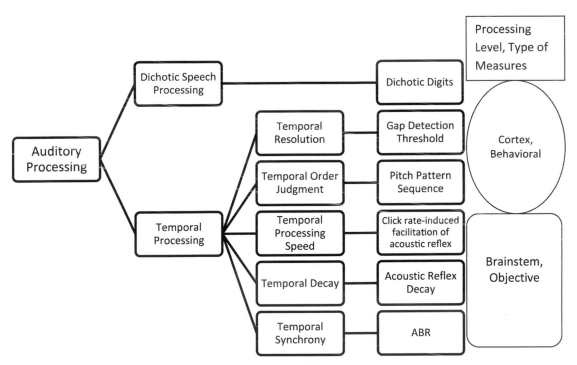

Fig. 5.14 Test battery for evaluation of auditory processing deficits.

Lille, Lesevre, Hazemann, Garnier, & Dally, 1990). Vigilance decrement has also been noted during methylene chloride exposure (Winneke, 1982).

◆ Use of subjective and objective measures: Acute low-level exposure to organic solvents can result in prenarcotic states of depression of the central nervous system (Winneke, 1982). This can negatively affect the ability to perform behavioral tasks. Therefore, some objective measures are included in the test battery.

◆ Control of patient fatigue and learning effects: The recommended tests involve simple behavioral tasks or no response from patients. In addition, the fatigue effects can also be controlled by interspersing objective measures among behavioral measures.

Dichotic Speech Processing

This type of processing involves simultaneous presentation of different stimuli to each ear, and the listener is expected to repeat the stimuli presented to both ears either in a particular order (say the words in the right ear first and then in the left) for a "directed listening" task or without specification of any order for a "free recall" task. The percentage of correctly repeated stimuli is calculated. Chronic solvent exposure can affect dichotic listening skills (Varney, Kubu, & Morrow, 1998). Although various stimuli including consonant-vowels and words can be used for testing dichotic processing skills, the best stimuli for testing in the context of hearing conservation probably are dichotic digits, which are least likely to be affected by hearing loss.

The dichotic digits test is performed by presenting one, two, three, or four digits simultaneously to each ear. The listener is asked to perform directed or free recall. The dichotic digits task with simultaneous presentation of two digits to each ear with free recall is least likely to be influenced by factors such as cognition and linguistic competency. Workers exposed to solvents perform poorly on the free recall dichotic digits task with the presentation of two digits to each ear (Fuente & McPherson, 2007).

Temporal Processing

Temporal processing refers to the processing of stimuli over time. Auditory temporal processing deficits can lead to difficulty in recognizing speech in quiet and noise (reviewed in Rawool, 2007a). Temporal processing skills can be divided into different categories and can be evaluated in a variety of ways using various stimulus configurations (Rawool, 2006a, 2007a). Some of the temporal processing measures are affected by the presence of a hearing loss (Rawool, 2006b).

Temporal Resolution

Temporal resolution refers to the lowest limits of the auditory system to resolve time. One way to measure temporal resolution is to determine the gap detection thresholds. This is the minimum time gap that is necessary to detect the gap between two stimuli. If the time gap is smaller than the gap detection threshold, the two stimuli are perceived as being one (**Fig. 5.15**). Various commercial tests are available for measuring gap detection, including the Random Gap Detection Test (RGDT), the Auditory Fusion Test Revised (AFT-R) test, and Gaps in Noise test. The exact procedures used in administering the tests vary, but all tests can be used to get an estimation of the gap detection thresholds. The AFT-R provides normative data for different age groups, including adults (Rawool, 2007a). Workers exposed to solvents show poorer performance on the RGDT compared with nonexposed individuals (Fuente & McPherson, 2007).

Temporal Order Judgment

Temporal order judgment involves the accurate perception of the sequence of stimuli. Two or three stimuli differing in pitch (e.g., high pitch, low pitch, low pitch) or duration (short, short, long) are presented with sufficient gaps between the stimuli. The patient's task is to accurately state or hum the sequence back. Two tests are available for temporal order judgment, including the Pitch Pattern Sequence (PPS) and Duration Pattern Sequence tests. Workers exposed to solvents show poor performance on the PPS task (Fuente & McPherson, 2007).

Temporal Processing Speed

The speed with which stimuli are processed over time can be referred to as temporal processing speed. Progressive increase of reaction time/speed has been previously noted at toluene exposures of

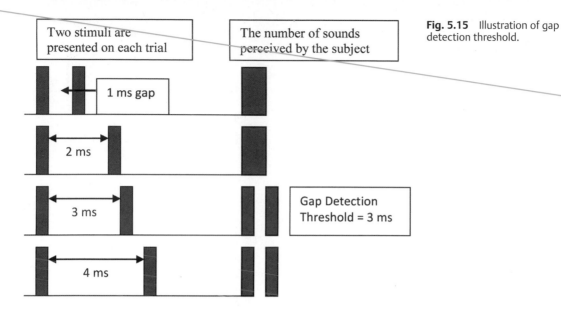

Two stimuli are presented on each trial

The number of sounds perceived by the subject

1 ms gap

2 ms

3 ms

Gap Detection Threshold = 3 ms

4 ms

Fig. 5.15 Illustration of gap detection threshold.

300 ppm for 30 minutes (Winneke, 1982). Thus, it is important to assess auditory processing speed in workers exposed to solvents.

ARTs evoked with clicks presented at faster rates are lower than those elicited with clicks presented at slow rates (Rawool, 1995, 1996a). This improvement in thresholds is shown in **Fig. 5.16**. ARTs obtained with a rate of 200 clicks/s (e.g., 80 dB pressure equivalent

sound pressure level [peSPL]) could be subtracted from those obtained at 50 clicks/s (e.g., 110 dB peSPL). The difference in the two thresholds (20 dB SPL) is the rate-induced facilitation (RIF) of the acoustic reflex. It appears that in the presence of reduced temporal processing speed, some of the clicks presented at higher rates are missed (**Fig. 5.17**), leading to a smaller RIF. Thus, in the presence of slower processing speed, the

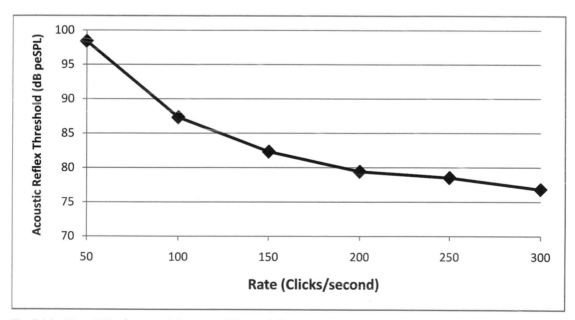

Fig. 5.16 Mean ARTs of young adults across different click rates.

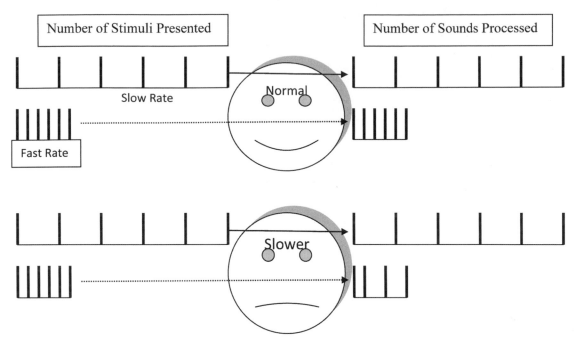

Fig. 5.17   Illustration of slower and faster temporal processing speed.

click RIF of ARTs is reduced (Rawool, 1996b). The click RIF has not been evaluated on individuals with auditory processing difficulties but is more objective than other potential tests of temporal processing speed such as recognition of time-compressed words and is not influenced by linguistic or cognitive factors.

Temporal Response Maintenance (Decay)

Temporal response maintenance can be thought of as the ability of the auditory system to continue to evaluate high-level stimuli without fatigue. This ability can be evaluated using an acoustic reflex decay test, which was described earlier in the nonorganic hearing loss section. Workers who are exposed to solvents can show significant reflex decay suggesting retrocochlear or brainstem pathology (Morata, Engel, Durão, et al., 1997).

Although traditionally reflex decay has been measured over a fixed time frame (10 seconds), it can also be measured using a fixed number of stimuli such as 1000 clicks (Rawool, 1996c). Furthermore, it can be measured at levels that approximate the exposure levels of workers exposed to impulse types of noises. The elicited response patterns (**Fig. 5.18**) may identify workers who are more susceptible to noise or ototoxin exposure.

When the reflex is recorded by presenting 1000 clicks at the rates of 50 or 100/s at 95 or 105 dB HL, the reflex decays in approximately 5 to 10% of the individuals, suggesting increased vulnerability to impulse noises. On the other hand, the reflex amplitude increases over time in approximately 5 to 10% of the individuals, suggesting tough ears. In the remaining subjects, the amplitude either remains steady or fluctuates over time.

Temporal Synchrony

Temporal synchrony can be referred to as the ability of the auditory neurons to simultaneously fire in response to a broadband stimulus. The integrity of the click-evoked ABR (**Fig. 5.13**) relies heavily on the synchronous firings of several auditory neurons. Thus, the previously described technique of ABR can be used as a measure of temporal synchrony. For this purpose, the ABR can be elicited using high-level stimuli such as 70 dB nHL and 80 dB nHL, and absolute and interpeak latencies, amplitudes, and morphology of the waveforms can be analyzed. It is best to record two waveforms at each presentation level using rarefaction and condensation clicks because of differences in resulting waveform morphology across individuals (Rawool, 1998b, 2007b;

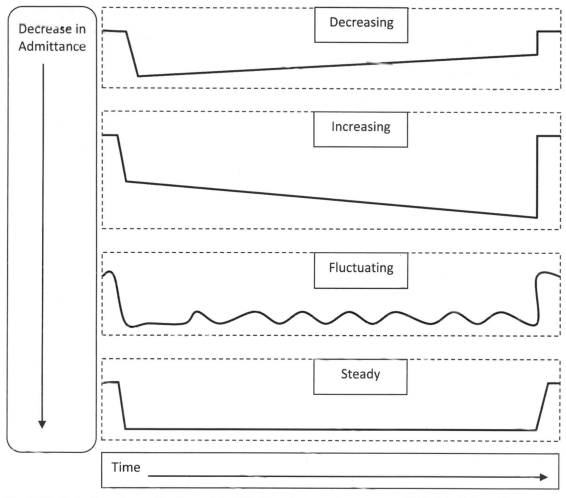

Fig. 5.18 Illustrations of acoustic reflex sustainability (decay) patterns in response to 1000 clicks (Adapted from Rawool, 1996c).

Rawool & Zerlin, 1988). Relatively higher click repetition rates (e.g., 30 clicks/s) that can increase the sensitivity of the ABR (Rawool, 2007b) without compromising the integrity of the waveforms are recommended for evoking the response.

Prolonged latencies and reduced amplitudes of the ABR have been noted previously in individuals exposed to solvents (Abbate, Giorgianni, Munaò, & Brecciaroli, 1993; Hirata, Ogawa, Okayama, & Goto, 1992; Kumar & Tandon, 1997; Nolfe, Palma, Guadagnino, Serra, & Serra, 1991; Vrca, Bozicević, Bozikov, Fuchs, & Malinar, 1997; Vrca, Karacić, Bozicević, Bozikov, & Malinar, 1996). For example, workers exposed to *n*-hexane show prolonged I to V interpeak latencies (Chang, 1987; Huang & Chu, 1989). Prolonged interpeak I to III latencies

have also been noted in some workers who are exposed to mercury and chlorinated hydrocarbons (Moshe, Frenkel, Hager, Skulsky, Sulkis, & Himelfarbe, 2002).

Binaural Interaction

Binaural interaction refers to comparative evaluation and/or fusion of the stimuli presented simultaneously to the two ears at a central auditory level. For example, a stimulus can be presented slightly earlier in time to the right ear compared with that presented to the left ear. The stimulus is perceived as a single or fused image that is lateralized to the right side. The phenomenon of masking level difference (MLD) also involves binaural interaction. In one version of the MLD test, thresholds are first obtained by presenting signals in phase to the two ears in noise that is also in phase (T1). The thresholds are then re-established by either presenting the signals or the noise out of phase at the two ears (T2). The thresholds are better for the condition where the signal or the noise is out of phase at the two ears compared with the condition where both the signal and the noise are in phase. The size of the MLD is determined by the difference between the two thresholds (T1-T2). MLDs appear to be normal in workers exposed to solvents (Fuente, McPherson, Muñoz, & Pablo Espina, 2006), suggesting normal binaural interaction. In future investigations, binaural interaction might be investigated using ABRs (Rawool & Ballachanda, 1990) to confirm the findings obtained using behavioral measures.

Review Questions

1. List the tests that could be included in the test battery used for evaluating an individual with nonorganic pathology. What is the best sequence for administering the tests?
2. Why is it important to not accuse a worker of malingering in the presence of suspected nonorganic pathology?
3. What types of findings on tonal threshold measures suggest the possibility of a nonorganic pathology?
4. Describe the Stenger test procedure for determining auditory thresholds in cases with suspected nonorganic unilateral hearing loss. What precautions are necessary in administering the tests?
5. How can you differentiate between AN and sensory hearing loss based on the results of a test battery?
6. List the tests that could be included in the test battery for evaluating tinnitus. Describe the purpose of each test.
7. How can you determine the severity of the tinnitus?
8. Describe test procedures for determining the loudness and pitch of the tinnitus, MML, and residual inhibition.
9. List the factors that should be considered in devising a test battery for assessing auditory processing disorders in industrial workers who are exposed to solvents.
10. List the tests that could be included in a test battery for assessing auditory processing disorders and the procedures used in administering the tests.

References

Abbate C, Giorgianni C, Munaò F, Brecciaroli R. (1993). Neurotoxicity induced by exposure to toluene. An electrophysiologic study. *Int Arch Occup Environ Health.* 64(6):389–392.

Alberti PW, Hyde ML, Riko K. (1987). Exaggerated hearing loss in compensation claimants. *J Otolaryngol.* 16(6):362–366.

Anari M, Axelsson A, Eliasson A, Magnusson L. (1999). Hypersensitivity to sound—questionnaire data, audiometry and classification. *Scand Audiol.* 28(4):219–230.

Andersson G, Lindvall N, Hursti T, Carlbring P. (2002). Hypersensitivity to sound (hyperacusis): a prevalence study conducted via the Internet and post. *Int J Audiol.* 41(8):545–554.

Aplin DY, Kane JM. (1985). Variables affecting pure tone and speech audiometry in experimentally simulated hearing loss. *Br J Audiol.* 19(3):219–228.

Attias J, Furst M, Furman V, Reshef I, Horowitz G, Bresloff I. (1995). Noise-induced otoacoustic emission loss with or without hearing loss. *Ear Hear.* 16(6):612–618.

Austen S, Lynch C. (2004). Non-organic hearing loss redefined: understanding, categorizing and managing nonorganic behaviour. *Int J Audiol.* 43(8):449–457.

Axelsson A. (1996). How severe is his tinnitus and what is its prognosis? In: Reich G, Vernon G, eds. *Proceedings of the Fifth International Tinnitus Seminar.* Portland, OR: American Tinnitus Association: 363–366.

Balatsouras DG, Kaberos A, Korres S, Kandiloros D, Ferekidis E, Economou C. (2003). Detection of pseudohypacusis: a prospective, randomized study of the use of otoacoustic emissions. *Ear Hear.* 24(6):518–827.

Balatsouras DG, Tsimpiris N, Korres S, Karapantzos I, Papadimitriou N, Danielidis V. (2005). The effect of impulse noise on distortion product otoacoustic emissions. *Int J Audiol.* 44(9):540–549.

Barrs DM, Althoff LK, Krueger WW, Olsson JE. (1994). Work-related, noise-induced hearing loss: evaluation including evoked potential audiometry. *Otolaryngol Head Neck Surg.* 110(2):177–184.

Bhagat SP, Davis AM. (2008). Modification of otoacoustic emissions following ear-level exposure to MP3 player music. *Int J Audiol.* 47(12):751–760.

Chaiklin JB, Ventry IM. (1965a). Introduction and research plan. *J Aud Res.* 3:79–190.

Chaiklin JB, Ventry IM. (1965b). Patient errors during spondee and pure-tone threshold measurement. *J Aud Res*. 5:219–230.

Chang YC. (1987). Neurotoxic effects of n-hexane on the human central nervous system: evoked potential abnormalities in n-hexane polyneuropathy. *J Neurol Neurosurg Psychiatry*. 50(3):269–274.

Coles RRA, Baskill JL. (1996). Absolute loudness of tinnitus: Tinnitus clinic data. In: Reich G, Vernon G, eds. *Proceedings of the Fifth International Tinnitus Seminar*. Portland, OR: American Tinnitus Association: 148–157.

Conn M, Ventry IM, Woods RW. (1972). Pure-tone average and spondee threshold relationship in simulated hearing loss. *J Aud Res*. 12:234–239.

Dorn PA, Piskorski P, Gorga MP, Neely ST, Keefe DH. (1999). Predicting audiometric status from distortion product otoacoustic emissions using multivariate analyses. *Ear Hear*. 20(2):149–163.

Durmaz A, Karahatay S, Satar B, Birkent H, Hidir Y. (2009). Efficiency of Stenger test in confirming profound, unilateral pseudohypacusis. *J Laryngol Otol*. 123(8):840–844.

Fuente A, McPherson B. (2007). Central auditory processing effects induced by solvent exposure. *Int J Occup Med Environ Health*. 20(3):271–279.

Fuente A, McPherson B, Muñoz V, Pablo Espina J. (2006). Assessment of central auditory processing in a group of workers exposed to solvents. *Acta Otolaryngol*. 126(11): 1188–1194.

Gaskill SA, Brown AM. (1990). The behavior of the acoustic distortion product, 2f1-f2, from the human ear and its relation to auditory sensitivity. *J Acoust Soc Am*. 88(2):821–839.

Gelfand SA. (1984). The contralateral acoustic reflex threshold. In: Silman S, ed. *The Acoustic Reflex: Basic Principles and Clinical Applications*. Orlando, FL: Academic Press: 137–186.

Gelfand SA. (2001a). Acoustic immittance assessment. In: Gelfand SA, ed. *Essentials of Audiology* (2nd ed.). New York: Thieme: 421–442.

Gelfand SA. (2001b). Nonorganic hearing loss. In: Gelfand SA, ed. *Essentials of Audiology* (2nd ed.). New York: Thieme: 219–255.

Gelfand SA, Silman S. (1985). Functional components and resolved thresholds in patients with unilateral non-organic hearing loss. *Ear Hear*. 6:151–158.

Gelfand SA, Silman S. (1993). Functional components and resolved thresholds in patients with unilateral nonorganic hearing loss. *Br J Audiol*. 27(1):29–34.

Gobba F. (2003). Occupational exposure to chemicals and sensory organs: a neglected research field. *Neurotoxicology*. 24(4-5):675–691.

Gold SR, Hunsaker DH, Haseman EM. (1991). Pseudohypacusis in a military population. *Ear Nose Throat J*. 70(10):710–712.

Gorga MP, Neely ST, Dorn PA. (1999). Distortion product otoacoustic emission test performance for a priori criteria and for multifrequency audiometric standards. *Ear Hear*. 20(4):345–362.

Gorga MP, Neely ST, Ohlrich B, Hoover B, Redner J, Peters J. (1997). From laboratory to clinic: a large scale study of distortion product otoacoustic emissions in ears with normal hearing and ears with hearing loss. *Ear Hear*. 18(6):440–455.

Gosztonyi RE Jr, Vassallo LA, Sataloff J. (1971). Audiometric reliability in industry. *Arch Environ Health*. 22(1): 113–118.

Hallam RS. (1996). *Manual of the Tinnitus Questionnaire (TQ)*. London: Psychological Corporation.

Helleman HW, Jansen EJM, Dreschler WA. (2010). Otoacoustic emissions in a hearing conservation program: general applicability in longitudinal monitoring and the relation to changes in pure-tone thresholds. *Int J Audiol*. 49(6):410–419.

Herdman AT, Stapells DK. (2003). Auditory steady-state response thresholds of adults with sensorineural hearing impairments. *Int J Audiol*. 42(5):237–248.

Hiller W, Goebel G. (2004). Rapid assessment of tinnitus-related psychological distress using the Mini-TQ. *Int J Audiol*. 43(10):600–604.

Hirata M, Ogawa Y, Okayama A, Goto S. (1992). A cross-sectional study on the brainstem auditory evoked potential among workers exposed to carbon disulfide. *Int Arch Occup Environ Health*. 64(5):321–324.

Huang CC, Chu NS. (1989). Evoked potentials in chronic n-hexane intoxication. *Clin Electroencephalogr*. 20(3): 162–168.

Jahner JA, Schlauch RA, Doyle T. (1994). A comparison of American Speech-Language Hearing Association guidelines for obtaining speech-recognition thresholds. *Ear Hear*. 15(4):324–329.

Jansen EJM, Helleman HW, Dreschler WA, de Laat JA. (2009). Noise induced hearing loss and other hearing complaints among musicians of symphony orchestras. *Int Arch Occup Environ Health*. 82(2):153–164.

Job A, Raynal M, Kossowski M, et al. (2009). Otoacoustic detection of risk of early hearing loss in ears with normal audiograms: a 3-year follow-up study. *Hear Res*. 251(1-2):10–16.

Johnson KO, Work WP, McCoy G. (1956). Functional deafness. *Ann Otol Rhinol Laryngol*. 65(1):154–170.

Kam AC, Cheung AP, Chan PY, et al. (2009). Psychometric properties of a Chinese (Cantonese) version of the Tinnitus Questionnaire. *Int J Audiol*. 48(8):568–575.

Kinstler DB, Phelan JG, Lavender RW. (1972). Efficiency of the Stenger test in identification of functional hearing loss. *J Aud Res*. 10:118–123.

Kuk FK, Tyler RS, Russell D, Jordan H. (1990). The psychometric properties of a tinnitus handicap questionnaire. *Ear Hear*. 11(6):434–445.

Kumar V, Tandon OP. (1997). Neurotoxic effects of rubber factory environment. An auditory evoked potential study. *Electromyogr Clin Neurophysiol*. 37(8):469–473.

Kvaerner KJ, Engdahl B, Aursnes J, Arnesen AR, Mair IW. (1996). Transient-evoked otoacoustic emissions. Helpful tool in the detection of pseudohypacusis. *Scand Audiol*. 25(3):173–177.

Lapsley Miller JA, Marshall L, Heller LM, Hughes LM. (2006). Low-level otoacoustic emissions may predict susceptibility to noise-induced hearing loss. *J Acoust Soc Am*. 120(1):280–296.

Laukli E, Hansen PW. (1995). An audiometric test battery for the evaluation of occupational exposure to industrial solvents. *Acta Otolaryngol*. 115(2):162–164.

Lim JJ, Lu PK, Koh DS, Eng SP. (2010). Impact of tinnitus as measured by the Tinnitus Handicap Inventory among tinnitus sufferers in Singapore. *Singapore Med J*. 51(7):551–557.

Lin YH, Ho HC, Wu HP. (2009). Comparison of auditory steady-state responses and auditory brainstem responses in audiometric assessment of adults with sensorineural hearing loss. *Auris Nasus Larynx*. 36(2):140–145.

Lin J, Staecker H. (2006). Nonorganic hearing loss. *Sem Neurol*. 26(3):321–330.

Lins OG, Picton TW. (1995). Auditory steady-state responses to multiple simultaneous stimuli. *Electroencephalogr Clin Neurophysiol*. 96(5):420–432.

Long GR, Talmadge CL, Lee J. (2008). Measuring distortion product otoacoustic emissions using continuously sweeping primaries. *J Acoust Soc Am.* 124(3):1613–1626.

Lonsbury-Martin BL, Martin GK. (1990). The clinical utility of distortion-product otoacoustic emissions. *Ear Hear.* 11(2):144–154.

Lutman ME, Qusem HYN. (1997). A source of audiometric notches at 6 kHz. In: Prasher D, Luxon LM, eds. *Advances in Noise Research Series. Vol. 1.* London: Whurr: 170–176.

Mahdavi ME, Mokari N, Amiri Z. (2011). Educational level and pseudohypacusis in medico-legal compensation claims: a retrospective study. *Arch Iran Med.* 14(1):58–60.

Marriage J, Barnes NM. (1995). Is central hyperacusis a symptom of 5-hydroxytryptamine (5-HT) dysfunction? *J Laryngol Otol.* 109(10):915–921.

Marshall L, Lapsley Miller JA, Heller LM, et al. (2009). Detecting incipient inner-ear damage from impulse noise with otoacoustic emissions. *J Acoust Soc Am.* 125(2):995–1013.

Martin FN, Champlin CA, McCreery TM. (2001). Strategies used in feigning hearing loss. *J Am Acad Audiol.* 12(2): 59–63.

Martin FN, Shipp DB. (1982). The effects of sophistication on three threshold tests for subjects with simulated hearing loss. *Ear Hear.* 3(1):34–36.

Massioui FE, Lille F, Lesevre N, Hazemann P, Garnier R, Dally S. (1990). Sensory and cognitive event related potentials in workers chronically exposed to solvents. *J Toxicol Clin Toxicol.* 28(2):203–219.

Mauermann M, Uppenkamp S, van Hengel PW, Kollmeier B. (1999). Evidence for the distortion product frequency place as a source of distortion product otoacoustic emission (DPOAE) fine structure in humans. II. Fine structure for different shapes of cochlear hearing loss. *J Acoust Soc Am.* 106(6):3484–3491.

Miller MH, Crane MA, Fox J, Linstrom C. (1998). Pseudohypoacusis: Worker compensation costs and professional implications. *Hear J.* 52(4):42–46.

Monro DA, Martin FN. (1977. Effects of sophistication on four tests for nonorganic hearing loss. *J Speech Hear Disord.* 42(4):528–534.

Morata TC, Engel T, Durão A, et al. (1997). Hearing loss from combined exposures among petroleum refinery workers. *Scand Audiol.* 26(3):141–149.

Moshe S, Frenkel A, Hager M, Skulsky M, Sulkis J, Himelfarbe M. (2002). Effects of occupational exposure to mercury or chlorinated hydrocarbons on the auditory pathway. *Noise & Health, 4*(16), 71–77.

Newman CW, Jacobson GP, Spitzer JB. (1996). Development of the Tinnitus Handicap Inventory. *Arch Otolaryngol Head Neck Surg.* 122(2):143–148.

Newman CW, Sandridge SA, Jacobson GP. (1998). Psychometric adequacy of the Tinnitus Handicap Inventory (THI) for evaluating treatment outcome. *J Am Acad Audiol.* 9(2):153–160.

Niklasson M, Arlinger S, Ledin T, et al. (1998). Audiological disturbances caused by long-term exposure to industrial solvents. Relation to the diagnosis of toxic encephalopathy. *Scand Audiol.* 27(3):131–136.

Nolfe G, Palma V, Guadagnino M, Serra LL, Serra C. (1991). Evoked potentials in shoe-workers with minimal polyneuropathy. *Electromyogr Clin Neurophysiol.* 31(3):157–162.

Odkvist LM, Arlinger SD, Edling C, Larsby B, Bergholtz LM. (1987). Audiological and vestibulo-oculomotor findings in workers exposed to solvents and jet fuel. *Scand Audiol.* 16(2):75–81.

Prasher D, Sułkowski W. (1999). The role of otoacoustic emissions in screening and evaluation of noise damage. *Int J Occup Med Environ Health.* 12(2):183–192.

Qiu WW, Yin SS, Stucker FJ, Welsh LW. (1998). Current evaluation of pseudohypacusis: strategies and classification. *Ann Otol Rhinol Laryngol.* 107(8):638–647.

Rabinowitz PM, Dobie RA. (2003). Use of the audiometric configuration to determine whether hearing loss is noise-induced: Can notch criteria help? *Spectrum (Lexington, Ky.).* 20(1):8–11.

Rawool VW. (1995). Ipsilateral acoustic reflex thresholds at varying click rates in humans. *Scand Audiol.* 24(3):199–205.

Rawool VW. (1996a). Click-rate induced facilitation of the acoustic reflex using constant number of pulses. *Audiology.* 35(4):171–179.

Rawool VW. (1996b). Effect of aging on the click-rate induced facilitation of acoustic reflex thresholds. *J Gerontol A Biol Sci Med Sci.* 51(2):B124–B131.

Rawool VW. (1996c). Acoustic reflex monitoring during the presentation of 1000 clicks at high repetition rates. *Scand Audiol.* 25(4):239–245.

Rawool VW. (1998a). Effect of probe frequency and gender on click-evoked ipsilateral acoustic reflex thresholds. *Acta Otolaryngol.* 118(3):307–312.

Rawool VW. (1998b). Effects of click polarity on the brainstem auditory evoked potentials of older men. *Audiology.* 37(2):100–108.

Rawool VW. (2006a). A temporal processing primer. Part 1. Defining key concepts in temporal processing. *Hear Review.* 13(5):30–34.

Rawool VW. (2006b). The effects of hearing loss on temporal processing. Part 2: Looking beyond simple audition. *Hear Review.* 13(6):30, 32, 34.

Rawool VW. (2007a). Temporal processing in the auditory system. In: Geffner D, Ross-Swain D, eds. *Auditory Processing Disorders: Assessment, Management and Treatment.* San Diego, CA: Plural Publishing: 117–137.

Rawool VW. (2007b). The aging auditory system, Part 1: Controversy and confusion on slower processing. *Hear Review.* 14(7):14–19.

Rawool VW, Ballachanda BB. (1990). Homo- and anti-phasic stimulation in ABR. *Scand Audiol.* 19(1):9–15.

Rawool VW, Zerlin S. (1988). Phase-intensity effects on the ABR. *Scand Audiol.* 17(2):117–123.

Rickards FW, De Vidi S. (1995). Exaggerated hearing loss in noise induced hearing loss compensation claims in Victoria. *Med J Aust.* 163(7):360–363. PubMed

Rintelmann WF, Schwan SA. (1999). Pseudohypacusis. In: Musiek FE, Rintelmann WF, eds. *Contemporary Perspectives in Hearing Assessment.* Boston: Allyn and Bacon: 415–435.

Sammeth CA, Preves DA, Brandy WT. (2000). Hyperacusis: case studies and evaluation of electronic loudness suppression devices as a treatment approach. *Scand Audiol.* 29(1):28–36.

Schechter MA, Henry JA. (2002). Assessment and treatment of tinnitus patients using a "masking approach." *J Am Acad Audiol.* 13(10):545–558.

Schlauch RS, Arnce KD, Olson LM, Sanchez S, Doyle TN. (1996). Identification of pseudohypacusis using speech recognition thresholds. *Ear Hear.* 17(3):229–236.

Shaffer LA, Withnell RH, Dhar S, Lilly DJ, Goodman SS, Harmon KM. (2003). Sources and mechanisms of DPOAE generation: implications for the prediction of auditory sensitivity. *Ear Hear.* 24(5):367–379.

Silman S, Silverman CA. (1991). *Auditory Diagnoses: Principles and Applications.* San Diego: Academic Press.

Snow JB Jr. (2006). Strategies of the Tinnitus Research Consortium. *Acta Otolaryngol. Suppl.* 556(556):89–92.

Stapells DR (2000). Threshold estimation by the tone evoked auditory brainstem response: A literature meta-analysis. *J Speech-Language Pathol Audiol.* 24(2):74–83.

Talmadge CL, Long GR, Tubis A, Dhar S. (1999). Experimental confirmation of the two-source interference model for the fine structure of distortion product otoacoustic emissions. *J Acoust Soc Am.* 105(1):275–292.

Torre P III, Cruickshanks KJ, Nondahl DM, Wiley TL. (2003). Distortion product otoacoustic emission response characteristics in older adults. *Ear Hear.* 24(1):20–29.

Van Maanen A, Stapells DR. (2005). Comparison of multiple auditory steady-state responses (80 versus 40 Hz) and slow cortical potentials for threshold estimation in hearing-impaired adults. *Int J Audiol.* 44(11):613–624.

Varney NR, Kubu CS, Morrow LA. (1998). Dichotic listening performances of patients with chronic exposure to organic solvents. *Clin Neuropsychologist.* 12:107–112.

Ventry, IM, Chaiklin, JB. (1965). Patient errors during spondee and pure-tone threshold measurement. *J Auditory Res.* 3:219–230.

Vernon J, Fenwick J. (1984). Identification of tinnitus: A plea for standardization. In Proceedings of the II International Tinnitus Seminar New York, 10 and 11 June 1983. *J Laryngol Otol Suppl.* 9:45–53.

Vrca A, Bozicević D, Bozikov V, Fuchs R, Malinar M. (1997). Brain stem evoked potentials and visual evoked potentials in relation to the length of occupational exposure to low levels of toluene. *Acta Medica Croatica.* 51(4-5):215–219.

Vrca A, Karacić V, Bozicević D, Bozikov V, Malinar M. (1996, Jul). Brainstem auditory evoked potentials in individuals exposed to long-term low concentrations of toluene. *Am J Ind Med.* 30(1):62–66.

Winneke G. (1982). Acute behavioral effects of exposure to some organic solvents -psychophysiological aspects. *Acta Neurol Scand Suppl.* 92:117–129.

Wolf M, Birger M, Ben Shoshan J, & Kronenberg J. (1993). Conversion deafness. *Ann Otol Rhinol Laryngol.* 102(5):349–352.

Chapter 6

Hearing Protection and Enhancement Devices

Although controlling noise at the source is the best strategy for protecting hearing, in some settings it is difficult to control noise levels (e.g., combat situations). Under such circumstances, hearing protection devices (HPDs), which are designed to reduce the noise level reaching the eardrum, can minimize the possibility of hearing loss. Use of earplugs can also reduce other effects of noise, including tinnitus, hyperacusis, annoyance, irritability, hypertension, etc. For example, earplugs may facilitate weight gains in very-low-birth-weight newborns in neonatal intensive care units (Abou Turk, Williams, & Lasky, 2009). Also, in the presence of high noise levels, use of HPDs is required by regulations. The U.S. Environmental Protection Agency (EPA; 2009) estimates the current legal hearing protector market to be approximately 4 billion units annually, comprising approximately 2.1 billion units sold to industrial users and 1.9 billion units sold to military and commercial users.

◆ Applicable Regulations/Standards

Occupational Health and Safety Administration (1983; 29 CFR 1910.95)

The Occupational Safety and Health Administration (OSHA) requires the use of HPDs when the noise exposure levels are equal to or above 8-hour time weighted average (TWA) of 90 dBA. The use of HPDs is recommended when the noise exposure levels are at or above 85 dBA TWA. The attenuation provided by HPDs must be sufficient to lower exposure levels to at least 90 dBA TWA; in the case of a worker with a standard threshold shift (see Chapter 4), the attenuation should be

sufficient to lower the levels to at least 85 dBA TWA.

Mine Safety and Health Administration (1999; 30 CFR Part 62)

These regulations are similar to OSHA except that when exposures exceed a TWA of 105 dBA, simultaneous use of both earplugs and earmuffs is required.

U.S. Department of Defense (2004; Instruction 6055.12, Hearing Conservation Program, March 5, 2004)

HPDs should be provided to all employees who are exposed to hazardous noise due to the use of noisy equipment or duties in noisy areas. Use of HPDs is required in the presence of hazardous noise regardless of exposure time. The HPDs must attenuate noise exposure below a TWA of 85 dBA. For exposures in the range of 108 to 118 dBA, both earplugs and earmuffs should be used. For exposures greater than 118 dBA, in addition to using both earplugs and earmuffs, exposure time should be limited (U.S. Department of Defense [DoD] form 2214, Jan 2000).

U.S. Navy and Marine Corps Public Health Center (2008; TM 6260.51.99–2)

Individuals exposed to sound levels of 85 dBA or above or 140 dB peak or above should wear HPDs regardless of duration of exposure. Lack of compliance with the mandatory and appropriate use of HPDs in noise-hazardous areas can lead to administrative or disciplinary action. In the presence of significant hearing loss, impulse/impact noise exposures above 165 dBP, TWAs above 104 dB(A), fitness for-duty evaluations, and duties in communication-critical situations, audiological consultation is recommended for selecting appropriate HPDs.

European Commission Directive 2003/10/EC (European Parliament and Council, 2003)

Use of HPDs is required at $L_{EX,8h}$ 85 dBA and/or peak levels of 137 dBC (140 Pa).

American National Standard for Construction Workers (American National Standards Institute/American Society of Safety Engineers, 2007; A10.46)

Instead of using noise exposure criteria or TWA for HPD use, a task-based method is recommended for HPD use. Construction and demolition workers should be required to use HPDs whenever they are performing tasks that cause noise exposure levels in excess of 85 dBA, regardless of the duration of the task. This eliminates the need for measuring noise exposure levels over the entire work shift. A sound level meter can be used to identify tasks that generate levels above 85 dBA, and signs can be posted near these tasks to remind workers to use HPDs.

◆ Classification of Hearing Protection Devices

A variety of HPDs are available for use in occupational and nonoccupational settings. The HPDs can be classified based on various characteristics, as shown in **Fig. 6.1**.

Physical Styles

HPDs are available in various physical styles including earplugs, semi-inserts, earclips, earmuffs, helmets, and earphones.

Earplugs

When inserted properly, earplugs are designed to fit inside the ear canal. A variety of materials are used in making earplugs, including vinyl, nylon, silicone, elastomeric formulations, slow recovery closed cell foam, spun fiberglass, and cotton wax. Some earplugs such as Joe's Ear Plugs® (Ashland, OR) are made of a combination of different materials such as pure beeswax, lanolin, and soft cotton.

Earplugs can be formable, thus allowing them to take the form of an individual ear canal (**Fig. 6.2**). They can also be preformed or premolded with a specific shape (**Fig. 6.3**) and often have a push-to-fit design, making it unnecessary to roll down the foam. This reduces any hand-to-foam contamination. One of the most commonly used earplugs are the roll-down foam earplugs (**Fig. 6.4**), which are made from slow recovery foam and can expand after insertion in the ear canal, thus allowing a tight seal.

Earplugs can also be custom made following ear impressions. For example, Phonak Communications AG (Murten, Switzerland) provides the serenity classic earplug, which is made from machine washable (up to 60°C) clinical nylon eShells. The eShells are very light and are linked by a silicone cord. Other serenity protection systems feature open eShells into which an earJack is fitted that includes either an acoustic or electronic filter (**Fig. 6.5**).

Semi-insert Device (Canal Cap)

This is an earplug-like HPD consisting of a soft pod or tip that is held in place by a lightweight band (**Fig. 6.6**). The pods are positioned in the conchae covering the entrances to the ear canals or are fitted to varying depths within the ear canals. Semi-inserts that cap the canal require the force of the band to retain their position and acoustic seal. Semi-inserts that enter the canal behave more like earplugs; they seal the ear to block noise with or without the application of band force.

Ear Clips

This is also an earplug-like HPD consisting of an ear clip chassis and replaceable foam pad (**Fig. 6.7**) that fits within the ear to block unwanted noise without intruding into the ear canal. The ear clip is lightweight and is designed to stay secured without relying on high-pressure bands or pressure inside the ear canal. The no-roll soft ear pads are designed to conform to the ear canal opening

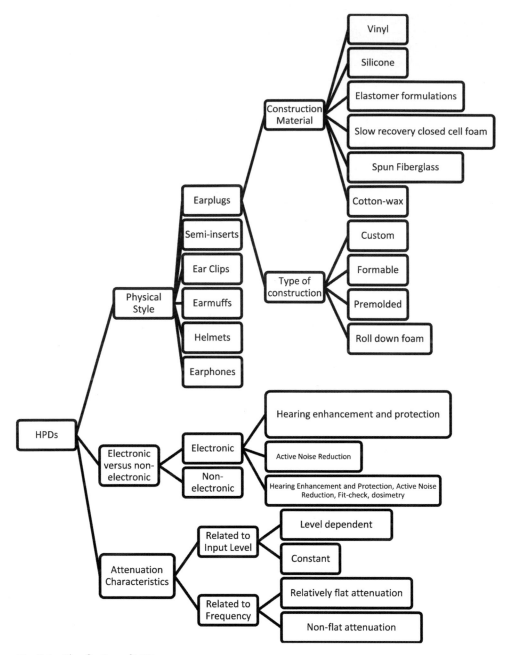

Fig. 6.1 Classfication of HPDs.

and concha. Individuals with sensitive ear canals might prefer the ear clips over earplugs.

Earmuff

This HPD is usually comprises a band that applies springlike force/pressure to two ear cups with soft cushions that seal against the external ear or pinna (supra-aural) or the sides of the head around the pinna (circumaural). The band can be designed for placement on the head, under the chin, or coupled to another piece of head gear. Some earmuffs are equipped with multiple position headbands. The ear cups may also be

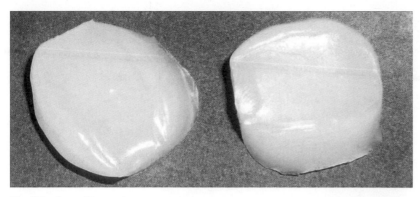

Fig. 6.2 Formable earplugs.

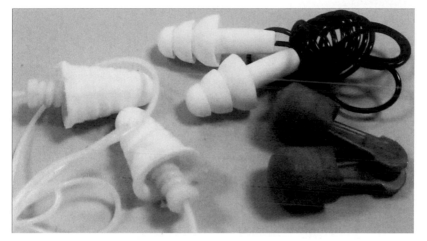

Fig. 6.3 Preformed or premolded earplugs.

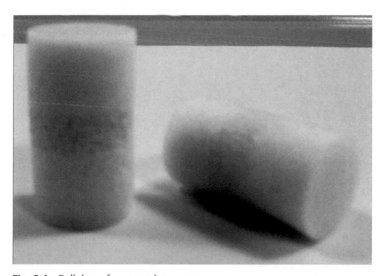

Fig. 6.4 Roll-down foam earplugs.

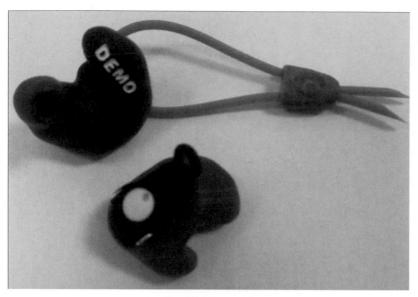

Fig. 6.5   Custom-made earplugs from Phonak Communications, AG.

held in position by attachment arms mounted on a hardhat or hardcap. The earcups are lined with sound-absorbing materials, usually foam, to absorb sound energy and to reduce reverberation within the cup.

One disadvantage of ordinary ear muffs during intense (190 dB sound pressure level [SPL], which is similar to high-level military exposures) blast exposure is that they tend to lift off the ear (Johnson & Patterson, 1992) when exposed to an improvised explosive device's shockwave, thus breaking the seal of the earmuff against the side of the head. This leads to exposure to both the hazardous noise and the shockwave. Another disadvantage of earmuffs is that localization of external sound sources is difficult. Removal of pinna cues for localization because of the position of the earmuffs cannot necessarily be offset by including dichotic cues.

Helmet

This type of HPD provides impact protection to the head or skull and is designed to also reduce

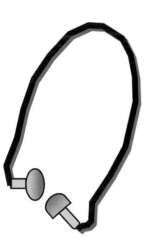
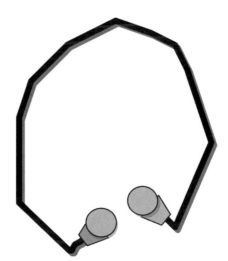

Fig. 6.6   Semi-insert devices.

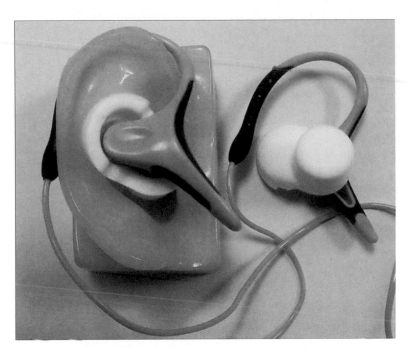

Fig. 6.7 Earclips.

the external sound through either structural elements and/or electronic means. Two-way communication systems can also be incorporated into helmets.

Earphones

Earphone-style HPDs are coupled to custom-made earphones and often incorporate electronic circuitry to control noise levels. Musicians often use these types of devices to allow good audibility during performance while reducing risk of hearing loss.

Electronic versus Nonelectronic

HPDs can also be classified based on the use of electronic and/or nonelectronic (structural) elements to reduce the sound reaching the eardrum.

Electronic or Active Hearing Protection Devices

Electronic manipulation of incoming sound is incorporated in some HPDs. These devices contain electronic components including microphones, circuitry to manipulate the incoming signal, and receivers. Electronic HPDs require the use of a battery and are more expensive.

Nonelectronic or Passive Hearing Protection Devices

This is a device that relies solely on its structural elements to block or otherwise control the transmission of sound into the ear canal; it does not use electronic circuits or acoustic elements to reduce the entry of external sound. These types of devices are less expensive, do not require batteries, and are widely used.

Electronic and Nonelectronic Hearing Protection Devices

Some devices use a combination of electronic and structural elements to reduce the sound transmitted to the ear canal through acoustic cancellation of the air-conducted and/or bone-conducted external sound and can also be referred to as active noise reduction HPDs.

Attenuation Characteristics Related to Input Level

HPDs can also be classified based on how the signal is attenuated by the HPDs. Most HPDs provide the same attenuation of noise level regardless of the input level. However, some HPDs are designed to produce a change in sound attenuation

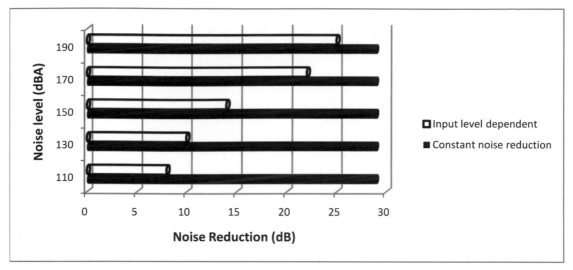

Fig. 6.8   Noise reduction provided by linear and input level–dependent HPDs.

as a function of the external sound level (**Fig. 6.8**) and can be referred to as amplitude-sensitive or input level–dependent HPDs. The change can be achieved using either electronic elements (compression) and/or nonelectronic elements.

Input level–dependent devices manipulate the loudness of sounds reaching the eardrum in such a way that soft sounds that are inaudible or are difficult to hear are amplified up to a specified safe level. Sounds that exceed these specified loudness levels are not amplified. Easily audible sounds that are nonhazardous are neither amplified nor attenuated. Hazardous sounds are attenuated. More specifically, the electronic (compression) circuit of the protector is set in such a way that the maximum loudness level that the worker is exposed to is limited to a safe level regardless of the loudness of the noise in the environment. An advantage of these protectors is that during quiet time and intermittent noise, there is no need to remove the hearing protector to hear well.

For example, the EB15 Electronic BlastPLG™ (Etymotic Research, Inc., Elk Groove Village, IL) earplugs provide gain or natural hearing for soft- and moderate-level sounds but provide attenuation at high-input levels (**Fig. 6.9**). Such devices can be useful for workers who work in noisy environments (Killion, Monroe, & Drambarean, 2011). Another example is the Combat Arms Earplugs (Aearo Technologies, Indianapolis, IN). In this earplug, the impacting sound is fed through

a filter by orifices at both sides. The small diameter of these orifices hampers the passage of sound levels above 110 dB SPL because of an increase in impedance with increase in the velocity of particles above such high levels.

Attenuation Characteristics Related to Frequency Response

Many commonly used HPDs provide more attenuation in the higher frequencies (nonflat or frequency-dependent attenuation). However, some devices such as those useful for musicians attempt to provide relatively equal or flat attenuation across the frequencies (**Fig. 6.10**). HPDs for musicians are discussed in greater detail in Chapter 9. Another example of relatively flat and nonflat attenuation is shown in **Fig. 6.11** for the two settings of the single-sided Combat Arms Earplugs (**Fig. 6.12**). At frequencies above the human hearing range (20 kHz), both earplugs and earmuffs can provide 30 dB or more attenuation (Behar & Crabtree, 1997).

Although infrasound (low-frequency sounds below the human hearing range) exposure can cause hearing loss at levels above 140 dB SPL, changes in blood pressure, respiratory rate, and balance can occur above 110 dB SPL. More specifically, infrasounds ranging in 95 to 125 dB SPL can cause increase in diastolic blood pressure and a decrease in systolic blood pressure and pulse rate in young healthy men, suggesting the

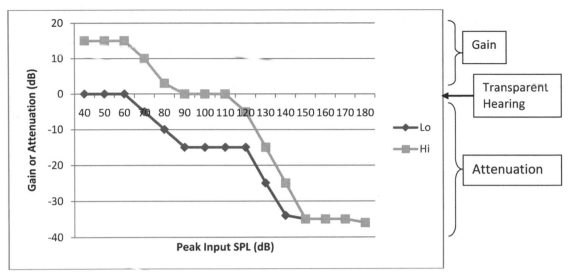

Fig. 6.9 Estimated gain, transparent hearing, and attenuation provided by the EB15 Electronic BlastPLG™ EB15 Electronic BlastPLG™ at Lo and Hi settings. The graph is based on data published by the manufacturer and Killion, Monroe, and Drambarean (2011).

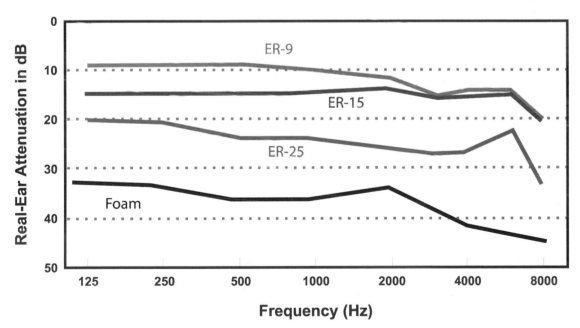

Fig. 6.10 Attenuation characteristics of the ER plugs (© Etymotic Research Inc. Used with permission).

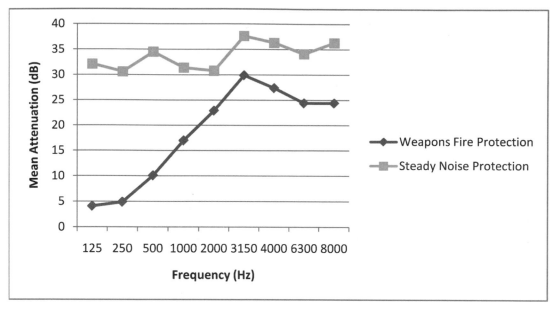

Fig. 6.11 Example of relatively flat and nonflat attenuation characteristics.

possibility of peripheral vasoconstriction with increased blood pressure (Danielsson & Landström, 1985). With 5 to 10 Hz infrasounds of 100 and 135 dB SPL, men can experience fatigue, apathy, and depression; pressure in the ears; loss of concentration; drowsiness; and vibration of internal organs (Karpova, Alekseev, Erokhin, Kadyskina, & Reutov, 1970; Slarve & Johnson, 1975). Even experienced U.S. Air Force officers report chest wall vibration when exposed to infrasounds (Mohr, Cole, Guild, & Vongierke, 1965).

Pääkkönen and Tikkanen (1991) evaluated the ability of earmuffs, helmets, and a prototype of a new noise helmet to attenuate low-frequency (4 to 250 Hz) noise. The noise levels inside the

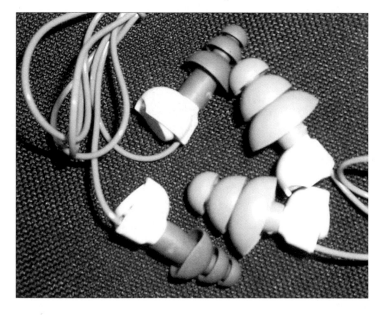

Fig. 6.12 Combat Arms Earplugs.

hearing protector at some frequencies were higher after the placement of the HPD, probably from a combination of the occlusion effect and physiological noise. The earmuffs attenuated noise levels by 1 to 20 dB in the 4 to 250 Hz frequency range. Commercial noise helmets provided less attenuation. New noise helmet prototypes attenuated low-frequency noise better than did earmuffs or commercial helmets (attenuation 5 to 39 dB).

In general, current HPDs do not appear to offer adequate protection against infrasounds. There is a need to devise active noise reduction devices capable of generating out-of-phase infrasounds to cancel incoming sounds and to evaluate their effectiveness. Other forms of protective gear should also be devised to offer better protection against other effects of infrasounds, including whole-body vibration, which can increase the noise reaching the cochlea, especially when the ear canals are partially occluded with HPDs.

Active Noise Reduction

Active noise reduction (ANR) is usually achieved via the use of electronic circuits that analyze the incoming sound, detect the main acoustic component in the sound, and generate a 180-degree out-of-phase signal that is played in the space under the protector. This signal, in theory, cancels the incoming signal. An error correction microphone is utilized to detect any remaining noise, and control parameters are adjusted to maximize the attenuation. ANR can be achieved using either digital or analog circuits and is available within earplugs and earmuffs. ANR is most effective for components below 900 Hz (Nixon, McKinley, & Steuver, 1992).

Communication Headset

This is a voice communication device (earplug, earmuff, semi-insert device, or helmet) that is designed also to reduce the level of sound at the users' ears by either structural elements and/or electronic means. These devices usually incorporate wireless (FM, infrared, or Bluetooth) or wired technology and associated electronic circuitry and signal processing for one- or two-way communication. Signal processing can include suppression of environmental noise. Some of the devices use specialized electronic circuits to limit the incoming sounds so that the earphones

themselves do not create sound levels that are hazardous to the wearer.

Hearing Enhancement Protection Systems

Hearing enhancement protection systems (HEPSs) are designed to provide hearing protection while at the same time providing ease of communication. For example, the communication enhancement protection system (CEPS), available from Communication and Ear Protection (Enterprise, AL; www.cep-usa.com), is compatible with existing equipment and is designed to protect soldiers from steady-state and impulse noise while maintaining the ability to identify enemy forces and to communicate effectively in noise. Sound levels can be adjusted so that they are audible but not hazardous. Microphones are placed at or near each ear, and sounds are processed separately to maintain the fidelity of the sounds. The CEPS is coupled with expanding foam earplugs that reduce hazardous noise and allow transmission of essential sounds.

Combined Fit-Check, Active Noise Reduction, Hearing Enhancement, Hearing Protection, Radio Communication, and Noise Dosimeter System

Some systems such as the QuietPro (Statoil ASA, Stavenger, Norway) are designed to perform several key elements of the hearing conservation program, including the following:

- Check if the fit of the HPD is adequate and provide an alerting signal for inaccurate fit.
- Actively reduce noise in the presence of significant low-frequency components.
- Provide hearing enhancement for soft, critical sounds through a selectable whisper mode. Provide the user the ability to lower ambient sounds in high-noise environments to reduce stress or to ensure rest.
- Attenuate high-noise levels.
- Allow radio communication without the use of a boom microphone. A microphone inside the earplug picks up speech signals through the skull, eliminating the need for a microphone in front of the user's mouth as well as associated background noise.
- Measure protected and unprotected noise exposure levels and provide an alerting signal

when protected noise exposure exceeds hazardous noise levels.

The system has a microphone outside the earplug for picking up ambient sounds that are digitally processed to filter out loud noises and are then sent to the speaker inside the earplug.

Effectiveness of Hearing Enhancement Protection Systems in Noisy, Hearing Critical Jobs

Casali, Ahroon, and Lancaster (2009) conducted a study to evaluate the operational performance of three different devices. Two of these were electronic HEPSs, including an ambient sound pass-through filtering and amplification circuit: a Peltor Comtac II (Aearo Technologies, Indianapolis, IN) circumaural headset (noise reduction rating [NRR] = 21; 16 dB maximum gain) and a CEPS (NRR = 29; 36 dB maximum gain). The third device was the Combat Arms Earplug with insertion to allow level-dependent attenuation, which begins around 110 dB (e.g., due to a gunshot) and increases with higher levels. It has an NRR of zero below such levels. Participants were U.S. Army Reserve Officers' Training Corps cadet soldiers. Their operational performance was evaluated in two training missions: reconnaissance of an enemy camp without full engagement and raid of an enemy camp with full engagement. In the raiding training mission, the CEPS allowed detection of auditory stimuli from 400 feet, followed by the Peltor from 233 feet. For the Combat Arms Earplug, the needed distance was 150 feet in comparison to the 220 feet required by a normal unprotected ear. There was a slight preference for electronic HEPS, depending on the particular mission. Ergonomics and usability of electronic HEPS might raise some concerns, but the preference for a particular device was related to the particular dimension that was being evaluated (e.g., comfort, ability to communicate, etc). All devices used in the study have been upgraded and thus the performance can be expected to be better.

Williams (2011) conducted a workplace trial to evaluate the performance of sound restoration, level-dependent, electronic HPDs. The participants were 15 very experienced trainers/instructors who worked at indoor and outdoor firing ranges instructing novice shooters and reassessing experienced shooters in safe handling and accurate use of weapons. They were also experienced users of passive HPDs. Seven of the participants probably had hearing loss and five had tinnitus. The results of the HPD trial were highly favorable. The ability to communicate both face-to-face and/or through the use of an electronic communications link allowed the HPDs to remain in place over the work duration, thus reducing the risk of noise injury from unexpected weapon discharges. The two concerns about the HPDs were that it was a hassle to carry or wear them all day and that they may not be comfortable over the entire duration of a workday.

There are often concerns about the increased cost of supplying high-performance, electronic, sound restoration, level-dependent HPDs over traditional passive HPDs. However, considering the many adverse effects of hearing loss (**Fig. 6.13**), the cost of potentially having to replace experienced workers because of hearing loss, and the possibility of fatal injuries resulting from miscommunication in hearing critical jobs, the increased cost of electronic HPDs may be insignificant.

Recreational Headsets

Some earmuffs or headsets are designed to serve as hearing protectors but have built-in radios to allow recreational listening. For workers who perform mechanical jobs, music can enhance performance. A risk in listening to music in noisy surroundings is that the workers may turn the music up to overcome background noise, leading to hazardous music exposure. Such a situation can not only cause hearing loss but may prevent the worker from hearing important signals including alarms. Thus, some agencies such as the DoD do not permit the use of HPDs with built-in radios. Some of the recreational headsets are equipped with maximum limits and do not allow the sound levels to exceed 80 or 85 dBA levels. Use of such recreational headsets might be permitted only under special circumstances.

Hearing Protection for Workers with Hearing Loss

In selecting hearing protection for workers with hearing loss, the following factors should be considered:

- Comfort
- The degree and configuration of hearing loss
- Ease of communication

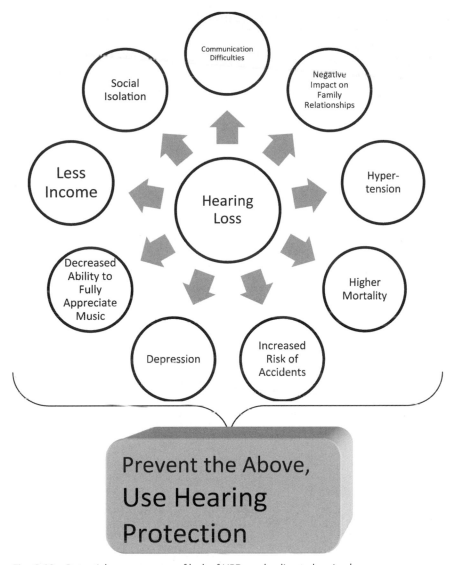

Fig. 6.13 Potential consequences of lack of HPD use leading to hearing loss.

- Job situation and the types of verbal or nonverbal signals the worker is expected to receive
- The noise exposure level and the amount of attenuation required

Use of Hearing Aids under Earmuffs

Hearing aids worn under an earmuff should be equipped with ANR, compression, and maximum output limits to ensure good speech audibility while minimizing noise exposure. The DoD allows the use of certain hearing aids with over-the-ear hearing protectors after evaluation and approval by a military audiologist or otolaryngologist, on an individual basis.

Combination Communication Enhancement and Hearing Protection Devices

Devices that provide enhanced hearing for soft sounds and protection from high-level sounds can be useful for workers with hearing loss, depending on the degree and configuration of hearing loss. Examples of such devices include the QuietPro and EB15 Electronic BlastPLG™ earplugs, which were discussed previously. Training in the appropriate use of these devices should be provided. Some workers may need an adaptation period for recognizing speech through the device and for localizing sounds.

Dual Hearing Protection with Electronic/ Communication Features

In extremely high noise levels, dual hearing protection (such as an earplug under an earmuff) equipped with electronic/communication features may permit clearer communication to workers with hearing loss while providing sufficient protection from noise.

Workers with High-frequency Hearing Loss

Many workers may have high-frequency hearing loss either due to exposure to noise or ototoxins, or due to age. These workers can benefit from Etymotic Research (ER) (Elk Grove Village, IL) earplugs that attenuate sounds relatively equally at all frequencies. They are also sometimes referred to as musician's earplugs and are described further in Chapter 9. ER makes "filter buttons" with 9, 15, and 25 dB attenuation that fit into custom-made ear molds (**Fig. 6.10**). Therefore, it is easy to replace a button for a different amount of attenuation depending on the setting and instrument. ER-20 is a preformed, low-cost HPD that provides more uniform (~20 dB) attenuation than the foam earplug. The NRR of ER-20 is 12 dB.

◆ Selection of Hearing Protection Devices

Several factors should be considered in selecting HPDs to ensure sufficient amount of hearing protection to prevent hearing loss and to improve worker acceptance and continued use (National Institute for Occupational Safety and Health [NIOSH], 1998). These factors include attenuation characteristics, comfort, ease of fit, convenience and availability, ability to hear important signals, compatibility with other work or protective gear, and many other factors that are specific to individual workers and specific work settings. Some of these factors are discussed below in greater detail.

Attenuation Characteristics

The HPD should allow sufficient attenuation without leading to overprotection. The attenuation must be sufficient to reduce the exposure levels to at least 85 dBA (OSHA, 1983) but preferably to 75 to 80 dBA. Noise levels should not be attenuated to below 70 dBA, as this will lead to overprotection.

Considering Noise Reduction Rating

EPA rules, found in 40 CFR Part 211, subpart B, which implement section 8 of the Noise Regulation Act (1972) were issued in 1979 (EPA, 1979; 44 FR 56120). These rules require manufacturers of HPDs to provide consumers with information on the labeling regarding the products' effectiveness in reducing the level of noise entering a user's ears at the time of its sale. More specifically, manufacturers are required to label HPDs with a NRR (**Fig. 6.14**). The NRR is currently obtained by the manufacturers using the procedure specified in ANSI S3.19-1974 (ANSI, 1974).

This standard specifies the experimenter-fit method, in which the experimenter (not the test subject) fits the hearing protector onto the head or into the ear of each test subject for each occluded test to derive the real ear attenuation at threshold (REAT). **Table 6.1** shows an example of open ear thresholds and occluded thresholds obtained with custom-made earplugs. The difference in the two sets of threshold is REAT and provides an estimation of the attenuation provided by the earplugs. REAT is determined three times for each subject using one-third octave bands of noise. Data are collected from at least 10 subjects for several frequencies. Mean attenuation and standard deviation is computed across several frequencies, and the NRR is calculated using the following equation:

$$NRR = 107.9 \, dBC - \left[10 \log \sum_{f=125}^{8000} [10^{0.1(L_{Af} - APV_{f98})}] - 3 \, dB \right]$$

where L_{Af} = A-weighted octave band level at frequency f of a pink noise spectrum with an overall level of 107.9 dBC, and APV_{f98} = mean attenuation value minus two standard deviations at frequency f (two standard deviations accounts for 98% of the variance in a normal distribution). The detailed procedure for calculating the NRR using this equation is shown in **Table 6.2**.

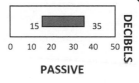

Noise Reduction Rating **26** DECIBELS (When used as directed)

The range of Noise Reduction Ratings for existing hearing protectors is approximately 0 to 30 (higher numbers denote greater effectiveness)

A. Portion of the Current Label

Noise Reduction Rating

15 — 35 | 0 10 20 30 40 50 DECIBELS

PASSIVE

PASSIVE NRR values indicate range of noise reduction when used as instructed by the manufacturer. When used in steady and intermittent noise environments, the difference between the noise level and respective NRRs is the user's estimated exposure level. The protector was not intended for impulse noise.

B. Portion of the Proposed Label for Passive HPDs

Noise Reduction Rating

ACTIVE

15 — 25 | 0 10 20 30 40 50 DECIBELS

10 — 20

PASSIVE

ACTIVE AND PASSIVE NRR values indicate range of noise reduction with and without electronic activation when used as instructed by the manufacturer. In steady and intermittent noise environments, the difference between the noise level and respective NRRs is the user's estimated exposure level. The protector was not tested for impulse noise.

C. Portion of the Proposed Label for ACTIVE Noise Reduction HPDs

Noise Reduction Rating

IMPULSIVE

10 — 25 | 0 10 20 30 40 50 DECIBELS

20 — 35

PASSIVE

IMPULSIVE and PASSIVE NRR values indicate range of noise reduction in impulsive and continuous noise environments when used as instructed by the manufacturer. The difference between the noise level and respective NRRs is the user's estimated exposure level.

D. Portion of the Proposed Label for IMPULSIVE Noise Reduction HPDs

Fig. 6.14 Relevant portions of the current and proposed NRR labels.

Table 6.1   REAT Measurements with Custom-made Earplugs

Condition	125	250	500	1000	2000	3000	4000	6000	8000
Occluded	10	5	5	20	30	55	65	65	50
Open	−5	−5	0	5	10	30	40	50	30
REAT	15	10	5	15	20	25	25	15	20

REAT, real ear attenuation at threshold.

Table 6.2   Computation of the NRR

	Freq (Hz)	125	250	500	1000	2000	3000	4000	6000	8000	
	dB										
1	Assumed pink noise	100	100	100	100	100		100		100	
2	Correction for conversion to C-weighted levels	−0.2	0	0		−0.2		−0.8		−3	
3	Unprotected dBC levels	99.8	100	100	100	99.8		99.2		97	dBC = 107.9
4	Corrections for conversion to A-weighted levels	−16.1	−8.6	−3.2	0	1.2		1.0		−1.1	
5	Unprotected dBA levels	83.9	91.4	96.8	100	101.2		101		98.9	
6	Average attenuation	32.1	30.6	34.5	31.4	30.8	37.3	36.3 (Ave = 36.8)	34.1	36.3 (Ave = 35.2)	
7	Standard deviation	5.9 × 2 = 11.8	6.1 × 2 = 12.2	6.5 × 2 = 13	5.5 × 2 = 11	4.1 × 2 = 8.2	5.3	6.1 → 5.3 + 6.1 = 11.4	6.7	6.9 → 6.7 + 6.9 = 13.6	
8	APV$_{98}$ (line 6 − line 7)	20.3	18.4	21.5	20.4	22.6		25.4		21.6	
9	Protected ear dBA (line 5 − line 8)	63.9	73	75.3	79.6	78.6		75.6		77.3	dBA = 84.91
10	NRR = Unprotected dBC − Protected dBA − 3										107.9 − 84.91 − 3 = 20

Note: dBA and dBC levels in the last column were calculated using the following formula discussed in Chapter 2:

$$L = 10 \log \sum_{i=1}^{n} 10^{\frac{Li}{10}}$$

where L = combined level in dB SPL, n = number of bands being combined, i = the ith band, and Li = the octave band level of the ith band.
NRR, noise reduction rating; SPL, sound pressure level.

The Original Proposed Use of Noise Reduction Rating

C-Weighted Noise Exposure Levels

When the noise is measured using the C-weighting network, the protected level that the worker is exposed to after using the HPD in theory could be estimated by using the following equation:

Protected dBA = unprotected dBC − NRR

where the protected dBA and the unprotected dBC are 8-hour TWAs determined according to the occupational noise standard, as discussed in Chapter 2. The protector in **Table 6.2** has an NRR of 20 dB. If this HPD was used in a 8-hour TWA of 94 dBC, in ideal cases the noise level entering the ear would be expected to be 94 − 20 = 74 dBA or lower in 98% of the workers if the protector is worn using the manufacturer's instructions.

A-Weighted Noise Exposure Levels

For A-weighted noise measurements:

protected dBA = unprotected dBA − (NRR − 7)

The 7-dB correction attempts to approximately account for the de-emphasis of low-frequency energy inherent to the A-weighting scale; in real-world situations, the difference in dBA and dBC measures is not always 7. If a protector has an NRR of 20 dB and it is used in an environmental noise level of 94 dBA, the noise level entering the ear is expected to be approximately 81 dBA [94 − (20 − 7) = 81] or less in 98% of the cases.

Relationship between the Labeled Noise Reduction Rating and Real-world Noise Reduction Rating

With the most accurate insertion depth, it is possible to get the labeled NRR in a few individuals. However, when workers use earplugs in the field, the actual attenuation is much less than the labeled NRR, and there is considerable variability in the achieved attenuation. The attenuation achieved from the use of the EAR foam earplugs in different investigations is shown in **Fig. 6.15** based on the data published by NIOSH (1998), which is based on the data compiled by Berger, Franks, and Lindgren (1996).

Using Noise Reduction Rating to Evaluate Noise Control

Because real-world NRR is much less than the labeled NRR, the Department of Labor/OSHA have instructed its inspectors to "derate" (reduce) a hearing protector's labeled NRR by 50% for evaluating the relative efficacy of HPDs and engineering noise controls. Thus, if the labeled NRR is 20 dB, and the unprotected 8-hour TWA is 94 dBC, then the protected 8-hour TWA is 84 dBA [94 − (20/2) = 84]. The protected exposure in this example meets the OSHA compliance regardless of whether or not the worker has a standard threshold shift. The steps for checking OSHA compliance for unprotected noise exposures measured in dBA are shown in **Table 6.3**.

National Institute for Occupational Safety and Health (1998) Recommendations for Using Noise Reduction Rating

NIOSH recommends using subject fit (not experimenter fit) data based on the ANSI S12.6–1997 (ANSI, 1997) standard. Some manufacturers provide this data on request. If subject fit

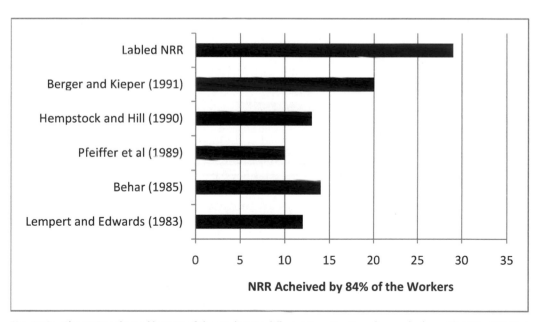

Fig. 6.15 The NRRs achieved by 84% of the workers in different investigations for an earplug with NRR of 29 (Behar, 1985; Berger & Kieper, 1991; Hempstock & Hill, 1990; Lempert & Edwards, 1983; Pfeiffer, Kuhn, Specht, & Knipfer, 1989).

Table 6.3   Steps for Checking OSHA Compliance Assuming Noise Exposures in dBA

Step number	Procedure	Result
1	Measure 8-hour TWA dBA	96 dBA
2	Labeled NRR of HPD	20 dB
3	Subtract 7 dB from the NRR (correction for dBA measures)	20 − 7 = 13 dB
4	Derate the corrected NRR in step 3 by 50% (divide by 2)	13/2 = 7.5
5	Subtract the expected HPD attenuation from the unprotected noise exposure to estimate protected noise exposure	96 − 7.5 = 88.5
6	Compare the estimated protected exposure to the permissible exposure limit	
	If the worker has no standard threshold shift (see Chapter 4), the protected levels should be at least 90 dB or lower	88.5 is below 90; the protected exposure in step 5 suggests effective noise control
	If the worker has a standard threshold shift, the protected level should be at least 85 dBA or lower	88.5 is above 90; in the presence of standard threshold shift, additional noise controls appear to be necessary

HPD, hearing protection device; NRR, noise reduction rating; TWA, time weighted average.

data are not available, NIOSH recommends subtracting 25% from the labeled NRR of earmuffs, 50% from the labeled NRR of foam earplugs, and 70% from the NRR of all other earplugs. **Figure 6.16** shows the difference between labeled and measured NRR84 for earmuffs (NIOSH, 1998), suggesting that subtracting 25% from the labeled NRR may be sufficient for earmuffs. The 50% subtraction for earplugs appears to be justified based on the data in **Fig. 6.15**. Steps for

following NIOSH recommendation are shown in **Table 6.4**.

For derating foam earplugs the following equations can be used:

$$\text{Protected exposure dBA} = \text{Unprotected exposure (dBA)} - [0.5\,(\text{NRR} - 7)]$$

$$\text{Protected exposure dBA} = \text{Unprotected exposure (dBC)} - 0.5\,(\text{NRR})$$

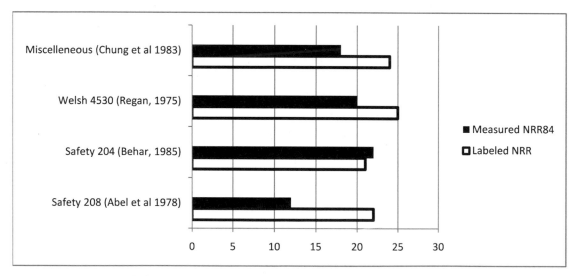

Fig. 6.16   Difference in labeled and measured NRR for earmuffs.

Table 6.4 Steps for Following NIOSH (1998) Recommendations Assuming Noise Exposures in dBA

Step number	Procedure	Result
1	Measure 8-hour TWA dBA	96 dBA
2	Labeled NRR of earplug (not foam)	20 dB
3	Subtract 7 dB from the NRR (correction for dBA measures)	20 − 7 = 13 dB
4	Subtract 70% from the corrected NRR in step 3	13 − (13 × 0.7) = 3.9
5	Subtract the expected HPD attenuation from the unprotected noise exposure to estimate protected noise exposure	96 − 3.9 = 92.1
6	Compare the estimated protected exposure to the permissible exposure limit	
	The protected exposure level should be below 85 dBA	92.1 dBA is above 85 dBA; thus the current HPD is inadequate

HPD, hearing protection device; NRR, noise reduction rating.

For derating earplugs other than foam earplugs the following equations can be used:

$$\text{Protected exposure dBA} = \text{Unprotected exposure (dBA)} - [0.3\,(\text{NRR} - 7)]$$

$$\text{Protected exposure dBA} = \text{Unprotected exposure (dBC)} - 0.3\,(\text{NRR})$$

For derating earmuffs using NIOSH recommendation, the following equations can be used:

$$\text{Protected exposure dBA} = \text{Unprotected exposure (dBA)} - [.75\,(\text{NRR} - 7)]$$

$$\text{Protected exposure dBA} = \text{Unprotected exposure (dBC)} - 0.75\,(\text{NRR})$$

Selecting the Necessary Attenuation Characteristics

In selecting the necessary attenuation characteristics, the worker's 8-hour TWA should be measured in dBA or dBC. The equations shown in **Table 6.5** can be used to determine the needed labeled NRR using a target-protected noise exposure level of 80 dBA. In theory, the labeled NRR values in **Table 6.5** should lower protected exposure levels to 80 dBA. In real practice, the actual attenuation the worker will receive from a foam earplug will vary from 0 to the highest labeled value depending on a variety of factors, including insertion depth, which can lead to under- or overprotection. Therefore, individual fitting checks are important.

New Proposed Noise Reduction Rating Requirements

The EPA (2009) has proposed new procedures for computing and labeling NRR values for HPDs. Some of the differences in the current and proposed procedures are shown in **Table 6.6**, and the key portions of the current and proposed labels are shown in **Fig. 6.14**. The new procedures

Table 6.5 Determination of the Needed Labeled NRR Obtained Using Experimenter Fit for dBA and dBC Measures Assuming Target-Protected Noise Exposure Level of 80 dBA

HPD type	8-hour TWA noise exposure	
	94 dBC	94 dBA
Foam earplugs	Labeled NRR= (Unprotected dBC − Target Protected dBA) × 2	Labeled NRR = [(Unprotected dBA − Target Protected dBA) × 2] + 7
	Labeled NRR = (94 − 80) × 2 = 28 dB	Labeled NRR = [(94 − 80) × 2] + 7 = 28 + 7 = 35 dB
Other earplugs (not foam)	Labeled NRR = (Unprotected dBC − Target Protected dBA)/.3	Labeled NRR = [(Unprotected dBA − Protected dBA)/.3] + 7
	Labeled NRR = (94 − 80)/0.3 = 46.67	Labeled NRR = [(94 − 80)/0.3] + 7 = 46.67 + 7 = 53.67
Earmuffs	Labeled NRR = (Unprotected dBC − Target Protected dBA)/0.75	Labeled NRR = [(Unprotected dBA − Target Protected dBA)/0.75] + 7
	Labeled NRR = (94 − 80)/0.75 = 18.67	Labeled NRR = [(94 − 80)/0.75] + 7 = 25.67

HPD, hearing protection device; NRR, noise reduction rating; TWA, time weighted average.

Table 6.6   Comparison of the Current and Proposed EPA Rules for Describing the Attenuation Characteristics of HPDs

Category	Current rule	Proposed rule
Number of participants	10	10 for earmuffs; 20 for earplugs and semi-inserts
Testing standard(s)	ANSI S3.19–1974	ANSI/ASA S12.6–2008 (2008); ANSI S12.42–1995 (2002; R2002) ANSI/ASA S12.68–2007 (2007); IEC 60711 (International Electrotechnical Commission, 1984)
Testing frequencies	Inclusion of 3150 and 6300 Hz	Exclusion of 3150 and 6300 Hz
Who fits the HPD?	Experimenter	Subject after training by the experimenter
Attenuation determination	Passive	Passive, active, and impulse attenuation testing
Test procedure	REAT	REAT, MIRE, and/or ATF depending on the types of devices
NRR	Single number based on mean and standard deviation data	Range based on the 20th and 80th percentile data; the low number represents the attenuation that can be achieved by at least 80% of test subjects; the high number represents the attenuation possible in at least 20 percent of test subjects. Two separate ranges for active and passive contributions.
Retest	No retesting/relabeling requirements	Recurrent testing is required based on the number of different hearing protector categories that are produced by a manufacturer. Relabeling is required if the product's NRR values differ by 3 dB or more compared with previous NRR values.

ANSI, American National Standards Institute; ASA, Acoustical Society or America; ATF, acoustical test fixture; EPA, U.S. Environmental Protection Agency; HPD, hearing protection device; MIRE, microphone in the real ear; NRR, noise reduction rating; REAT, real ear attenuation at threshold.

were proposed by EPA by considering the following factors:

- The NRR should be mainly based on the sound attenuation provided by the device.
- The variability in the attenuation induced by individual differences in humans, the training provided to them, and the testing protocols must be accounted for in the labeled rating.
- The test method should yield a rating of product effectiveness that is as close as possible to the one expected when used under real-world conditions.
- The method should provide a reliable and repeatable means for measuring product performance, with minimal variability due to non-product–related factors.

Because the objective of the hearing protector labeling program is to provide an assessment of the acoustic performance of only the product, the EPA (2009) has proposed adoption of the ANSI S12.6–2008 Method A protocol for all hearing protectors in their passive mode (ANSI/Acoustical Society of America [ASA], 2008). The assumption underlying Method A is that other essential elements of hearing conservation such as training in the use of HPDs and engineering controls of noise will be in place. The subjects used in collecting the laboratory data must have pure tone air conduction thresholds better than 25 dB HL, and they need to be proficient in obtaining hearing thresholds with 5 dB test-retest reliability. Selection criteria can be used to identify a population of test subjects that produces high attenuations and has a narrow range of attenuations across subjects. Subjects can be rejected for various physical reasons during the *pretest* process to meet these criteria. However, once selected, participants cannot be removed from the pool of tested subjects because of their poor attenuation results. The experimenter can train the subject on how to best fit and use the specific hearing protector before the subject enters the booth. Once the subject enters the test room, the experimenter cannot provide further instruction. This fitting protocol can be referred to as experimenter-trained subject fit.

The current federal (EPA) NRR procedures do not permit the testing of electronic devices that incorporate varying strategies such as ANR, sound restoration, and hearing protection along with communication enhancement. Similarly, current NRR procedures do not apply to HPDs that rely on acoustical and mechanical elements to change attenuation. Consequently, these devices cannot be labeled as HPDs. For these reasons, the EPA (2009) has proposed incorporation of the microphone in the real ear (MIRE) and acoustical test fixture procedures for testing special types of devices.

Microphone in the Real Ear

As suggested by the name, MIRE relies on placement of a microphone in the ear canal of the participant. The SPL in the ear canal near the eardrum can be measured with and without the HPD in place. The difference in the two measures provides an estimate of the attenuation provided by the HPD and is referred to as insertion loss. Alternatively, the SPL at the entrance of the ear canal can be measured and compared with the SPL near the eardrum with the HPD in place to estimate the transmission loss provided by the HPD.

The EPA (2009) has proposed the MIRE technique to evaluate the active contribution to the total HPD noise reduction provided by ANR devices. Both earmuffs and earplugs would be assessed with the electronics or the ANR turned on and off in a broadband noise field. The difference between the noise levels measured in the on and off conditions will provide an estimation of the active attenuation contribution. The active contribution is then added to the attenuation measured with the REAT method

in the passive mode. For earmuffs, the REAT and MIRE data will be obtained from the same participants.

For earplugs, placement of the miniature microphone in the occluded ear can adversely affect the operation of control circuits. If a probe microphone is used, then the probe needs to be placed between the wall of the ear canal and the earplug (**Fig. 6.17**), which can create a potential leakage path. **Figure 6.18** shows attenuation measured using the REAT procedure and the MIRE (insertion loss) procedure by placing a probe microphone on the floor of the right and left ear canals. For both procedures, data was averaged across two test trials. The two measures yield somewhat similar results at 1, 2, 3, and 4 kHz, but differences are apparent at other test frequencies. Alternatively, the probe can be passed through a sound bore in the earplug (**Fig. 6.16**), which also can create a leakage path and reduce potentially useful space for additional circuitry for specialized sound modifications. Thus, the EPA has proposed the use of acoustic text fixtures for obtaining the MIRE data for ANR earplugs.

Acoustic Test Fixture

This procedure is very similar to the MIRE procedure, but the microphone is placed in the ear canal of the acoustic test fixture, which is an anthropometrically correct mannequin with an embedded ear simulator. The ear simulator can be suspended inside a capsule within a relatively solid acrylic body. Incorporation of replaceable

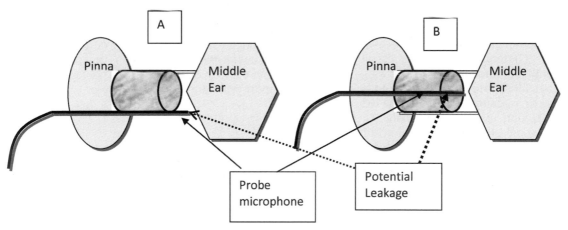

Fig. 6.17 Potential leakage paths during MIRE measurements for earplugs.

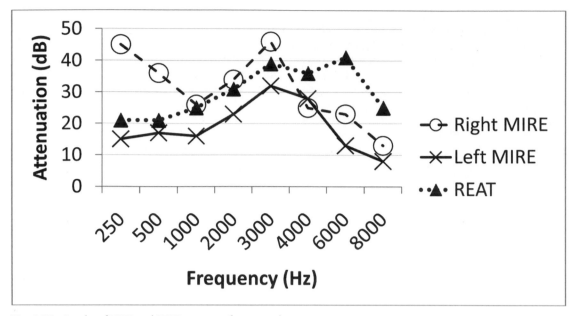

Fig. 6.18 Results of MIRE and REAT measures for an earplug.

ear canals and pinna sets in the fixture can allow testing of both muffs and plugs. Anthropometrically correct mannequins allow simulation of sound diffraction effects around the head (Parmentier, Dancer, Buck, Kronenberger, & Beck, 2000). The EPA has proposed the use of an impulse acoustic test fixture for evaluating performance of HPDs in high sound level impulse environments to prevent the risk of hearing loss in human subjects.

Attenuation Provided by Double Protection

Double protection usually adds only 5 to 10 dB to the maximum attenuation provided by the use of a single HPD. Thus, if the earmuff provides 40 dB attenuation and the earplug provides 20 dB attenuation, dual protection will provide 45 to 50 dB attenuation. It should be noted that when exposure levels exceed 105 dBA, dual protection may be inadequate (NIOSH, 1998) and should be supplemented by administrative controls to allow reduction of duration of exposure. In the presence of high-level impulse noise, dual protection consisting of low-profile sound restoration earmuffs along with earplugs may be necessary for providing sufficient protection and allowing situational awareness (Murphy & Tubbs, 2007).

Factors that Minimize or Limit Attenuation

Four factors impose a limit on the amount of attenuation provided by HPDs (**Fig. 6.19**) including sound transmission through the HPD barrier, the extent of the airtight seal against the ear canal wall for earplugs or in the circumaural area for earmuffs, HPD vibrations, and conduction of sounds through bone (Berger, 1980).

Structural Transmission

Some sound is expected to pass through the barrier formed by earplugs depending on the mass, stiffness, and internal damping of HPD materials. Similarly, some sound will pass through earmuffs depending on the absorption characteristics of the earcups, the cushion liner, and bladder. Structural transmission effects are most pronounced above 1000 Hz.

Loose Seal

Loose seals can minimize the attenuation by 5 to 15 dB over a wide range of frequencies. To minimize this, it is important to ensure that earcups of earmuffs are making an airtight seal in the circumaural region of each ear, and that devices like earplugs are making an airtight sear in the ear canal.

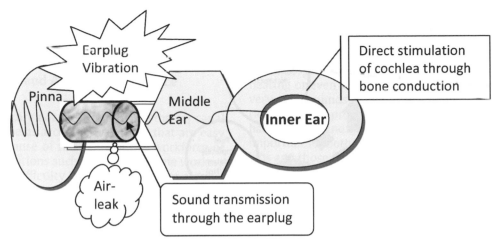

Fig. 6.19 Factors that limit the attenuation provided by HPDs.

Hearing Protection Device Vibration

At high noise levels, the inner third bony walls of the ear canal can vibrate; this vibration can be transmitted to earplugs that are located within the ear canals. Because of the flexibility of the outer cartilaginous two-thirds of the ear canal, earplugs can vibrate in a pistonlike manner. Earmuffs also vibrate as a mass-spring system. The stiffness of the spring element depends on the volume of air trapped inside the earcup, the absorption characteristics of the earmuff cushion, and the characteristics of the individual circumaural region. Vibrations usually limit the possible amount of attenuation for low frequencies such as 125 Hz or infrasounds.

Bone and Tissue Conduction

At high stimulus levels of above 40 to 50 dBA, the noise can reach the cochlea through bone and tissue conduction. At high levels, the skull begins to vibrate, thus stimulating the cochlea. This transmission imposes a limit on the maximum attenuation possible through HPDs, as most HPDs attenuate sounds transmitted through air conduction. This issue becomes an important factor when a high amount of attenuation is needed, such as when wearing dual protection.

Comfort

If a worker experiences discomfort due to the use of HPDs, that worker is not likely to wear the HPD, thus reducing its effectiveness. HPDs that are more comfortable and thus are more acceptable are more efficient protectors than HPDs that have higher attenuation characteristics. Comfort and attenuation appear to be inversely related (Byrne, Davis, Shaw, Specht, & Holland, 2011; Park & Casali, 1991a). Thus it is important to achieve a balance between attenuation characteristics and comfort to maximize HPD effectiveness (Arezes & Miguel, 2002).

The concept of comfort is complex (Davis, 2008) and may have a physical dimension (canal irritation or tight feeling) and a psychological dimension (e.g., feeling of isolation). HPD comfort can be assessed using bipolar comfort rating scales or comfort index ratings (Casali, Lam, & Epps, 1987). Some dimensions related to comfort (Arezes & Miguel, 2002; Park & Casali, 1991b) are shown in **Fig. 6.20**. In assessing comfort, it is important to allow the worker to try the HPD for a few days in real work conditions to get a true impression of some of the comfort dimensions such as softness and earmuff weight (Ivergård & Nicholl, 1976). Characteristics of a comfortable earmuff (Bhattacharya, Tripathi, & Kashyap, 1993; Ivergård & Nicholl, 1976; Nixon, McKinley, & Steuver, 1992) are shown in **Fig. 6.21**. Significant buildup of heat and humidity under the cup of earmuffs can occur even in a low physical effort, environmentally controlled situation with a simultaneous decline in comfort ratings (Davis & Shaw, 2011). Comfort cannot be modified through counseling (Franks, Davis, & Murphy, 2005). Thus, when a worker reports

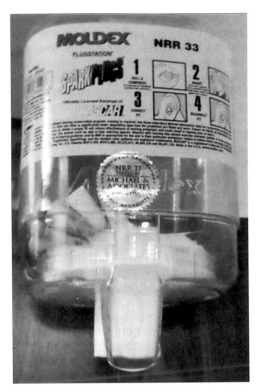

Fig. 6.22   Earplug dispenser.

the pinna back and upward can straighten adult ear canals; pulling it slightly downward can straighten children's ear canals. A slightly different direction for pulling may be necessary for some ears. The ear canal should be free of excessive cerumen or any other objects. If there is excessive cerumen, it should be removed before proceeding with ear impressions. In the presence of any pathological conditions, a referral should be made to an otolaryngologist and the ear impression should not be made until the condition is treated. The worker should be informed about any major deformities in the ear canal that can make regular use of a custom mold difficult. The shape of the ear canal should be carefully observed, and this information should be used in selecting and placing the otoblock and in directing the syringe for depositing ear impression material in the ear canal.

Otoblock

An otoblock attached to a thread or dental floss (**Fig. 6.23**) should be placed near the eardrum to prevent any ear impression material from touching the eardrum.

to expose workers to hazardous noise levels, workers need to understand that even though they may not get complete protection, the risk and the degree of hearing loss can be reduced by wearing available protection.

◆ Making Ear Impressions for Customized Hearing Protection Devices

The quality of an ear impression can partially determine the ease of insertion and removal, the attenuation characteristics, and ear canal comfort. Thus it is important to make a good ear impression with a relatively long ear canal. The following steps can help in ensuring a good ear impression.

Otoscopy

The ear canal should be straightened to carefully observe the ear canal and the eardrum. Pulling

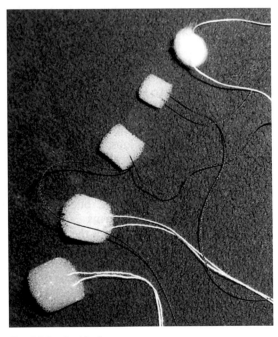

Fig. 6.23   Otoblocks.

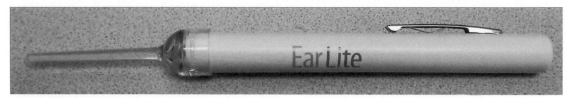

Fig. 6.24   Earlight.

Choosing the Size of the Otoblock

It is important to choose an otoblock that is suited to each individual ear canal. An undersized otoblock can allow ear impression material to go beyond the otoblock. An oversized otoblock can prevent deep placement of the block in the ear canal and can occupy too much of the ear canal space that should be occupied by the impression material.

Placement of the Otoblock

The otoblock should be placed in the ear canal using an ear light (**Fig. 6.24**) at least beyond the first bend of the ear canal and when possible, beyond the second bend of the ear canal. Deep impressions are recommended for all customized molds, including those with frequency-dependent attenuation. To achieve this goal, the otoblock should be placed as close to the eardrum as possible. The string of the otoblock should be placed on the floor of the ear canal.

Preparing the Impression Material

Either silicon (**Fig. 6.25**) or powder (polymer) and liquid (monomer) impression materials can be

used. In preparing these materials for placement in the ear canal and using them, the directions provided by manufacturers should be followed as closely as possible. The material should be used as quickly as possible after it is prepared.

Placing the Impression Material in the Syringe

After preparing the impression material, it should be quickly placed in the barrel of the syringe (**Fig. 6.26**). The material should be pushed with the plunger to minimize air pockets.

Depositing the Impression Material in the Ear

The ear canal should be straightened with one hand, and the ear canal should be filled with the impression material by placing the nozzle of the syringe in the ear canal with the other hand. The nozzle should be slowly pulled out while filling the ear canal, and then the helix, concha, and tragus should be filled with the material. The material should be pressed gently in the concha and helix areas. The outer surface of the impression should be smoothed gently by using a finger (a controversial recommendation), which makes it easier to glue it to the box for shipping and also is helpful in removing minor air pockets. It is important to not press hard. Sufficient curing time should be allowed, which is usually 10 to 15 minutes.

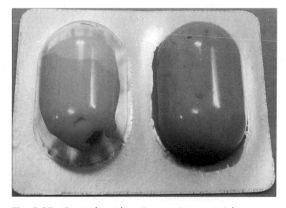

Fig. 6.25   Prepackaged ear impression material.

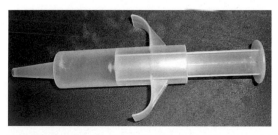

Fig. 6.26   Syringe for depositing ear impression material in the ear canal.

Removal of the Ear Impression

The ear impression seal should be broken by removing the helix curl slightly while pulling the pinna away and back from the ear impression. The rest of the ear impression should be slowly pulled out while simultaneously holding on to the string of the otoblock to prevent the otoblock from staying in the ear canal. The otoblock string should remain attached to the ear impression. The impression should be removed primarily by pulling out the body of the impression and not the otoblock string.

Reexamination of Ear Canals

The ear canal should be reexamined to ensure that all impression material has been removed from the ear canal. Some ear canals may show signs of irritation with the use of silicon materials. In rare cases, bleeding may be apparent when the patient is on prescription blood thinners, which may require medical referral.

Examination of Ear Impressions

The ear impression should be carefully examined to ensure sufficient length of the ear canal portion and that there are no missing portions or distortions. If the ear impression does not appear adequate, another impression should be made. An inadequate ear impression can change the attenuation characteristics of the customized HPD and make the HPD ineffective or uncomfortable to wear. As previously mentioned, if the HPD does not make an airtight seal against all walls of the ear canal, the attenuation can be reduced by 5 to 15 dB over a broad frequency region.

Shipping Ear Impressions

Impressions made from the powder and liquid materials should be glued to the bottom of the box. The order form should be placed in such a way that it will not press against the ear impressions or distort or damage the impressions during shipping. If the ear or ear canal has any unusual characteristics (e.g., surgically altered ear canal or relatively short ear canal), this information should be provided to the manufacturer.

◆ Checking the Physical Fit of Hearing Protection Devices

After the HPD type and size has been selected or after receiving the custom-molded HPD, it is important to ensure that the HPDs fit comfortably and adequately in the worker's ears. In some cases, it may be necessary to grind down the length of the ear canal if the worker reports pain, which can result from the HPD touching the ear drum. In other cases, discomfort can arise from other rough spots on the HPD. It is important to not do too much grinding, as it will reduce the possibility of achieving an airtight seal.

◆ Checking the Adequacy of Hearing Protection Device Attenuation

Although the equations in **Table 6.5** can be used to determine the needed labeled NRR, the actual attenuation achieved in real field situations can vary from 0 to the labeled NRR. Therefore, it is important to check the attenuation provided by the HPDs for each worker and preferably for each ear. Individual fit testing of HPDs has been recommended for several reasons (Occupational Safety and Health Administration, National Institute of Occupational Safety and Health, and National Hearing Conservation Alliance, 2008):

- ◆ It can be used to train workers in proper use of their HPDs.
- ◆ It can be used to train occupational hearing conservationists and other professionals in efficient fitting of HPDs.
- ◆ If an employee develops a standard threshold shift, individual fit testing can be useful in evaluating the amount of attenuation of the HPDs and can point to any need for HPDs with different attenuation or need for retraining for correct insertion of the HPDs.
- ◆ It can provide an objective record of the adequacy of attenuation provided by the HPDs.
- ◆ It can assist in documenting the overall effectiveness of the hearing conservation program.
- ◆ It can allow selection of HPDs that have attenuation characteristics appropriate for the worker's noise exposure level to minimize under- or overprotection. A variety of

protectors can be tested in a short amount of time using the field MIRE (F-MIRE) technique, allowing the selection of the appropriate model.

Procedures for Checking the Adequacy of Attenuation

A variety of procedures (**Fig. 6.27**) are available to determine if target attenuation is provided by the selected HPD. The resulting attenuation characteristics determined for each worker can be summarized using a personal attenuation rating (PAR), which is computed using techniques similar to those used for computing NRR (Berger, Voix, Kieper, & Cocq, 2011). Currently, such procedures are not standardized. Thus, the precision and accuracy of the procedures and PAR values derived from the use of different protocols can vary. For a better estimate of the personal attenuation characteristics, the procedure should be repeated at least twice after reinserting or replacing the HPD.

Some procedures check the fit at only one frequency, while other procedures incorporate three or more frequencies. With the use of single frequency, an error of 3 to 6 dB is expected in the estimated attenuation. When three or more frequencies are used for evaluation, the error is reduced to approximately 0.5 to 1 dB (Murphy, 2011). When possible, attenuation characteristics should be determined for each ear. Differences in ear canal symmetry might lead to a well-fitted HPD in one ear and a loose HPD in the other ear, causing a unilateral significant threshold shift (Rawool & Davis, 2010).

Each of the fit check procedures describes the attenuation characteristics of the specific HPD for the specific individual ear, using the specific protocol, under the environmental conditions in which it was tested, and with the specific procedures used for insertion and the achieved insertion depth. When explaining the PAR data to workers, emphasis should be placed on the fact that the attenuation provided by their HPDs can vary depending on the accuracy of insertion or placement of the HPD and the resiliency of the HPD. To get attenuation values similar to those obtained during the fit check procedures, it is important to insert the earplug correctly and

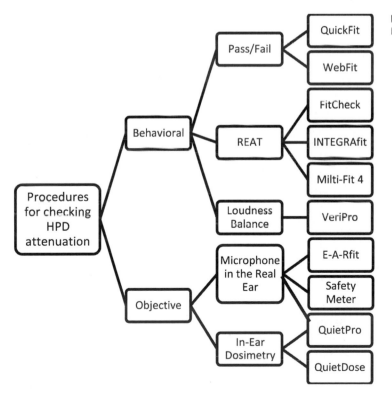

Fig. 6.27 Procedures for checking HPD attenuation.

deeply or to place the earmuff properly. It is also important to replace earplugs and cushions of the earmuffs as needed. The best opportunity for providing individual training to workers is at the time of individual fit testing. Specific errors made by the individuals in inserting or removing the HPDs can be observed and corrected by showing attenuation data and by carefully observing the worker. A private space that is free from intrusions should be used while checking the fit and providing personal training.

Behavioral Test Procedures

Behavioral test procedures require the subject to listen to sounds and to respond in some way.

Pass-Fail Procedures

During these procedures, the worker is expected to listen to certain sounds with and without earplugs. If the difference in the thresholds meets a predetermined attenuation criterion, the fit is considered adequate. An example of pass-fail procedures is the QuickFit procedure developed by NIOSH (Department of Health and Human Services [DHHS]/NIOSH, 2009). The QuickFit test device provides a pulsing one octave band noise centered around 1000 Hz. The signal sounds like a whooshing sound. The device should be placed over the ear after turning the power on, and the user should be asked to adjust the volume control until the sound is barely audible or is at threshold. The device is then set aside and the earplug is inserted in the ear. The QuickFit device is then placed against the protected ear while pressing the boost button. If the boosted test sound cannot be heard through the earplug, the user has achieved at least a 15 dB attenuation, thus passing the fit check. If the boosted test sound remains audible through the earplug, the fit is inadequate. The earplug either needs to be reinserted correctly or a different type of HPD might be appropriate for the specific user. A web-fit variation of the QuickFit procedure is available online as QuickFitWeb for users. The users listen to the same narrowband noise centered at 1000 Hz through the computer's speakers with and without the earplugs to see if the HPD is providing at least 15 dB attenuation around 1000 Hz. The tool is available at www.cdc.gov/niosh/mining/topics/hearingloss/quickfitweb.htm.

Real Ear Attenuation at Threshold–Based Procedures

The REAT procedure can be conducted in the sound field using the procedure similar to that described in the ANSI standard (ANSI/ASA, 2008; S12.6). Service providers who are equipped with an audiometer, loudspeakers, and a sound-treated booth can get a good idea about the fit of the earplug by obtaining thresholds with and without the HPD using pulsed narrowband noises. It can also be performed by presenting pulsed one-third octave band noises through large circumaural earphones instead of loudspeakers. The test-retest variability in REAT measures can be expected to be ± 5 dB if a 5-dB step size is used in obtaining thresholds. If the step size is reduced to ± 2 dB near the threshold, the test-retest variability may be reduced to ± 2 dB. REAT-based measures are more time-consuming than MIRE-based measures, especially when a smaller step size is used and data are obtained individually for each ear.

NIOSH has developed a system called Multifit4 that allows simultaneous testing of four subjects using the REAT procedure. The subjects are seated in a sound-isolated chamber, and the test stimuli are delivered through circumaural headphones. Subjects track their thresholds with and without the HPD in place. The difference in the two thresholds provides the REAT values, which can be saved automatically in a database (Kwitowski, Carilli, & Randolph, 2010). One potential disadvantage of this procedure is that it may not allow individualized training for each worker.

Other fit-testing systems that use REAT-based procedures are commercially available as FitCheck™ for insert type hearing protectors (Michael and Associates, State College, PA) and IntegraFit™ for insert type HPDs (Workplace INTEGRA, Inc., Greensboro, NC).

Loudness Balance Procedure

The VeriPRO system (Howard Leight by Sperian, Sperian Hearing Protection, LLC, San Diego, CA) uses the loudness balance procedure to check the personal attenuation and provides a PAR value. The audio processor in the system converts digital signals from the VeriPRO software, calibrates it to specially designed high-output headphones, and amplifies the sounds. During the complete check mode, five frequencies (250, 500, 1000, 2000, and 4000 Hz) are evaluated. For a quick fit check, loudness balance testing is conducted only at 500 Hz. Initially, without the earplugs, the user is asked to adjust the volume of the sounds in the headphones to be equally loud in both ears. Then the earplug is inserted in one ear and the loudness balance is reestablished by increasing the volume in the earphone with the earplug. The amount of increase in the volume in the plugged ear gives an estimation of the attenuation provided by the earplug in that ear. The attenuation in the other ear is then determined by plugging that ear and repeating the loudness balance procedure. Some workers, especially those with hearing loss, may have difficulty in establishing loudness balance, and this procedure can be performed only on insert-type HPDs.

Objective Test Procedures

The objective test techniques do not require any response from the subject.

Microphone in the Real Ear

As mentioned previously, these techniques all require the placement of a microphone in the ear canal and are referred to as F-MIRE. For use of the F-MIRE technique, specially equipped earphones are used to simultaneously measure the noise outside the earmuff and inside the ear canal to estimate the attenuation provided by earmuffs. The SonoPass systems developed by Sonomax Technologies Inc. (Motreal, Quebec, Canada [the software is sold by the brand name SonoPass by Sonomax and by the name E-A-Rfit by Aero Technologies, a subsidiary of 3M [St. Paul, MN]) use specially probed test earplugs to allow MIRE testing for frequencies ranging from 125 to 8000 Hz and yield a PAR value. The SafetyMeter fit testing system from Phonak uses a special ear jack to allow MIRE testing and PAR determination of their custom-fitted earplugs (see **Fig. 6.5**). F-MIRE testing is incorporated within the QuietPro HPDs, which provide an alerting signal if the fit is inadequate.

F-MIRE procedures can be performed much more quickly than REAT-based procedures. Because no response is required from the subject, training is unnecessary and test-retest variability is less. The 95% confidence level of the PAR values as a function of the number of fits for earplugs for one of the F-MIRE protocols varies from ±4.4 dB to ±6.3 dB, depending on plug type. A single repeat measurement can reduce the variability to ±3.1 to ±4.5 dB. The variability is mainly related to variability in fitting the earplugs (Berger, Voix, Kieper, & Cocq, 2011).

In-ear Dosimetry

In these procedures, a microphone placed inside the ear canal measures the noise exposure levels of workers. If the protected exposure levels are safe, the fit of the HPD or the HPD can be considered adequate for the worker. This approach is the best approach for employees who are exposed to high-level impulse-type noises and wear dual protection. In-ear dosimetry is incorporated in the QuietPro device. The QuietDose system (Howard Leight by Sperian, Sperian Hearing Protection, LLC, San Diego, CA) also allows measurement of the protected exposure through the use of a variety of earplugs. FitCheck for earmuffs from Michael and Associates also provides noise exposure levels under earmuffs.

◆ Reevaluation of Hearing Protection Device Attenuation

OSHA (1983) requires reevaluation of HPD attenuation whenever there is an increase in noise exposure leading to the possibility that the attenuation may be insufficient. More effective protection should be provided when necessary.

◆ Training Workers for Accurate Hearing Protection Device Use

Interventions that are designed specifically for an individual or a group of workers with the goal of changing behavior are effective in improving the use of HPDs (El Dib & Mathew, 2009; Joseph, Punch, Stephenson, Paneth, Wolfe, & Murphy, 2007). After receiving individual instruction to ensure that the subject is capable of achieving a visually acceptable fit, poorly performing participants can insert earplugs properly and achieve sufficient attenuation. Such individualized instruction is better than just written or videotaped instructions (Murphy, Stephenson, Byrne, Witt, & Duran, 2011). As mentioned previously, training the worker in the use of HPDs at the time of the fitting and fit checking procedures can allow

Table 6.7   Components of Worker Training for Using Earplugs

Insertion	Consequences of inaccurate insertion
	Accurate insertion procedure
Seal check	Consequences of inadequate seal
	Checking adequacy of seal
Insertion depth check	Need for deep insertion
	Visual and auditory checks
Removal	Consequences of quick removal
	Accurate removal procedure
Cleaning	Consequences of dirty earplugs
	Following manufacturer's instructions and storing in a clean box
Replacement	Recognizing worn out earplugs
	Replacing worn out earplugs

individualized training and an opportunity for the worker to ask questions or express any concerns about the use of HPDs. Workers need to understand that improper HPD use can lead to insufficient protection and subsequent hearing loss.

Worker Training for Use of Earplugs

Major components of training workers in the use of earplugs are outlined in **Table 6.7**, including insertion, seal-check, insertion-depth check, removal, cleaning, and replacement.

Insertion of Earplugs

Workers need to understand the consequences of inadequate insertion, including discomfort, irritation of the ear canal, and inadequate hearing protection. Workers should be informed about the correct procedures for inserting earplugs. Steps involved in insertion of roll-down–type foam ear plugs (DHHS/NIOSH, 2004) are outlined in **Table 6.8**. The worker should be requested to practice the insertion. The trainer should observe the worker and provide any feedback on achieving correct insertion. Images of correct and incorrect insertion should be provided and the impact of each type of insertion should be discussed. A videotoscope can be very useful in showing the worker how the inserted earplug is seating in the ear canal and how it should ideally be seated in the ear canal. This is especially useful during any retraining activities.

Checking Adequacy of Seal

It is important to check the adequacy of the seal of HPDs because inadequate seals can lead

Table 6.8   Steps Involved in Inserting a Foam Earplug (DHHS/NIOSH, 2004)

Step	Goal	Procedure	Possible error
1	Roll the earplug into a very thin crease-free cylinder	Initially squeeze the earplug lightly while rolling it between the forefinger and thumb. Gradually increase the pressure as the plug becomes thinner. In the presence of small or thin fingers, it is better to use the palms to ensure the cylinder shape.	Rolling the earplug into a ball or cone shape that will not reach deep in the ear canal thus minimizing the effectiveness of the HPD.
2	Straighten the ear canal	Reach one hand around the back of the head and pull the pinna up and back. In some cases, the pinna needs to be pulled back in a slightly different direction. For young children, pulling the pinna slightly downward straightens the ear canal.	Not straightening the ear canal before insertion of earplug can lead to shallow insertion due to a natural curve in the ear canal.
3	Insert the earplug	During insertion, try to feel that the earplug is far enough in the ear canal.	Shallow insertion
4	Ensure best possible fit	Place a finger on the outer side of the foam earplug for ~10–20 s until it expands. Then, release and push again for another 5 s.	Pushing on an earplug that is not properly inserted is not going to be effective. If insertion is shallow, the earplug should be removed and reinserted correctly.

HPD, hearing protection device.

to a significant reduction in the attenuation. A loosely fitted earplug can also work out of the ear canal during regular work activities, thus leading to additional reduction in attenuation. The seal can be checked using one of the following procedures.

Noise Attenuation Test

The worker can place his hands cupped over the inserted earplugs. If the earplugs are inserted correctly, there should be no further reduction of noise (Royster & Royster, 1994).

Tug Resistance Test

The worker can tug very gently on the handle of the earplug. If the employee feels a sensation of gentle suction on the eardrum and it feels that the earplug will not come out easily, then the seal is most likely adequate (Royster & Royster, 1994).

Occlusion Hum Test

After the insertion of one earplug, the worker can hum or say a prolonged "ahh...." If the voice sounds louder in the ear with the plug, the seal is likely adequate (Royster & Royster, 1994). The increased loudness in the plugged ear is caused by the occlusion effect. The occlusion effect is created by enhancement of the low-frequency content of one's own voice due to vibration of the unoccupied bony portion of the ear canal. These vibrations generate airborne sounds that cannot escape if the ear canal is properly sealed by the earplug, and vibrate the eardrum. The occlusion effect is expected to be minimal for a deeply inserted earplug because the earplug will occupy most of the bony portion and minimize its vibration. Therefore, this test is probably not the best test for checking the seal.

Perceptual Noise Attenuation Test

Some workers can be trained to recognize the required amount of attenuation by listening to a noise with and without a properly inserted earplug. A wideband noise available from most audiometers can be used for such training. Alternatively, the relatively inexpensive QuickFit test device can be used for training. As mentioned previously, the device yields a narrowband noise centered around 1000 Hz.

Ensuring Proper Insertion Depth

Deep fitting is necessary to minimize the occlusion effect and to improve comfort. Deep fitting also provides maximum attenuation. The workers should visually examine the earplugs. The outer edge of the earplugs should be aligned with the tragus. By changing the insertion depth, a change in the amount of occlusion effect can be perceived. Less occlusion effect suggests a better insertion depth.

Removal of Earplugs

Hasty removal of the earplugs can lead to discomfort. If discomfort is felt, the worker is less likely to use the earplug in the future. Workers need to understand the correct procedures for removing the earplugs without causing any discomfort or harm. Earplugs that create an airtight seal should not be suddenly pulled out of the ear. The airtight seal should be broken gently by slowly twisting the earplug before pulling it out of the ear canal. The worker can listen to noise or music while breaking the seal; increase in sound level indicates that the seal is broken.

Fitting Earmuffs

The headband needs to be centered directly on the top of the head, and the center of the muff cushion needs be aligned with the center of the ear canal. Occlusion effect can also be tested with earmuffs.

Hearing Protection Device Hygiene

Workers need to understand the importance of clean earplugs. Dirty or poorly maintained earplugs can cause ear canal irritation and infections. Manufacturers' instructions should be followed in care, use, and maintenance of HPDs. Earplugs can be often washed with warm water and soap and dried, but some earplugs such as those made from spun fiberglass, silicone resin, and putty are not designed for washing. Workers should be provided with a carrying case for HPDs when the HPDs are not in use, and the carrying case should be clean. Earmuff cushions should be periodically cleaned.

Hearing Protection Device Replacement

Examples of worn out earplugs and earmuff cushions should be shown to workers. Workers need to understand that after multiple uses, both earplugs and earmuff cushions lose their original appearance or resiliency and the ability to form an airtight seal. Worn out earplugs and earmuff cushions should be replaced to ensure continued adequate hearing protection.

Training in the Use and Care of Electronic Hearing Protection Devices

Electronic HPDs are costly to replace but with proper use and care can be used for a relatively long period. Although written instructions are usually provided about the use and care of electronic HPDs in the manufacturer's manual, individual training should be provided to workers to ensure proper use and a long life. The training should include all of the following material:

◆ Insertion and removal: Insertion and removal of the device should be demonstrated, and the worker should be allowed to practice. Improper insertion can irritate the ear canal and may lead to partial or little use of the device.

◆ The function of any controls switches (e.g., on or off) or buttons should be discussed. Practice in operating any controls (e.g., low versus high noise surroundings) should be provided. For example, an illustration such as **Fig. 6.9** can be useful in showing how the two switches (Hi and Lo) on the EB15 Electronic BlastPLG™ earplugs work. More specifically, information such as the fact that the device provides some gain for soft sounds and natural hearing for moderately loud sounds and attenuation for very high sounds on the "Hi" setting can be useful for workers with hearing loss and may boost their confidence in using the device correctly as required for their surroundings. The illustration can also be used to show that at very high noise levels, the HPDs provide limited attenuation and that workers can suffer hearing loss if they engage in recreational shooting because of assumed complete protection with these devices. More specifically with high noise exposures, the workers will continue to be exposed to levels of approximately 115 dB SPL, which are hazardous to hearing. Such information provided using illustrations may encourage workers to limit nonoccupational impulse noise exposures (see Chapter 10).

◆ For devices that provide radio communication along with hearing protection, the noise exposure may mainly come from radio communication. The importance of and the ways to control such exposures should be discussed if there is no maximum safe limit set on the radio transmitted signals.

◆ Any means of controlling wind noise should be discussed.

◆ Removal of wax at the end of the day with the cleaning tool and use of a brush to clean off any debris from the device should be demonstrated.

◆ Replacement of any wax filters should be demonstrated.

◆ Some electronic devices require proper attachment and replacement of the tip. The technique for attachment and replacement should be provided. Some tips can be washed and reused until they lose their original shape and ability to form a tight seal in the ear canal. Other tips cannot be washed. Appropriate information should be provided, depending on the selected tip.

◆ Workers need to be asked to open the battery door when the device is not in use to extend battery life. Battery insertion and removal should be shown, and information about the appropriate type of battery should be provided. Any low battery warning on the device should be discussed. Workers should be informed that batteries are dangerous if swallowed and should not be stored along with medicine tablets. Batteries should be kept away from children and pets and should not be replaced in front of children.

◆ Workers should be informed that electronic devices cannot be used while taking a shower or swimming and that hairsprays should not be used while the devices are in ears.

◆ Electronic devices should not be exposed to extreme heat or humidity.

◆ Workers should be asked to slowly increase the duration of device use over time to get accustomed to the physical presence of the device in the ear canal and to get used to any sound modifications performed by the device.

◆ If any irritations develop in the ear canal, the use of the device should be discontinued and the worker should seek audiological consultation to improve the fit of the devices if needed and medical advice to treat any persistent pathology of the ear canal.

◆ Warranty information should be provided.
◆ Annual device evaluation should be recommended and could be performed at the time of annual audiological monitoring.

◆ Motivating Workers to Use Hearing Protection Devices

In motivating workers to use HPDs, the factors that are associated with high HPD use should be considered (**Fig. 6.28**). For example, workers who believe that they can use HPDs for a long period (self-efficacy) are more likely to consistently use HPDs (Melamed, Rabinowitz, Feiner, Weisberg, & Ribak, 1996). Self-efficacy can be enhanced by providing HPDs that are comfortable, that are easy to fit, and that are compatible with other work gear. Experience with tinnitus is associated with higher HPD use. Thus, allowing workers to experience simulated tinnitus through the presentation of high-pitched tones, broadband noises, or

clicks may facilitate the use of HPDs (Rawool & Colligon-Wayne, 2008).

Protector use is highest when hearing loss prevention programs were most complete, indicating that underuse of protection, in substantial part, is attributable to incomplete or inadequate company efforts. Protector use shows significant associations with a percentage of employees specifically required to use protection, management score, and average employee time spent in noise over 95 dBA ($R^2 = 0.65$). (Daniell, Swan, McDaniel, Camp, Cohen, & Stebbins, 2006). In addition to the provision of initial baseline training, use of a personal noise level indicator and subsequent brief refresher training designed to reinforce the key messages provided during initial training can lead to some improvement in HPD use (Seixas, Neitzel, Stover, et al., 2011). Tightened hearing protection regulations may preserve hearing, especially in the high frequencies among soldiers, suggesting better use of HPDs (Mrena, Ylikoski, Kiukaanniemi, Mäkitie, & Savolainen, 2008).

In addition to the required signs about hazardous noise levels and HPD use, reminder signs for ways of conserving hearing (**Fig. 6.29**) and consequences of hearing loss (see **Fig. 6.12**) might motivate workers to use HPDs.

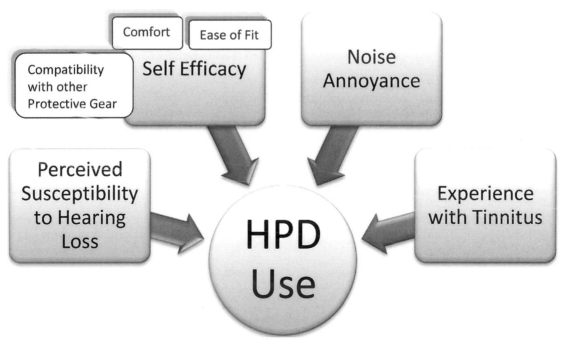

Fig. 6.28   Factors associated with HPD use.

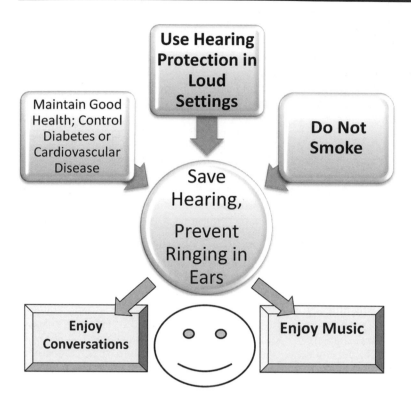

Maintain Good Health; Control Diabetes or Cardiovascular Disease

Use Hearing Protection in Loud Settings

Do Not Smoke

Save Hearing, Prevent Ringing in Ears

Enjoy Conversations

Enjoy Music

Fig. 6.29 Example of sign to promote hearing conservation and HPD use.

◆ Measuring Overall Effectiveness of the Hearing Protection Device Component of the Hearing Conservation Program

Otoacoustic Emission Testing

Bockstael and colleagues (2008) evaluated the effectiveness of two HPDs designed for protection of impulse noise by measuring otoacoustic emissions (OAEs) before and after noise exposure. They found no difference in emissions before and after the noise exposure, suggesting that the protection offered by the HPDs was effective. One potential limitation of this approach is that the OAEs may not be present at higher frequencies in all workers prior to noise exposure.

Frequency of Hearing Protection Device Use

Inconsistent use of HPDs will not provide effective hearing protection. The frequency of HPD use can be used as an indicator of overall effectiveness of HPDs. Workers have a tendency to report more HPD use than actual use on a questionnaire

(Seixas, Neitzel, Stover, et al., 2011). A task card filled out on the day of use may provide more accurate measure of frequency of use (Reeb-Whitaker, Seixas, Sheppard, & Neitzel, 2004), although workers may fail to use the card on a consistent basis (Seixas, Neitzel, Stover, et al., 2011).

Percentage of Employees Using Hearing Protection Devices in Hazardous Noise

Many workers do not use HPDs even when the use is required and the noise levels are hazardous. Therefore, the percentage of workers with required HPD use and those with recommended HPD use can provide some insight into the overall effectiveness of HPDs. Enquiries into the reasons for lack of use might lead to possible solutions for improving the number of individuals using HPDs.

Personal Attenuation Data

Personal attenuation data collected from randomly selected workers can provide an estimate of the number of workers who are inserting or using their HPDs correctly and who are receiving adequate attenuation.

Protected Noise Exposure Data

These levels can be estimated by using the noise exposure levels and personal attenuation data. HPDs that provide in-ear dosimetry can automatically provide this type of data for all workers. If the exposure levels are below the hazardous noise levels, the HPD component can be considered effective.

Audiometric Database Analysis

Analysis of audiometric data can provide several kinds of data, including the number of employees that show a threshold shift, and is described in detail in Chapter 8. The analysis can provide some insight into the overall effectiveness of a hearing conservation program, including the effectiveness of HPDs.

Review Questions

1. Under what circumstances are workers required to wear hearing protection? When is dual protection required? When are administrative controls in addition to dual protection necessary?
2. Discuss the various classifications of HPDs. Review the need for protection from infrasounds and the potential shortcomings of available protection devices.
3. What types of HPDs can be used by workers with hearing loss?
4. Discuss the concept of NRR and the differences between the current and proposed NRR labeling schemes of the EPA for HPDs.
5. Discuss the various factors that should be considered during the selection of HPDs for individual workers.
6. Outline the procedure for taking ear impressions for custom-made HPDs.
7. Discuss the potential advantages of individual fit testing and review various procedures for determining attenuation characteristics of the HPDs for individual ears.
8. Discuss the essential elements of training in the use and care of earplugs and electronic HPDs.
9. What strategies can be used to motivate workers to use HPDs?
10. What outcome measures can be used to evaluate the overall effectiveness of the HPD component of the hearing conservation program?

References

Abou Turk C, Williams AL, Lasky RE. (2009). A randomized clinical trial evaluating silicone earplugs for very low birth weight newborns in intensive care. *J Perinatol.* 29(5):358–363.

American National Standards Institute. (1974). *American National Standard for the Measurement of Real-Ear Hearing Protector Attenuation and Physical Attenuation of Earmuffs* (ANSI S3.19–1974). New York: American National Standards Institute.

American National Standards Institute. (1997). *Methods for Measuring the Real-ear Attenuation of Hearing Protectors* (ANSI S12.6-1997). New York: American National Standards Institute.

American National Standards Institute. (2002). *Microphone-in-Real-Ear and Acoustic Test Fixture Methods for the Measurement of Insertion Loss of Circumaural Hearing Protection Devices* (ANSI S12.42–1995 (R2002). New York: American National Standards Institute.

American National Standards Institute/Acoustical Society of America. (2007). *Methods of Estimating Effective A-weighted Sound Pressure Levels When Hearing Protectors are Worn* (ANSI/ASA S12.68–2007). New York: American National Standards Institute.

American National Standards Institute/Acoustical Society of America. (2008). *Methods for Measuring the Real-Ear Attenuation of Hearing Protectors* (ANSI/ASA S12.6–2008). New York: American National Standards Institute.

American National Standards Institute/American Society of Safety Engineers. (2007). *Hearing Loss Prevention in Construction and Demolition Work. American National Standard for Construction and Demolition Operations* (ANSI/ASSE A10.46–2007). New York: American National Standards Institute.

Arezes PM, Miguel AS. (2002). Hearing protectors acceptability in noisy environments. *Ann Occup Hyg.* 46(6): 531–536.

Behar A. (1985). Field evaluation of hearing protectors. *Noise Control Engineering J.* 24(1):13–18.

Behar A, Crabtree RB. (1997). Measurement of hearing protector attenuation at ultrasonic frequencies. In: Burroughs CD, ed. *Proceedings of Noise-Congress 97.* Poughkeepsie, NY: Noise Control Foundation: 97–102.

Berger EH. (1980). *EARlog-5.* Indianapolis, IN: Aero Company.

Berger EH, Franks JR, Lindgren F.(1996). International review of field studies of hearing protection attenuation. In: Axelsson A, Borchgrevink H, Hamernik RP, Hellstrom

PA, Henderson D, Salvi RJ, eds. *Scientific Basis of Noise-Induced Hearing Loss.* New York: Thieme: 361–377.

Berger EH, Kieper RW. (1991). *Measurement of the Real World Attenuation of E-A-R Foam and ultraFit Brand Earplugs on Production Employees.* Indianapolis, IN: Cabot Safety Corporation, E-A-R 91–30/HP.

Berger EH, Voix J, Kieper RW, Cocq CL. (2011). Development and validation of a field microphone-in-real-ear approach for measuring hearing protector attenuation. *Noise Health.* 13(51):163–175.

Bhattacharya SK, Tripathi SR, Kashyap SK. (1993). Assessment of comfort of various hearing protection devices (HPD). *J Hum Ergol (Tokyo).* 22(2):163–172.

Bockstael A, Keppler H, Dhooge I, et al. (2008). Effectiveness of hearing protector devices in impulse noise verified with transiently evoked and distortion product otoacoustic emissions. *Int J Audiol.* 47(3):119–133.

Byrne DC, Davis RR, Shaw PB, Specht BM, Holland AN. (2011). Relationship between comfort and attenuation measurements for two types of earplugs. *Noise Health.* 13(51):86–92.

Casali JG, Ahroon WA, Lancaster JA. (2009). A field investigation of hearing protection and hearing enhancement in one device: for soldiers whose ears and lives depend upon it. *Noise Health.* 11(42):69–90.

Casali JG, Lam ST, Epps BW. (1987). Rating and ranking methods for hearing protector wearability. *Sound Vibration.* 21(12):10–18.

Daniell WE, Swan SS, McDaniel MM, Camp JE, Cohen MA, Stebbins JG. (2006). Noise exposure and hearing loss prevention programmes after 20 years of regulations in the United States. *Occup Environ Med.* 63(5):343–351.

Danielsson A, Landström U. (1985). Blood pressure changes in man during infrasonic exposure. An experimental study. *Acta Med Scand.* 217(5):531–535.

Davis RR. (2008). What do we know about hearing protector comfort? *Noise Health.* 10(40):83–89.

Davis RR, Shaw PB. (2011). Heat and humidity buildup under earmuff-type hearing protectors. *Noise Health.* 13(51):93–98.

Department of Health and Human Services/National Institute for Occupational Safety and Health. (2004). *Wearing Hearing Protection Properly.* Information Cicular No. 9472. Atlanta, GA: Centers for Disease Control and Prevention.

Department of Health and Human Services/National Institutes of Occupational Safety and Health. (2009). *QuickFit Earplug Test Device.* (NIOSH) Publication No. 2009-112. 534, 1–2. www.cdc.gov/niosh/mining/pubs/pdfs/2009-112.pdf. Accessed July 7, 2011.

El Dib RP, Mathew JL. (2009). Interventions to promote the wearing of hearing protection. *Cochrane Database Syst Rev.* 4:CD005234.

European Parliament and Council. (2003). *Directive 2003/10/EC on the Minimum Health and Safety Requirements Regarding the Exposure of Workers to the Risks Arising from Physical Agents (Noise).* (Seventeenth individual Directive within the meaning of Article 16(1) of Directive 89/391/EEC). *Off J Eur Union.* L42/38–L42/44.

Franks JR, Davis RR, Murphy WJ. (2005). "Field measurement of hearing protection device performance." Proceedings of Inter-noise, 2005, August 7–10.

Hempstock TI, Hill E. (1990, Oct). The attenuations of some hearing protectors as used in the workplace. *Ann Occup Hyg.* 34(5):453–470.

International Electrotechnical Commission, Technical Committee 29, Electoacoustics. (1984). *Occluded-ear Simulator for the Measurement of Earphones Coupled to the Ear by Ear Inserts.* IEC 60711. [Replaced by IEC 60318-4 ed1.0 (2010-01).]

Ivergård TB, Nicholl AG. (1976). User tests of ear defenders. *Am Ind Hyg Assoc J.* 37(3):139–142.

Johnson DL, Patterson J Jr. (1992). Rating of hearing protector performance for impulse noise. In: *Proceedings of Hearing Conservation Conference.* Lexington, KY: Office of Engineering Services, University of Kentucky: 103–106.

Joseph A, Punch J, Stephenson MR, Paneth N, Wolfe E, Murphy WJ. (2007). The effects of training format on earplug performance. *Int J Audiol.* 46(10):609–618.

Karpova NI, Alekseev SV, Erokhin VN, Kadyskina EN, Reutov OV. (1970). Early response of the organism to low-frequency acoustical oscillations. *Noise Vibration Bull.* 11(65):100–103.

Killion MC, Monroe T, Drambarean V. (2011). Better protection from blasts without sacrificing situational awareness. *Int J Audiol.* 50(Suppl 1):S38–S45.

Kwitowski, A. J., Carilli, A. M., & Randolph, R. F. (2010). MultiFit4: An Improved System for hearing protector fit-testing. *Spectrum (Lexington, Ky.), 27*(2), 17–25.

Lempert BL, Edwards RG. (1983). Field investigations of noise reduction afforded by insert-type hearing protectors. *Am Ind Hyg Assoc J.* 44(12):894–902.

Melamed S, Rabinowitz S, Feiner M, Weisberg E, Ribak J. (1996). Usefulness of the protection motivation theory in explaining hearing protection device use among male industrial workers. *Health Psychol.* 15(3):209–215.

Mine Safety and Health Administration. (1999). Health standards for occupational noise exposure: Final rule (30 CFR Part 62, 64). *Federal Register.* 64(176):49548–49634, 49636–49637).

Mohr GC, Cole JN, Guild E, Vongierke HE. (1965). Effects of low frequency and infrasonic noise on man. *Aerosp Med.* 36(9):817–824.

Mrena R, Ylikoski J, Kiukaanniemi H, Mäkitie AA, Savolainen S. (2008). The effect of improved hearing protection regulations in the prevention of military noise-induced hearing loss. *Acta Otolaryngol.* 128(9):997–1003.

Murphy WJ. (2011). Personal attenuation ratings for fit-testing: Estimation and application. Paper presented at the 36th annual Hearing Conservation Conference. Mesa, Ariszona, USA. *Spectrum (Lexington, Ky.).* 28(Supplement II):31.

Murphy WJ, Stephenson MR, Byrne DC, Witt B, Duran J. (2011). Effects of training on hearing protector attenuation. *Noise Health.* 13(51):132–141.

Murphy WJ, Tubbs RL. (2007). Assessment of noise exposure for indoor and outdoor firing ranges. *J Occup Environ Hyg.* 4(9):688–697.

National Institute for Occupational Safety and Health. 1998. *Criteria for a Recommended Standard: Occupational Noise Exposure—Revised Criteria 1998.* (Publication No. 98–126). Atlanta, GA: National Institute for Occupational Safety and Health.

Nixon CW, McKinley RL, Steuver JW. (1992). Performance of active noise reduction headsets. In: Dancer AL, Henderson D, Salvi RJ, Hamernik RP, eds. *Noise Induced Hearing Loss.* St. Louis, MO: Mosby-Year Book: 389–400.

Occupational Safety and Health Administration, National Institute of Occupational Safety and Health, and National Hearing Conservation Alliance. (2008). *Best Practice Bulletin: Hearing Protection-Emerging Trends: Individual Fit Testing.* http://www.hearingconservation.org/associations/10915/files/AllianceRecommendationForFitTesting_Final.pdf. Accessed July 5, 2011.

Occupational Safety and Health Administration. (1983). 29 CFR 1910.95. *Occupational Noise Exposure; Hearing*

Conservation Amendment; Final Rule, effective 8 March 1983. Federal Register. 48:9738–9785.

Pääkkönen R, Tikkanen J. (1991). Attenuation of low-frequency noise by hearing protectors. *Ann Occup Hyg.* 35(2):189–199.

Park MY, Casali JG. (1991a). A controlled investigation of in-field attenuation performance of selected insert, earmuff, and canal cap hearing protectors. *Hum Factors.* 33(6):693–714.

Park MY, Casali JG. (1991b). An empirical study of comfort afforded by various hearing protection devices: Laboratory versus field results. *Applied Acoustics.* 34: 151–179.

Parmentier G, Dancer A, Buck K, Kronenberger G, Beck C. (2000). Artificial head (ATF) for evaluation of hearing protectors. *Acustica.* 86(5):847–852.

Pfeiffer BH, Kuhn HD, Specht U, Knipfer C. (1989). *Sound Attenuation by Hearing Protectors in the Real World.* Sankt Augustin, Germany: Berufsgenossenschaftliches Institutfur Arbietssicherheit, BIA Report 5/89.

Rawool VW, Colligon-Wayne LA. (2008). Auditory lifestyles and beliefs related to hearing loss among college students in the USA. *Noise Health.* 10(38):1–10.

Rawool VW, Davis J. (2010, April). "Unilateral Threshold Shift and Asymmetric HPD Attenuation." Poster presentation at the American Academy of Audiology's annual meeting, AudiologyNOW! 2010, San Diego, CA.

Reeb-Whitaker CK, Seixas NS, Sheppard L, Neitzel R. (2004). Accuracy of task recall for epidemiological exposure assessment to construction noise. *Occup Environ Med.* 61(2):135–142.

Royster JD, Royster LH. (1994). Practical tips for fitting hearing protection. *Hearing Instruments.* 45(2):17–18.

Seixas NS, Neitzel R, Stover B, et al. (2011). A multicomponent intervention to promote hearing protector use among construction workers. *Int J Audiol.* 50(Suppl 1):S46–S56.

Slarve RN, Johnson DL. (1975). Human whole-body exposure to infrasound. *Aviat Space Environ Med.* 46(4 Sec 1):428–431.

U.S. Army Center for Health Promotion and Preventive Medicine. (2004). Pub No. 51–004–0204 *Hearing Conservation.* Aberdeen Proving Ground, MD: U.S. Army Center for Health Promotion and Preventive Medicine.

U.S. Department of Defense. (2004). Instruction 6055.12. *Department of Defense Hearing Conservation Program.* Washington, DC: U.S. Department of Defense.

U.S. Environmental Protection Agency. (1972). Noise Regulation Act. Public Law 92–574, Section 8 [42 U.S.C. 4907] Labeling. p 8. www.nonoise.org/epa/Roll15/roll15doc44.pdf. Accessed July 6, 2011.

U.S. Environmental Protection Agency. (1979). Noise labeling requirement for hearing protectors. *Federal Register.* 44(190)40CFR Part 211:56130–147.

U.S. Environmental Protection Agency. (2009). 40 CFR Part 211 [EPA-HQ-OAR-2003-0024; FRL-8934-9] RIN 2060-A025. Product noise labeling hearing protection devices. *Federal Register.* 74(149):39150–39196.

U.S. Navy and Marine Corps Public Health Center. (2008). *Navy Medical Department Hearing Conservation Program Procedures* (NMCPHC – TM 6260.51.99–2). Portsmouth, VA: U.S. Navy and Marine Corps Public Health Center.

Williams W. (2011). A qualitative assessment of the performance of electronic, level-dependent earmuffs when used on firing ranges. *Noise Health.* 13(51):189–194.

Chapter 7

Training and Motivating Workers to Follow Hearing Conservation Procedures

Although noise control is the most effective means of hearing conservation, the knowledge of workers regarding the effects of noise, the need to conserve hearing, the ways of conserving hearing, and the consequences of carelessness or noncompliance is equally important. Effective education of workers regarding all aspects of hearing conservation is highly critical to the overall success of a hearing conservation program (HCP). Factors outlined in **Fig. 7.1** should be considered in designing the education and motivation component of the HCP.

◆ Applicable Standards

Occupational Safety & Health Administration (1994; 29 CFR 1910.1200)

This standard is titled "Hazards Communication" and requires employers in the manufacturing sector to offer a comprehensive hazard communication program that includes a worker training program. The intent of this standard is to inform workers of health hazards, including the effects of hazardous noise exposure.

Occupational Safety & Health Administration (1983b; 29 CFR 1910.95)

The Occupational Safety and Health Administration (OSHA) requires employers to offer annual training programs to all employees whose noise exposure is 85 dBA time weighted average (TWA) and ensure employee participation. In addition, the information offered during the training sessions must be updated on a regular basis to be consistent with changes in protective equipment and work processes. The employer must ensure that each employee is informed of the effects of noise on hearing; the purpose of hearing protectors; the advantages, disadvantages, and attenuation offered by the various devices; and is instructed on selection, fitting, use, and care of hearing protection devices (HPDs). Employees should also be informed about the purpose of audiometric testing and test procedures. The employees should also have access to the noise standard and any information provided by OSHA about the noise standard. In addition, OSHA should have access to all material relating to an employer's training and education program.

Federal Railroad Administration (2008; 71 FR 63123, Oct. 27, 2006, as amended at 73 FR 79702, Dec. 30, 2008)

The Federal Railroad Administration (FRA) requires railroads to offer an HCP at least once each calendar year and requires employees to complete the training at least once every 3 years. In addition to the information required by OSHA, FRA requires information on noise monitoring, noise levels associated with major categories of equipment and operations, noise operational controls, hazardous noise exposure levels, and procedures for filing an excessive noise report.

U.S. Navy (U.S. Navy and Marine Corps Public Health Center, 2008)

The U.S. Navy requires training before assigning personnel to duties in hazardous noise. Civilians are required to obtain the training from

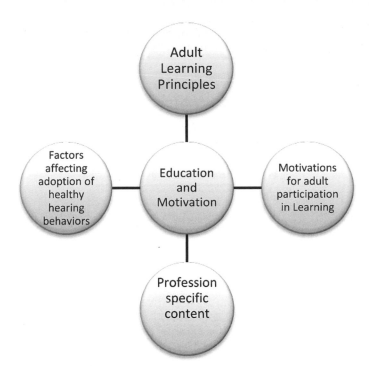

the command during an orientation module. Participation in training has to be documented on the baseline/reference audiogram or in the individual health record.

Initial Training

Initial training should be comprehensive to ensure familiarity with the following topics:

- The physical and psychological effects of noise and hearing loss
- Recognition of posted and unposted space and equipment where hazardous noise is possible
- Audiometric testing and its purpose
- The proper selection, fitting, use, and care of HPDs
- The responsibilities of both supervisors and employees in preventing hearing loss
- Hazards of noise exposure during recreational activities
- Potential impact of hearing loss on job performance and fitness for duty

Refresher Training

Provision of refresher training in conjunction with the annual monitoring audiogram may be more effective.

The U.S. Navy requires documentation of the effectiveness of initial and refresher training via follow-up surveys or other means. Sources for hearing conservation training materials and information are available at www.nmcphc. med.navy.mil/occupational_health/audiology/hearingconservation_toolbox.aspx.

◆ Theoretical Construct and Model for Promoting Preventative Health Behaviors

It is insufficient to provide only knowledge. Even with knowledge, people may not adopt protective behaviors. For example, one study reported that although 75% of the individuals were aware that exposure to loud sounds could cause hearing loss, 50% of them were exposing themselves to loud music. Several factors can influence the adoption of protective or healthy hearing behaviors (Rawool & Colligon-Wayne, 2008), as shown in **Fig. 7.2**. The knowledge of these factors can be helpful in designing educating and motivating sessions that are tailored to meet each worker's unique needs.

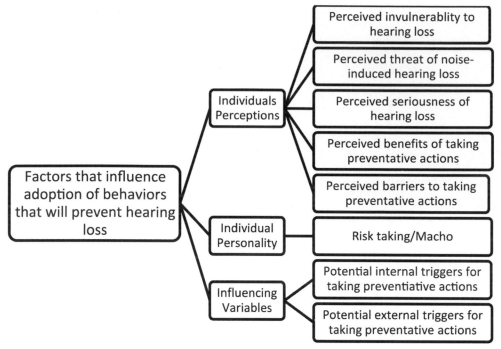

Fig. 7.2 Factors that influence adoption of behaviors that can prevent hearing loss.

◆ Individual Perceptions or Beliefs

Every individual has some perceptions about their work environment, the effect of noise or other ototoxins on them, and the hearing conservation efforts. These perceptions are likely to influence their actions toward preserving hearing.

Perceived Invulnerability to and Threat of Noise-induced Hearing Loss

Some workers may consider themselves invulnerable to hearing loss for a variety of reasons, including those described in the following sections.

Belief That the Noise Levels Are Not High Enough to Damage Hearing

The presence of very high or continuous noise levels leads to higher use of hearing protection (Daniell, Swan, McDaniel, Camp, Cohen, & Stebbins, 2006). If workers perceive the noise as not being too loud or loud enough to cause hearing loss, they may not adopt protective behaviors. Depending on the degree of hearing loss, individuals with hearing loss may actually not hear the noise as well and perceive it as not being too loud.

Belief That Effective Noise Controls Are In Place

Some workers may believe that the noise controls that have been implemented are helping them to protect their hearing. In reality, noise controls may not have reduced the noise exposure sufficiently to protect hearing or in some cases might be ineffective (Reeves, Randolph, Yantek, & Peterson, 2009).

Knowledge about the Percentage of Workers Likely to Suffer Hearing Loss

With a TWA of 90 dBA, 29% of the workers may suffer from hearing loss. Therefore, approximately 71% are not expected to experience hearing loss. Some workers may believe that they will be among those who will not suffer from hearing loss.

Belief That the Worker Is Too Young to Suffer from Hearing Loss

Some workers may believe that only older individuals are prone to having hearing loss.

Belief That Noise Exposure Will Toughen Ears

Some workers may believe that by exposing themselves to noise, they can toughen their hearing and prevent further hearing loss, and that use of hearing protection will prevent toughening from occurring.

Perceived Seriousness of Hearing Loss

Hearing loss is an invisible disability, and full awareness of the implication of the disability may not occur until the disability becomes advanced. Some individuals may also believe that hearing aids will be able to fix their hearing.

Perceived Benefit of Taking Preventative Action

If workers do not strongly believe that noise control procedures or HPDs will help them protect their hearing, they may not adopt the preventative action. Such misconceptions may arise from older workers who might convey the message that they suffered from hearing loss in the presence of noise control or use of HPDs. Such workers may not have been fitted with proper HPDs or may not have used them correctly or efficiently.

Perceived Barriers to Taking Preventative Action

If workers perceive barriers to taking preventative action, they may not use HPDs. For example, some workers may believe that they will not be able to hear important warning signals or may not be able to communicate properly in critical situations with the use of HPDs. If they believe that implementation of noise control procedures reduces their productivity with a potential negative impact on their income, they may not maintain the noise controls. Some workers may hide their dosimeters in lunch boxes if they believe that the company may be shut down and that they will lose their jobs if others become aware of how much noise that they are really

exposed to. Other true barriers may include persistent irritation or infection of the ear canal or middle ear infections. As an example, barriers to the use of hearing protector use by musicians are described in Chapter 9.

Risk-taking or Macho Personality

A few individuals may perceive the use of HPDs as a sign of weakness or not being "manly enough" to tolerate the noise. Some of these behaviors may arise from peer pressure.

Potential Internal Triggers for Taking Preventative Action

Tinnitus: Individuals who have previously experienced tinnitus or are currently suffering from tinnitus are more likely to use HPDs (Rawool & Colligon-Wayne, 2008).

Hearing loss: Previous experience with temporary hearing loss resulting from ear infections can serve as an internal trigger for taking preventative action (Rawool & Colligon-Wayne, 2008).

Difficulty understanding speech following loud sound exposure: This may serve as an internal trigger for those workers who have to communicate regularly following noise exposure perhaps due to another part-time job.

Potential External Triggers for Taking Preventative Action

Requirement for Taking Preventative Action with Vigilant Implementation

Use of HPDs is more prevalent in companies that have a more complete HCP in place.

Media Campaigns

In some cases, the use of media campaigns can be helpful in promoting healthy hearing behaviors.

Example of a Training Program Incorporating Some of the Previously Mentioned Factors

Intervention mapping is an example of a systematic approach to intervention development aimed to improve hearing protection among farm workers and managers. The approach specifies 12 performance objectives (e.g., "monitor hearing with regular testing") that are cross-referenced with six relevant determinants (knowledge and behavioral capability; perceived exposure and susceptibility and noise annoyance; outcome expectations; barriers; social influence; skills and self-efficacy) to create a matrix of objectives for farm workers and their managers. The objectives are divided into five categories: two for both farm workers and their managers, including noticing exposures and taking action, and three only for the managers (surveying and planning, implementation and evaluation, and communication) (Fernandez, Bartholomew, & Alterman, 2009).

◆ Considering Motivations for Adult Participation in Learning

Boshier (1991) listed seven factors that motivate adults to participate in the learning process:

1. Communication improvement
2. Social contact: make friends and meet others
3. Educational preparation
4. Professional advancement or job requirement: they wish to seek advanced job opportunities or it is required to maintain the job
5. Family togetherness
6. Social stimulation: they are trying to escape regular routines and seek stimulation or escape from boredom
7. Cognitive interest: they are learning for the sake of learning itself

The most prevalent factor for participation in training sessions for workers who are enrolled in an HCP is that they are required to do so, or the "external expectation" factor (4). However, some of the seven listed factors can be considered in designing the delivery of the information related to hearing conservation. For example, some social interaction can be inserted in training sessions to capitalize on the social relationships and social welfare factors. As a more specific example, participants could check the accuracy of insertion of HPDs of other workers. For capitalizing on the escape/stimulation factor (6), it is important to revise training materials on a regular basis and to make them as stimulating as possible. Inclusion of challenging problem-solving opportunities can engage and stimulate participants

at the same time and minimize the possibility of boredom.

◆ Consideration of Principles of Effective Adult Learning

Vella (1994) described the following principles of adult learning, which can be applied to the training component of the HCP.

Needs Assessment

It is important to involve participants in deciding what is to be learned. For example, at the beginning of refresher training sessions, it may be useful to ask participants to decide which of the areas of hearing conservation training they feel most deficient in and to emphasize these areas in more detail. For more formal needs assessment and for those participants who might be reluctant to share their needs, it may be useful to provide a checklist of the content of the program and ask participants to check those areas that they would like to be emphasized. At the bottom of the checklist, there should be a place for them to write concerns about other areas that may not necessarily be covered by the checklist. The instructor needs to be flexible in delivering the content to meet the participants' needs. The participants could also provide their input into the overall HCP and how it could be improved.

Safe and Secured Learning Environment

Learners should feel free to express their concerns and issues without having to worry that management or supervisors may not like their comments, causing them to miss promotion opportunities. In the presence of such fears, true learning may be hampered. For example, if they are not wearing HPDs because of discomfort and other types of HPDs are not available, they need to feel free to ask for a trial with other HPDs. Encouraging discussions about concerns with a fellow worker, obtaining a consensus at the beginning about confidentiality of the learning session, or allowing a way to anonymously share concerns online are some of the helpful ways to create a safe environment for the hearing conservation training sessions. Although part of the training should occur in the presence of managers and supervisors to encourage a collaborative effort for the implementation of the HCP, it is also important to offer training in the absence of authority figures.

A Sound Relationship between Instructor and Learner

The instructor should spend some time getting to know each participant (including any hearing difficulties) before beginning the session. In addition, the instructor needs to spend some time in establishing rapport with workers at the beginning of training sessions. Ice-breaking activities such as stating hobbies or sharing some humorous stories without trivialization of the learning session or sharing specific hearing-related concerns at the beginning of the session may be helpful. During group and individual education sessions such as those offered at the end of an annual hearing evaluation, the instructor needs to convey a genuine interest in the well-being of the worker(s) and avoid a mechanical approach, suggesting that the training is being conducted to fulfill the legal requirements.

Well-designed Sequence of Content and Reinforcement

In terms of content, it is important to start with simple content before moving to more complex content. The most important take-home messages should be presented at the beginning of the session for better retention. It is important to provide multiple kinds of reinforcement and feedback to learners about how well they know or learn the material.

Action with Reflection

Learners should have an opportunity to reflect on and apply or implement the information they learn.

Respect for Learners as Subjects of Their Own Learning

It is important to allow participants to learn and master the subject they learn in their own ways. For example, some adults are fast-paced learners who learn more effectively on their own without actively involving themselves in the learning process. If they can demonstrate 100%

knowledge level on a prerefresher training test, and show no threshold shifts on annual evaluations, they might be excused from having to attend the entire training session. This approach may also allow the instructor to focus on those workers who truly need the refresher training.

Cognitive, Affective, and Psychomotor Involvement

Use of projects such as making up creative signs for areas with hazardous noise can allow participants to involve cognition and psychomotor aspects. Simulation of hearing loss or tinnitus, and role-playing workers with hearing loss can allow workers to feel what it might be like to have hearing loss.

Immediacy of the Learning

Although all of the content within the hearing conservation training program is important, workers need to know what the most useful information is and how to apply that information in their everyday work context. Brainstorming sessions on this topic can be helpful.

Clear Roles

The role of the person in charge of the instruction should be clearly defined. There should be written policies about what the instructor's role is and what the worker's role is in the learning process. Companies may adopt disciplinary policies for those workers who either do not show up for training sessions or disrupt the training sessions in any way.

Teamwork

Using small groups for discussions, brainstorming sessions, or collaborative projects can encourage teamwork and enhance learning.

Engagement of Learners

It is important to engage learners in what they are learning. The content should be delivered in an interactive fashion so that all participants have opportunities to engage themselves in the learning process by asking or answering questions, sharing comments, and by commenting or expanding on comments made by other participants. A continuous lecture format without involvement of the audience should be avoided.

Accountability

It is important to determine if the content was delivered completely and effectively, if the learners learned sufficient information about hearing conservation, and if they have the necessary skills such as correct insertion of earplugs or recognizing when noise levels are potentially hazardous to hearing.

◆ Pretraining Preparation

Gather Knowledge about the Target Audience

Examine the target audience, including their specific profession, their specific work environments, their work styles, their relationships with supervisors, and any hobbies including noisy and non-noisy hobbies. Consider any barriers for use of noise control measures and HPDs specific to the work settings. This will allow the trainer to capitalize on the interests of specific individuals and is important for establishing rapport and gaining cooperation

Involve All Related Personnel in Training

Find out the main person responsible for overall worker safety and find out all personnel besides workers or employees whose attendance at the hearing conservation training sessions has the potential for improving the effectiveness of the program, including management, consultants, and all members of the hearing conservation team, including noise control engineers, supervisors, union officials, and vendors of manufacturing equipment.

Collaborate with All Members of the Hearing Conservation Team

Discuss the specific roles of various team members in the HCP—and specifically in the different aspects of the training program—to ensure that all aspects are properly covered. Members need to be aware of the important roles played by each member of the team.

Schedule the Group Training Sessions Efficiently

Select the most suitable days and time for the training program in consultation with managers and supervisors to minimize any negative impact on or interference with production. Arrange for different training activities through the year to ensure that hearing conservation remains in the forefront and is not lost or forgotten in the daily rigors of work-related duties.

Prepare an Outline of the Content of the Program

Outline the general content of the program with the most information delivered at the beginning of the program. Tailor the content of the program to meet the needs of the specific target audience. Also, adjust the content by taking into account the context in which the training is being offered.

Consider the Context in Which Training is Being Offered

Small Employee Group Sessions

The attenuation performance of HPDs is similar for young adults regardless of whether they receive individual or group (five participants) training. Thus, group training for proper HPD insertion may be more cost-effective, at least for young adults (Joseph, Punch, Stephenson, Paneth, Wolfe, & Murphy, 2007).

Part of Regular Safety Meetings

In this context, the possibility of hearing loss needs to be made very obvious because of the invisible nature of hearing loss. The message about hearing conservation should not get masked by other obvious safety concerns such as visible physical injuries, including eye injuries.

Self-education through Videotapes, DVDs, or Computer Software

This type of training should be used as an adjunct to in-person training because the needs of individuals workers may not be met through this type of training.

Individual Training Sessions

The best time to provide individual training sessions is immediately after annual/periodic monitoring audiograms. During the baseline audiogram session, full explanation of the audiogram and the audiometric test procedures should be provided. During annual monitoring, workers can be questioned about what they remember about the audiogram and test procedures, and any missing information should be repeated. For example, a worker can be asked to compare the baseline thresholds to the new audiogram to see if there are any changes in thresholds. The worker can be asked to evaluate if there is any difference in the right or left ear thresholds. During this session, the effectiveness of the worker's HPD can also be assessed by considering noise exposure and any changes in hearing. Any needs for changing the specific type of device used depending on discomfort or any other factors can also be assessed during this session. A worker can be asked to demonstrate the insertion of the HPDs and explain care, maintenance, and/or replacement procedures.

Prepare/Collect Training Aids

Effective educational aids can help in keeping the training sessions lively and motivating the workers to adopt hearing conservation strategies. The types of educational aids that can be used are PowerPoint slides that incorporate animations, video or short movie clips, and Internet sites that can demonstrate simulated hearing loss and tinnitus. Additionally, handouts, pamphlets, and other materials such as a copy of the relevant regulations should also be made available. Some pamphlets are readily available from the National Institute of Occupational Safety and Health (NIOSH) website. Other useful pamphlets can be obtained from the National Hearing Conservation Association. A variety of HPDs including worn or abused devices, assistive listening devices for workers with hearing loss, various hearing aids, and different types of alerting devices, dosimeters, and sound level meters should also be available for demonstrations.

Prepare or Plan for Pre- and Postassessments

Preassessments can assist in determining the content that workers seem to be less knowledgeable about and thus need to be highlighted during training. Postassessments can allow determination of the efficacy of the training sessions and aid in determining the efficacy of the HCP.

The NIOSH Hearing Loss Prevention Attitude-Belief survey (Franks & Stephenson, 1994) was designed with the assumption that to achieve positive noise-protective behaviors in workers, their beliefs and intentions need to change. The survey has 26 items representing 10 content areas. Four of the content areas evaluate the barriers perceived by the workers for the use of HPDs, including comfort, muffling of important sounds, communication difficulty, and convenience. Four additional content areas evaluate workers' perception about susceptibility to hearing loss, severity of the consequences of hearing loss, benefits of preventative actions, and barriers to preventative action. Workers' behaviors are assessed through the social norms and behavioral intentions scales. In addition, a self-efficacy scale is incorporated in the survey. Individuals are expected to respond using a five-point Likert scale: (1) strongly agree, (2) disagree; (3) neither agree nor disagree, (4) agree, and (5) strongly agree. An improvement in the scores on the attitude scale of the survey may reflect that the training or parts of training were effective (Joseph, Punch, Stephenson, Paneth, Wolfe, & Murphy, 2007).

Goals of Training

The training should be designed to achieve the following goals:

1. Workers will review all effects of occupational and nonoccupational noise on hearing.
2. Workers will discuss the effects of ototoxins on hearing.
3. Workers will recognize exposure to hazardous noise and ototoxins and will report the exposure to safety personnel or management.
4. Workers will fully and truthfully participate in the measurements of noise levels and exposures.
5. Workers will participate in developing a plan for noise control and take all measures to implement and maintain noise control procedures.
6. Workers will undergo annual audiometric monitoring and will understand the results of audiometric testing.

7. Workers will properly use and maintain their HPDs or any other protective devices designed to reduce exposure to ototoxins.
8. Workers will fully participate in assessing the effectiveness of the HCP.

Content of the Program

Although the general content should include elements required by OSHA or the U.S. Navy, somewhat different content can be presented to management and supervisors versus workers to address the information and motivation needed by each entity.

Outline of Content Specific to Management and Supervisors

- Different components of an effective HCP
- Compliance with regulations and potential fines for lack of compliance
- Estimated cost of the HCP
- Potential for workers' compensation and any related legal costs
- Results and benefits of the current HCP
  ◇ Annual report of percentage of workers with and without standard or NIOSH threshold shifts
  ◇ Report on the effectiveness of any noise control measures

Motivational Aspects of Training

Several strategies discussed previously can be helpful in motivating workers. In addition to those strategies, examples of permanent and temporary hearing loss can be shown on the audiograms, and the consequences of hearing loss can be explained. Similarly, examples of tonal and noisy tinnitus can be demonstrated, and the potential consequences can be explained to workers.

Helping Workers Understand the Potential Impact of Future Hearing Loss

Videos or DVDs with vivid nature pictures and nature sounds can be played with full sound, minimal sound, and minimum treble to partially mimic high-frequency loss. During this demonstration, workers with hearing loss should be provided with some amplification or FM devices to ensure full understanding of the material. Similarly, videos of social conversations with full, minimal, or filtered sounds can also be helpful. Several suitable video clips are available on the Internet that can be downloaded free of charge. Shorter clips interspersed with interactive discussions may be more effective depending on the audience. Multimedia programs such as the NIOSH hearing loss prevention (HLP) training program, which consists of a short instructional mini-movie, a HLP program motivational video, and a prerecorded slide presentation showing HPD fitting and verification procedure, can be effective in promoting effective insertion of HPDs (Joseph, Punch, Stephenson, Paneth, Wolfe, & Murphy, 2007).

◆ Ensuring Transference of Learning

It is important to ensure that learning is transferred to the work environment. Incorporation of the following elements (**Fig. 7.3**) in the training session can enhance transference:

Association: Present new information in the context of what workers already know. For example, if they report that they remember that hazardous noise exposure results in hearing loss, ask them to discuss the potential impact of noise-induced hearing loss or other effects of noise. If they have experienced temporary thresholds shifts or tinnitus, it is better to discuss permanent hearing loss in this context.

Similarity: Use material that is similar to what workers already know. For example, if workers have previously seen normal and noise-exposed cochlear structures, use of similar pictures can enhance learning. The picture can be enhanced by adding different colors or animations to avoid boredom. Instead of lecturing with the visual aids, workers can be asked to observe and discuss the differences in the normal and damaged cochlea.

Degree of original learning: It is important to plan for and offer very effective baseline training sessions. What the workers learn during the baseline session and how well they apply that information is going to have a strong effect on how well they continue to adopt healthy hearing behaviors to accommodate any changes in their work environment.

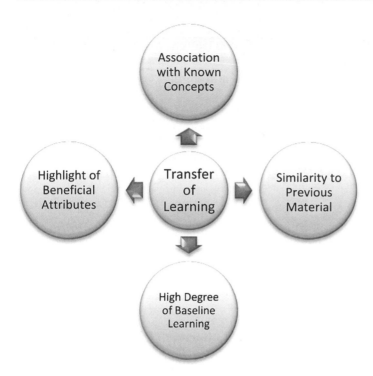

Fig. 7.3 Elements that can enhance transfer of learning.

Highlight beneficial attributes: It is important to include elements in training that are extremely beneficial or critical to the worker's specific profession or work environment. For example, if hearing is critical to the job and if hearing loss can compromise work efficiency, this should be emphasized. If there are incentives for proper use of HPDs, these should be emphasized.

◆ Computer-based Interventions

Computer-based interventions can be a cost-effective way of providing training. As an example, a multimedia program has been developed to increase the use of HPDs among workers exposed to hazardous noise (Eakin, Brady, & Lusk, 2001). The program appears to have been effective in increasing HPD use among construction (Lusk, Hong, Ronis, Eakin, Kerr, & Early, 1999) and factory (Lusk, Ronis, Kazanis, Eakin, Hong, & Raymond, 2003) workers. Computer-based audiometric testing, attitude testing through a questionnaire, and tailored feedback and education based on the audiometric results and responses to the questionnaire through

multimedia technology appears to be feasible and is liked by workers (Hong & Csaszar, 2005).

The National Center for Rehabilitative Auditory Research has developed a multimedia, computer-based, self-administered HLP program that will be available in two forms: one targeting active duty military personnel and the other targeting veterans to minimize the progression of hearing loss resulting from social, recreational, and nonmilitary occupational noise exposure (Saunders & Griest, 2009). The program incorporates the principles of the Health Belief Model (Rosenstock, 1966) and the Health Promotion Model (Pender, Murdaugh, & Parsons, 2002). Potential advantages and disadvantages of computer-based training are shown in **Table 7.1**.

Steps for Developing Computer-based Training

Hong and Csaszar (2005) outlined the following steps for developing a computer-based training program:

1. Determine objectives and related material to be included in the training.

Table 7.1   Advantages and Disadvantages of Computer-based Training

Advantages	Limitations	Possible techniques for addressing disadvantages
Cost-effective delivery of instruction to a large group of individuals	High costs for developing computer-based training programs.	Seek funding support from industries, as the training cost may be reduced later.
Individuals can complete the training at their own convenience	Individuals must have access to a computer and any attached hardware if audiometric testing is performed simultaneously.	Provide access to some computers and hardware on the industry premises in sound-isolated areas.
There is no need for an educator or trainer to be present	A skilled multidisciplinary team is required to develop computer-based training.	The same team can be employed to develop computer-based training in other areas of safety.
Individuals may feel a sense of confidentiality about their learning pace or ability	Impersonal training; the software may not necessarily gear to the specific profession of the worker.	During development and testing, build flexibility to allow insertion of profession-specific comments on video clips.
Individuals complete the training at their own pace (slow or fast)	Extended design and production hours for developing effective computer-based training.	Build adequate funding sources.
Active involvement of participants in the learning process through higher interaction	Individuals vary in terms of how they react to audiometric test results or any questionnaires. The unique reactions require unique responses in terms of psychosocial support and motivation, which can be provided by an experienced trainer. The tailored intervention offered by computers is likely to be limited.	Do not rely solely on computer-based training. Always supplement it with an individual training session.
Easy insertion of video or media clips allows enhancement of interest in the training	Any video clips used within computer-based interventions can get outdated in terms of the fashion trends (clothing, hair, etc.), the current or local language structures, or technical advances. Under such circumstances, workers may not be able to relate to individuals in the video clip.	During development and design, build flexibility to allow insertion of current video clips.
Efficient recordkeeping for meeting the requirements of regulations	The records may generate a false impression of an efficient training component.	Do not rely solely on records.
Efficient collection of data for evaluating the effectiveness of training	Although immediately after the end of the training participants may respond to questions correctly, this may not necessarily translate into better protective behaviors. The records may give false impressions of use of HPDs.	Augment the evaluation of the knowledge base of workers by onsite observation of noise controls and use of HPDs. Include pre- and post-training tests. Several questions should be devised and should be randomly presented so that workers cannot memorize answers.

2. Create detailed scripts (the material that will appear on each screen from beginning to end).
3. Seek feedback from external reviewers on the scripts and make necessary modifications.
4. Develop decision algorithms (rules) for providing feedback and information to workers.
5. Design graphics and record any audio and video clips to be included in the training.
6. Develop computer software and database.
7. Pilot test the software and seek reviews from external content experts or experienced educators.
8. Based on the results of the pilot test and feedback from external experts, make necessary changes to remove glitches and to enhance the software.

◆ Effectiveness of a Hearing Conservation Training

Participation in a hearing conservation training program can increase knowledge about hearing health and can increase the use of HPDs (Chesky, Pair, Yoshimura, & Landford, 2009; Cunningham, Curk, Hoffman, & Pride, 2006; Ewigman, Kivlahan, Hosokawa, & Horman, 1990; Joseph, Punch, Stephenson, Paneth, Wolfe, & Murphy, 2007; Knobloch & Broste, 1998). The auditory thresholds of employees who participated in HCPs, including training at five fabrication plants, showed less deterioration after 5 years than a control group not exposed to occupational noise (Lee-Feldstein, 1993). Such findings suggest that hearing conservation training has the potential to conserve hearing of workers exposed to hazardous noise.

Review Questions

1. Discuss OSHA requirements in reference to the education or training component of an HCP.
2. Review the factors that can influence the adoption of protective or healthy hearing behaviors in the context of hearing conservation.
3. Outline factors that motivate adults to participate in the learning process.
4. Review the principles of effective adult learning.
5. What type of pretraining preparation is necessary before offering training to workers enrolled in the HCP?

6. What should be the goals of training that is offered as a part of the HCP?
7. What specific content will you include for supervisors and managers?
8. What type of strategies will you use to help workers understand the potential impact of hearing loss?
9. Discuss the advantages and disadvantages of computer-based training.
10. Outline the steps involved in designing computer-based training.

References

Boshier R. (1991). Psychometric properties of the alternative form of the educational participation scale. *Adult Education Quarterly.* 41(3):150–167.

Chesky K, Pair M, Yoshimura E, Landford S. (2009). An evaluation of musician earplugs with college music students. *Int J Audiol.* 48(9):661–670.

Cunningham DR, Curk A, Hoffman J, Pride J. (2006). Despite high risk of hearing loss, many percussionists play unprotected. *Hearing J.* 59(6):58–66.

Daniell WE, Swan SS, McDaniel MM, Camp JE, Cohen MA, Stebbins JG. (2006). Noise exposure and hearing loss prevention programmes after 20 years of regulations in the United States. *Occup Environ Med.* 63(5):343–351.

Eakin BL, Brady JS, Lusk SL. (2001). Creating a tailored, multimedia, computer-based intervention. *Comput Nurs.* 19(4):152–160, quiz 161–163.

Ewigman BG, Kivlahan CH, Hosokawa MC, Horman D. (1990). Efficacy of an intervention to promote use of hearing protection devices by firefighters. *Public Health Rep.* 105(1):53–59.

Federal Railroad Administration. (2006). *71 FR 63123, (Oct. 27, 2006). As amended at 73 FR 79702, Dec. 30, 2008. Part 227. Occupational Noise Exposure.* Washington, DC: Federal Railroad Administration.

Fernandez ME, Bartholomew LK, Alterman T. (2009). Planning a multilevel intervention to prevent hearing loss among farmworkers and managers: a systematic approach. *J Agric Saf Health.* 15(1):49–74.

Franks JR, Stephenson MR. (1994). *The Development of a Hearing Conservation Attitude Survey: Final Report.* NIOSH contract 211-93-0006. Atlanta, GA: National Institute for Occupational Safety and Health.

Hong O, Csaszar P. (2005). Audiometric testing and hearing protection training through multimedia technology. *Int J Audiol.* 44(9):522–530.

Joseph A, Punch J, Stephenson M, Paneth N, Wolfe E, Murphy W. (2007). The effects of training format on earplug performance. *Int J Audiol.* 46(10):609–618.

Knobloch MJ, Broste SK. (1998). A hearing conservation program for Wisconsin youth working in agriculture. *J Sch Health.* 68(8):313–318.

Lee-Feldstein A. (1993). Five-year follow-up study of hearing loss at several locations within a large automobile company. *Am J Ind Med.* 24(1):41–54.

Lusk SL, Hong OS, Ronis DL, Eakin BL, Kerr MJ, Early MR. (1999). Effectiveness of an intervention to increase construction workers' use of hearing protection. *Hum Factors.* 41(3):487–494.

Lusk SL, Ronis DL, Kazanis AS, Eakin BL, Hong O, Raymond DM. (2003). Effectiveness of a tailored intervention to increase factory workers' use of hearing protection. *Nurs Res.* 52(5):289–295.

Occupational Safety and Health Administration. (1994). 29 CFR 1910.1200. Hazard communication; Final rules. *Federal Register* 59:6126–6184.

Occupational Safety and Health Administration. (1983). 29 CFR 1910.95. Occupational noise exposure; hearing conservation amendment; final rule, effective 8 March 1983. *Federal Register.* 48:9738–9785.

Pender NJ, Murdaugh CL, Parsons MA. (2002). *Health Promotion in Nursing Practice*, 2nd ed. Upper Saddle River, NJ: Prentice Hall.

Rawool VW, Colligon-Wayne LA. (2008). Auditory lifestyles and beliefs related to hearing loss among college students in the USA. *Noise Health.* 10(38):1–10.

Reeves ER, Randolph RF, Yantek DS, Peterson JS. (2009). *Noise Control in Underground Metal Mining.* Information Circular 9518, DHHS (NIOSH) Publication No. 2010–111. Atlanta, GA: National Institute for Occupational Safety and Health

Rosenstock IM. (1966). Why people use health services. *Milbank Mem Fund Q.* 44(3):94–127.

Saunders GH, Griest SE. (2009). Hearing loss in veterans and the need for hearing loss prevention programs. *Noise Health.* 11(42):14–21.

U.S. Navy and Marine Corps Public Health Center. (2008). *Navy Medical Department Hearing Conservation Program Procedures* (NMCPHC – TM 6260.51.99–2). Portsmouth, VA: U.S. Navy and Marine Corps Public Health Center.

Vella J. (1994). *Learning to Listen, Learning to Teach.* San Francisco: Jossey-Bass, 3–22.

Chapter 8

Evaluating and Improving the Effectiveness of Hearing Conservation Programs

It is insufficient to have a hearing conservation program (HCP) in place. It is important to evaluate whether or not the program is effectively preventing hearing loss. All components of the HCP should be thoroughly and carefully evaluated to determine the degree to which the HCP is in compliance with the relevant or applicable regulation and whether or not it is successful in conserving hearing. An important subcomponent of the evaluation is to make changes for correcting deficiencies in a timely and cost-effective manner. If the outcomes of the evaluation are not used to correct deficiencies, the evaluations are of no value.

◆ Sample of Applicable Regulations

Occupational Safety & Health Administration (1983; 29 CFR 1910.95)

The standard requires employers to administer a continuing effective HCP. The best way to ensure that the program is effective as required by the Occupational Safety and Health Administration (OSHA) is to perform an ongoing assessment of the HCP.

U.S. Department of Defense (2004; Instruction 6055.12, Hearing Conservation Program, March 5, 2004)

The U.S. Department of Defense (DoD) requires annual evaluation of the effectiveness of an HCP based on the prevalence of standard threshold shifts (STSs) during annual audiograms and the

percentage of employees enrolled in the HCP receiving annual audiograms.

U.S. Navy Hearing Conservation Program Requirements (U.S. Navy and Marine Corps Public Health Center, 2008)

The U.S. Navy requires at least annual evaluations of program effectiveness using the percentage of employees enrolled in the HCP receiving annual audiograms, the percentage of employees with STS, and the percentage of employees with OSHA-recordable hearing loss.

◆ Frequency of Hearing Conservation Program Evaluations and Improvements

Ideally, all components of the HCP should be evaluated on an ongoing basis. For example, if a worker notices an increase in noise in a particular area, he should take the initiative to notify his supervisor and/or the HCP team. The HCP implementers should then measure the noise levels and take appropriate steps to control the noise (see Chapters 2 and 3). Similarly, when an STS is apparent in a worker, the cause of the STS should be determined through careful program evaluation. If the STS is due to a poorly fitted hearing protection device (HPD), it should be corrected. Besides ongoing program evaluations and correction of deficiencies, the entire program should be evaluated at least annually. Such evaluations will reveal deficiencies that are not obvious but can negatively affect the outcomes of the HCP.

◆ Individuals Responsible for Assessing Effectiveness

Management, program implementers, or the HCP team should conduct periodic program evaluations.

Responsibilities of Management

The responsibilities of management in assessing program effectiveness during the two phases of program evaluations are as follows (Franks, Stephenson, & Merry, 1996):

Evaluation of Effectiveness Phase

◆ Dedication of adequate resources for a comprehensive program evaluation
◆ Hiring and maintaining individuals who are qualified and trained to collect and analyze relevant data and to evaluate the HCP
◆ Attending to comments and reactions of noise-exposed workers and making use of the comments to evaluate any program deficiencies
◆ Ensuring that the HCP is evaluated on a regular basis

Using the Outcomes of the Evaluation Phase

◆ Commitment to accept and correct any deficiencies revealed by the periodic evaluation
◆ Dedication of financial and personnel resources to correct any deficiencies
◆ Determination to institute and carry out any necessary disciplinary measures for noncompliance (e.g., not using HPDs)

Responsibilities of the Program Implementer or the Hearing Conservation Program Team

Evaluation of Effectiveness Phase

◆ Commitment of sufficient time and other resources to conduct a comprehensive evaluation
◆ Performance of the audiometric database analyses with or without assistance of an outside conductor or contractor to complete the analyses
◆ Commitment to detect problems or deficiencies sooner following best practices. For example, detection of National Institute of Occupational Safety and Health (NIOSH) STS and correction of related deficiencies is better than waiting until the OSHA STS is apparent
◆ Willingness to ask questions, not being afraid to seek out elusive information, and interacting with all members of the hearing loss prevention program team. For example, if removal of some noise control measures is apparent, it is important to find out who removed the measures and why and when they were removed

Using the Outcomes of the Evaluation Phase

◆ Effective communication of findings to management and to affected employees
◆ Willingness and persistence in taking steps to correct any detected deficiencies

Responsibilities of the Employees during the Evaluation of Hearing Conservation Program Effectiveness

Evaluation of Effectiveness Phase

◆ Provision of feedback to the management and the HCP team
◆ Willingness to communicate problems, concerns, and difficulties related to implementing and maintaining required changes such as noise control measures or use of HPDs. If a particular HPD is uncomfortable or is causing communication difficulties, the HCP team and management needs to know about such issues
◆ Paying attention to the noise levels in the environment and reporting any perceived changes in levels

Using the Outcomes of the Evaluation Phase

◆ Cooperating in correcting all deficiencies and maintaining any noise control measures

Basic Approaches to Program Evaluation

Some examples of basic approaches that can be used in evaluating the HCP are as follows:

◆ To assess if the program is in compliance with the related regulation (e.g., OSHA, Mine Safety and Health Administration [MSHA], Federal Railroad Administration, DoD, etc.)
◆ To detect deficiencies in the implementation of the program's components

- To quantify improvements in the HCP
- To evaluate the audiometric thresholds of workers
- To evaluate the effectiveness of each component of the HCP

◆ Assessment of Program Compliance with Related Regulations

To evaluate the compliance of the program, the relevant regulations should be carefully read by the HCP team. Preparation of a checklist for any relevant regulations along with best practices can help in efficient evaluation of the program against the relevant standard. An example of a list for assessing if the noise measurement and engineering noise control components of the HCP are in compliance (partially based on the U.S. Navy HCP requirements [U.S. Navy and Marine Corps Public Health Center, 2008]) is shown in **Table 8.1**. Other checklists for OSHA and MSHA compliance are readily available at the NIOSH website (Franks, Stephenson, & Merry, 1996).

Potential Limitations of Checklist Audits

In checking whether or not various portions of the HCP are in compliance, the evaluator has to often rely on the information provided by the program implementers. The information needs to be accurate and not simply provided to give the appearance that the program is in compliance. A careful evaluation of all records along with the checklist can be useful in confirming the validity of answers provided by program implementers. It should be noted that compliance based on checklists does not necessarily mean that the program is effective. The rates of STSs may be high in the presence of high compliance reported on checklists (Wolgemuth, Luttrell, Kamhi, & Wark, 1995).

◆ Seeking Feedback from Management and Employees

Feedback from management and workers can provide unique insights into HCP deficiencies, reasons for such deficiencies, and potential solutions for correcting the deficiencies that may not be apparent using other assessment procedures. The feedback can be obtained by using structured interviews or focus groups.

Interviews of Management and Employees

Structured interviews of management and employees using the types of lists shown in **Table 8.1** can provide information about discrepancies in perception of managers and employees and areas that need further closer evaluations. Such areas could be explored along with the related records to find the reasons for discrepancies. Any program deficiencies revealed through such evaluations should be addressed.

As an example, some of the HCP deficiencies revealed by one study (Daniell, Swan, McDaniel, Stebbins, Seixas, & Morgan, 2002) using structured interviews of management and employees with lists of questions, noise monitoring, and audiometric record evaluations were as follows:

- Noise exposure: The mean full-shift time weighted average (TWA) for noise exceeded 95 dBA in 22% of the sample. Peak levels were higher than 140 dBA in 66% of samples, and the maximum sound pressure level exceeded 115 dBA in 72% of the sample. Only 1 of the 10 companies had planned any new engineered noise controls, and no company had planned any new administrative controls.
- Hearing protectors: Five of the ten companies reported evaluating hearing protector attenuation but only by using manufacturer's specifications without derating the noise reduction rating and without considering noise exposure levels.
- Education and training: Annual training was never or intermittently provided at 3 of the 10 companies. Training at the other 7 companies usually comprised only a noninteractive video presentation in English to all workers, including those who did not have English language fluency.

Advantages and Limitations of Interviews

The advantages of interviews are that programs or program components that do not have optimum effectiveness can be quickly identified. The limitation of interviews is that there could be a reporting bias, which can lead to underestimation of program deficiencies (Daniell, Swan, McDaniel, Stebbins, Seixas, & Morgan, 2002). For example, workers may show reporting bias due to fear of business closure due to lack of compliance with subsequent loss of their jobs or fear of negative consequences in terms of lack of

Table 8.1 Example of a Checklist for Assessing the Compliance of the Noise Level and Engineering Noise Control Components of the HCP

Program component	Implemented?		
	Yes	No	Comment

Noise levels and exposure measurements

Are individuals making the noise and exposure measurements trained/qualified?

Who made the measurements?

- Industrial hygienist
- Audiologist
- Safety specialist
- Exposure monitor
- An individual who is adequately trained by taking the Exposure Monitoring course or other training approved by the U.S. Navy and Marine Corps Public Health Center

Is the equipment used for noise measures functioning adequately?

- Was the calibration of sound level meters and dosimeters checked prior to each measurement?

Are records available for noise measures?

Dosimetry: The 8-h TWA

- With 3 dB exchange rate (U.S. Navy)
- With 5 dB exchange rate (OSHA)

Sound level meter:

- Real time SPL in dBA
- Real time SPL in dBC
- Impulse measures using the peak response option
- Are sources with loudest sound emissions identified in areas where noise exceeds 84 dBA?

Are all unusual noise exposures measured and recorded?

- Greater than 16 h of continuous or intermittent noise exposure per day
- Intense low-frequency noises with difference in A- and C-weighted levels of greater than 15 dB
- Noises above 140 dBA
- Impulse noises above 165 dB peak SPL

Were all involved parties informed about the performance and result of noise measures?

- Workers
- Managers
- Noise control engineers
- Individuals conducting auditory monitoring/medical surveillance

Are all areas with potentially hazardous noise identified with signs?

Are all workers exposed to potentially hazardous noise levels identified and enrolled in HCP using relevant criteria?

For example, exposure to 8-h TWA exceeding 84 dBA on average for more than 2 days a month or impact or impulse noise of 140 dB peak SPL or greater peak SPL.

For personnel that are not enrolled in the HCP, was the decision made by qualified individuals (industrial hygienist, audiologist, or occupational medicine physician) after evaluating noise surveys and audiometric history?

Frequency of noise measures

Are noise measures performed at least initially?

Are noise measures made within 30 days following notification of potential changes in noise levels?

Engineering noise control

Are attempts made to eliminate or reduce hazardous noise levels?

Were the noise controls effective and to what extent?

Is there a periodic schedule for maintenance of noise control measures and equipment to minimize noise?

HCP, health conservation program; OSHA, Occupational Safety and Health Administration; SPL, sound pressure level; TWA, time weighted average.

promotion by the management if their responses did not match with those provided by management. For example, Daniell and colleagues (2002) reported that none of the 10 companies they evaluated had a copy of the hearing conservation standard or related informational materials and no interviewed representative had ever read the standard. However, 35% of the interviewed employees reported availability of the standard as well as other information materials.

◆ Focus Groups

A focus group is a qualitative research tool that is frequently used in social research, business, and marketing. Focus groups are valuable in gauging opinions and attitudes, in assessing effectiveness of procedures, and in generating recommendations.

Prince, Colligan, Stephenson, and Bischoff (2004) conducted focus groups of employees, supervisors, and managers with four goals: (1) to obtain a historical viewpoint of hearing conservation practices and policies over time, (2) to gain an in-depth understanding of the actual implementation of the various program components, (3) to gauge actual worker acceptance of the program, and (4) to spot ongoing employee training/informational needs related to hearing conservation. The focus groups in this study provided valuable information in areas where paper documentation was sparse or where onsite observations did not agree with initial paper audits. For example, the study revealed that implementation of engineering noise controls, which were only partially effective in reducing hazardous noise levels, may have led to contentment, reduced HPD use in the presence of hazardous noise levels, and thus more hearing loss.

Advantages and Limitations of Focus Groups

The advantages of focus groups are that they are good for groups with lower literacy levels (e.g., migrant workers), they can provide in-depth data through the direct interactions between facilitators and workers, the generated comments are spontaneous, and workers are able to build on other worker's responses.

Limitations of the use of focus groups for assessing effectiveness of HCPs are that group facilitators need to have excellent skills including the ability to handle various personalities such as experts, quiet persons, outsiders, friends, hostile persons, etc. The facilitator needs to listen attentively with sensitivity and empathy and be able to think at the same time. The facilitator also needs to have adequate knowledge of the topic of hearing conservation. Another limitation is that analyses of the unstructured data may be time-consuming or cumbersome. In addition, workers may try to conform to the opinions of supervisors or managers due to fears of lack of confidentiality of statements made during the focus groups even after initial instructions that include the statement that what is discussed within the focus group should not leave the room.

◆ Use of Task-based Statistics

Task-based statistics can provide useful information to program implementers and managers and alert them of the need for any changes. Two examples of these types of statistics are as follows.

Compliance with Audiometric Testing

This is calculated by taking the number of individuals enrolled in the HCP who have a current audiogram (obtained within last 12 months), dividing it by the number of individuals enrolled, and multiplying the number by 100. Thus, if there are 100 individuals enrolled in the HCP and 78 have a current audiogram, the compliance is 78%. Program implementers then could explore the reasons for lack of current audiograms for 22% of employees and address any deficiencies. For example, consequences could be implemented for those who do not show up for audiometric testing without valid reasons (e.g., prolonged illness).

Compliance with Hearing Protection Device Use

This can be calculated by taking the number of individuals in an area where HPD use is required who are observed (through random checks) using HPDs, dividing it by the number of individuals required to use HPDs, and multiplying the number by 100. Thus if 10 employees in an area are required to use HPDs and 6 were observed using the HPDs, then the compliance is 60%. In this case, the reasons for low compliance rates should be investigated, and measures should be implemented to correct the deficiency. This approach can be strengthened by determining the number of workers who are using their HPDs correctly with proper insertion depth and proper replacement of worn out devices as needed.

◆ Use of Noise Exposure Statistics

Noise exposure statistics can provide useful information about the noise measurement and noise control components of the HCP. Examples of noise exposure statistics are as follows:

- Percentage of workforce in potentially hazardous noise based on dosimetry (8-hour TWA above 84 dBA with a 3 dB exchange rate)
- Percentage of workforce in potentially hazardous noise based on hazardous impact noise exposure measures (peak SPLs of 140 dB or higher)
- Percentage of workforce exposed to hazardous noise during certain tasks, although the daily noise dose may be low
- Number of areas or machines where engineering noise controls were implemented
- Effectiveness of noise control measures in dB in terms of the difference between precontrol noise levels and postcontrol noise levels
- Percentage of employees removed from the HCP due to reduction in noise dose

◆ Evaluation of Audiometric Data

Evaluation of audiometric data can provide useful information about the effectiveness of HCPs by revealing whether or not the hearing of workers is being preserved.

Evaluation of Program Effectiveness Based on the Variability in Serial Monitoring Audiometry (American National Standards Institute S12.13 TR-2002)

This approach to the evaluation of HCP effectiveness involves the following steps:

1. Compile the audiograms including demographic information.

2. Retain the first valid monitoring audiogram per person per year. Drop baseline audiograms and any retest audiograms unless retesting was conducted for reasons unrelated to noise-induced temporary threshold shift.

3. Choose a restricted database for analysis. Ideally, a sample size of at least 30 employees is recommended to generate reliable results. The selection of the restricted database will depend on the desired outcome.
   ◇ For assessing the effect of recent hearing conservation efforts on senior employees, choose employees who have at least 10 monitoring audiograms and then evaluate the variability in the 4 latest monitoring audiograms.
   ◇ For assessing the effect of recent hearing conservation efforts on newly hired employees, choose employees who have at least three monitoring audiograms and then evaluate the variability in these audiograms.
   ◇ For evaluating the effectiveness of the HCP since the time it was initiated, select the audiograms of employees who have a baseline audiogram during the year the HCP was initiated and also have all annual/monitoring audiograms through the current year.
   ◇ If audiometric data are available for a matching control group of non-noise–exposed employees, use the control group data for comparison to the noise-exposed restricted group.

4. Plot the average auditory thresholds of the restricted groups for each year and test frequency to visually examine any aberrations in the data. If the data appears to be reliable, proceed with analysis.

5. Calculate the following two indicators of variability for the control and the restricted groups:
   ◇ Percent worse sequential ($\%W_s$): This is the percentage of workers who show 15 dB worsening of thresholds at any test frequency in either ear between two sequential audiograms.
   ◇ Percent better or worse sequential ($\%BW_s$): This is the percentage of workers who show 15 dB improvement or worsening of thresholds at any test frequency in either ear between two sequential audiograms.

Table 8.2　Example of Determination of Whether or Not an Individual (Female, Age in 1997: 47 years) will be Included in the Percent Worse (%W$_s$) or Percent Better or Worse Sequential (%BW$_s$) Statistics

Test year/no.	Right ear thresholds (dB) at each frequency (kHz)						Left ear thresholds (dB) at each frequency (kHz)						Include in		
	0.5	1	2	3	4	6	0.5	1	2	3	4	6	Test compared	%W$_s$	%BW$_s$
1993/5	25	45	55	55	45	60	10	40	25	35	45	50			
1994/6	30	50	55	55	55	55	15	35	40	40	40	40	5–6	Yes	Yes
1995/7	30	50	55	55	50	55	15	45	45	45	50	45	6–7	No	No
1996/8	30	50	45	45	45	60	10	40	40	45	50	45	7–8	No	No
1997/9	30	50	55	45	45	60	15	50	55	50	50	40	8–9	No	No

6. If the analysis is being conducted based on comparisons of tests 4 and 5 and any later tests, use both %W$_s$ and %BW$_s$ statistics (see example in **Table 8.2**) along with the following criteria to determine HCP rating:
   ◇ %W$_s$: Less than 17 is acceptable, 17 to 27 is marginal, and greater than 27 is unacceptable
   ◇ %BW$_s$: Less than 26 is acceptable, 26 to 40 is marginal, and greater than 40 is unacceptable
7. If the first four sequential tests are being utilized for analyses, use only the %W$_s$ statistic to determine the rating of the HCP performance (example in **Table 8.3**). This is because threshold improvements can appear initially due to the learning effect. If the %W$_s$ values are less than 20, the HCP performance is rated as being acceptable; for values between 20 and 30, the performance is rated as being marginal; for values greater than 30, the performance is rated as being unacceptable.
8. From year to year, the rating may fall into two different ranges, in which case the HCP performance can be described using the two ratings such as marginal to acceptable (**Tables 8.4** and **8.5**).

9. If the rating is unacceptable, search for sources of high variability including inadequate use of HPDs or audiometric testing conducted using poorly controlled procedures.

Limitations of the Use of Variability in Serial Monitoring Audiometry for Assessing Hearing Conservation Program Effectiveness

♦ Individuals with poor auditory sensitivity may show greater threshold variability than individuals with better hearing. This may not be necessarily connected to poor performance of an HCP (Amos & Simpson, 1995).
♦ Although the variability rating may be marginal or acceptable, some individuals may suffer significant threshold shifts from the baseline. For example, the individual whose thresholds are shown in **Table 8.3** is showing a consistent and significant threshold shift at 2, 3, 4, and 6 kHz from the baseline in the right ear and a consistent significant threshold shift at 6 kHz in the left ear. Also, he is showing some fluctuations at 2 kHz in the left ear. The individual whose thresholds are shown in **Table 8.2** is also showing a significant threshold shift at 2 and 3 kHz in the left ear.

Table 8.3　Example of Determination of Whether or Not an Individual (Male, Age in 1996: 59 years) will be Included in the Percent Worse (%W$_s$) Statistics

Test year/no.	Right ear thresholds (dB) at each frequency (kHz)						Left ear thresholds (dB) at each frequency (kHz)						Include in	
	0.5	1	2	3	4	6	0.5	1	2	3	4	6	Test compared	%W$_s$
Baseline	10	15	25	30	40	55	15	25	25	35	45	50		
1993/2	15	20	30	35	45	65	15	25	35	45	45	55		
1994/3	30	25	40	45	50	60	20	25	40	45	50	55	2–3	Yes
1995/4	15	20	45	50	60	70	15	20	35	40	45	55	3–4	No
1996/5	10	20	45	55	60	70	25	20	35	45	55	65	4–5	No

Table 8.4   Percent Worse (%W$_s$) Statistics from 10 Employees at a Hypothetical Small Manufacturing Shop

Employee no.	To be included in %W$_s$ statistics based on year to year comparison?			
	2006–2007	2007–2008	2008–2009	2009–2010
1	No	No	No	Yes
2	Yes	No	No	No
3	Yes	Yes	No	No
4	No	No	Yes	No
5	No	No	No	Yes
6	No	Yes	No	No
7	No	No	Yes	No
8	No	No	No	No
9	Yes	No	No	No
10	No	No	No	No
Number of employees to be included in %W$_s$ statistic	3	2	2	2
Percentage of employees to be included in %W$_s$ statistic	30%	20%	20%	20%
Rating	Unacceptable	Marginal	Marginal	Marginal

Evaluation of Individual Effectiveness

The baseline and annual audiograms of each worker can be compared to evaluate if there are any significant changes in thresholds (**Tables 8.2** and **8.3**). Significant changes in auditory thresholds in the absence of other contributing factors suggest the possibility of an ineffective HCP (National Institute of Occupational Safety and Health [NIOSH], 1998).

The success of smaller HCPs can be judged by the lack of changes in audiometric thresholds related to workplace or solvent exposure in each worker. If all workers show no effect of occupational noise

on their hearing, then the program can be judged to be highly effective (NIOSH, 1998).

Evaluation of Overall Program Effectiveness

When it is not possible to examine each worker's audiometric results to judge the effectiveness of the HCP, then evaluation of overall program effectiveness is considered (NIOSH, 1998). NIOSH suggests a two-step protocol for evaluating program effectiveness. The first step is to evaluate the integrity of the audiometric data. The second step is to compare the rate of threshold shifts

Table 8.5   Percent Better Worse (%BW$_s$) Statistics from 10 Employees at a Hypothetical Small Manufacturing Shop

Employee No.	To be included in % BW$_s$ statistics based on year to year comparison?			
	2006–2007	2007–2008	2008–2009	2009–2010
1	No	No	No	Yes
2	Yes	No	No	No
3	Yes	Yes	No	No
4	No	No	Yes	No
5	No	No	No	Yes
6	No	Yes	No	No
7	No	No	Yes	No
8	Yes	No	No	No
9	Yes	No	No	No
10	Yes	No	No	No
Number of employees to be included in %W$_s$ statistic	5	2	2	2
Percentage of employees to be included in %W$_s$ statistic	50%	20%	20%	20%
Rating	Unacceptable	Acceptable	Acceptable	Acceptable

of noise-exposed workers to that of individuals who are not exposed to occupational noise.

Step 1: Evaluation of the Integrity of the Audiometric Data

Integrity of audiometric data can be evaluated by using the procedure described by the American National Standards Institute (ANSI) which was outlined previously (ANSI, 2002). High variability in sequential thresholds can occur because of insufficient control of audiometric test procedures, poor control of test environment, poor calibration procedures, or poor recording of audiometric information. Low variability in sequential thresholds suggests a well-controlled program that is producing accurate and reliable audiometric test records.

Step 2: Consideration of the Rate of Threshold Shifts due to Occupational Noise or Solvent Exposure

Ideally, the rate of STSs in noise-/ototoxin-exposed workers should be compared with age-matched workers who are not exposed to noise/ototoxins in the same company. The disadvantages of this approach include the requirement of audiometric testing of all workers, including those who are not exposed to noise.

In the absence of availability of audiometric data from workers who are not exposed to noise, an STS rate of 3% or less in noise-exposed workers indicates an effective HCP (NIOSH, 1998). The 3% criterion was calculated by NIOSH by using the data from a population not exposed to noise, which is included in Annex C of ANSI S3.44–1996 (ANSI, 1996). Other recommended criteria vary from 3 to 6% (Franks, Davis, & Kreig, 1989; Morrill & Sterrett, 1981; Simpson, Stewart, & Kaltenbach, 1994). HCPs that show higher rates of significant threshold shifts can be considered ineffective.

In considering such threshold shifts without a matched control group, workers who have other significant contributing factors probably should not be included. They should be counseled and followed up separately, as noted in Chapters 4 and 5. Software such as the NoiseScan software (Pyykkö, Toppila, Starck, Juhola, & Auramo, 2000; Finnish Institute of Occupational Health, Laajaniityntie, FIN-01620, Vantaa, Finland) may be useful for easy consideration of all other contributing factors. The software provides the ISO 1999 (International Organization for Standardization, 1990)

and the noise scan models for prediction of hearing loss. The ISO 1999 model takes into account age, noise exposure, and gender in predicting hearing loss using the equal-energy principle (see Chapter 2). The noise scan model takes into account several other factors. History about medical conditions, cardiovascular risk factors, hearing loss, drugs, hereditary factors, hearing loss, etc., can be entered in the NoiseScan model database. The NoiseScan model is based on the ISO 1999 model but assumes that a worker with a lower number of other confounding risk factors is less vulnerable to noise than is a person with a larger number of contributing factors (Toppila, Pyykkö, & Starck, 2001; Toppila, Pyykkö, Starck, Kaksonen, & Ishizaki, 2000). Accounting for variables such as smoking and recreational use of firearms can significantly decrease the hearing loss attributable to occupational noise exposure (Agrawal, Niparko, & Dobie, 2010). In the NoiseScan model, the probability of noise-induced hearing loss (NIHL) is based on the number of contributing risk factors. For workers with zero or one risk factors, the 80% fractile of the database A in ISO 1999 (ontologically normal population with no reported history of excessive noise exposure) gives the best prediction; for those with two or three risk factors, the 50% fractile gives the best prediction; and for those with more than three risk factors, the 25% fractile gives the best prediction of hearing loss (Kuronen, Toppila, Starck, Pääkkönen, & Sorri, 2004).

Limitations of the Use of Standard Threshold Shift Rates

The presence of high STS rates suggests deficiencies in the HCP. However, low STS rates can result from a variety of other reasons than an effective HCP. In the presence of a low STS rate, the following factors should be ruled out as a cause (ANSI, 2002):

◆ *High employee turnover:* If the employee turnover is high, STS rates may appear low because the employees do not continue with the job for a long enough period to show the occurrence of the STS.
◆ *Prior baseline revisions in a high percentage of the population:* If the baselines of a high portion of the population have already been revised because of previous occurrences of STS, the current STS rate may appear to be low.

◆ *Changes in audiometric testing practices or instruments from the baseline to current audiograms:* Such changes may mask a significant deterioration in hearing, yielding low STS rates.

Confounding Factors Causing High Standard Threshold Shift Rates in the Presence of Effective Noise Controls or Hearing Protection Device Use

Ototoxic substances can cause hearing loss or can increase the risk of NIHL, as described in Chapters 1 and 4. In such cases, reduction to exposure to such substances can reduce the rate of STS.

◆ Prevention Index

Two steps are involved in calculating the prevention index (PI; Silverstein, 2010):

1. All industries with HCPs are rank-ordered by the incidence rate (high to low) for worker compensation claims. They are also ranked based on the number of worker compensation claims.
2. The two rankings are then averaged to generate the PI.

This measure is useful for governing agencies to identify industries that are showing poor performance in terms of reducing injuries and to focus attention on industries that may need more assistance in improving their performance (Silverstein, Viikari-Juntura, & Kalat, 2002). For example, in reference to NIHL, an industry with a higher incidence rate and a higher number of workers' compensation claims will have a lower PI and can be targeted for studying the reasons for ineffective HCP (Daniell, Swan, McDaniel, Camp, Cohen, & Stebbins, 2006).

◆ Use of Surveillance Data

One approach to evaluating the effects of hearing conservation efforts is to examine available surveillance data to identify high-risk industries and target these for evaluation and correction of deficiencies. Kock and colleagues (2004) used a database of 840 companies in selected high-risk industries based on the national register in Denmark. They measured the A-weighted equivalent sound level (LAeq) for a full shift of 830 manual workers recruited from 91 randomly selected workplaces in each industry using dosimeters. Approximately 50% of the workers were exposed to more than 85 dBA and approximately 20% were exposed to more than 90 dBA.

Reilly, Rosenman, and Kalinowski (1998) reported the use of a state-based surveillance system to identify and correct deficiencies in the implementation of HCPs. They interviewed 1378 individuals with occupational NIHL reported to the Michigan Department of Consumer and Industry Services by Michigan's audiologists and otolaryngologists from 1992 to 1997. Based on these interviews, 43 companies were inspected because of reported lack of audiometric monitoring and hearing protection in the presence of hazardous levels of noise. Twenty three of these investigated companies had noise levels above 85 dBA, and seventeen of these either lacked an HCP or had an incomplete HCP. Because all individuals with NIHL may not seek audiologists or otolaryngologists, the true magnitude of NIHL may be underestimated by the surveillance system. However, the surveillance system was successful in detecting some of the absent or deficient HCPs, thereby potentially preventing future hearing deterioration in 758 similarly exposed coworkers.

Middendorf (2004) used OSHA's Integrated Management Information System (IMIS) to gauge temporal and industrial trends of noise exposure. The author noticed a decreasing trend in 50% and 100% dose exposures in manufacturing during the 1985 to 1994 period, which predicts lower incidence of NIHL. The noise exposures documented in IMIS from the agriculture and construction industries suggested high exposure to workers in these sectors. Middendorf (2004) noted that OSHA's IMIS data must be interpreted with consideration of the sampling strategies used to collect it. The author further noted that the small number of noise records from sectors other than manufacturing makes it difficult to examine trends in these sectors and reduces the usefulness of the data for surveillance. The author made the following suggestions for improving the usefulness of the data for surveillance:

◆ Check the data for accuracy
◆ Include all measured noise exposures even if the permissible exposure limit and action level exposures were measured on the same worker

◆ Include additional noise exposure parameters, such as sample durations and frequency of exposure
◆ Include information about engineering controls
◆ Include information about the use of hearing protection
◆ Include standardized job codes and processes

◆ Use of Database Software

Currently available database software can generate several types of statistics that can be used for checking compliance and effectiveness of the HCP. Examples of these statistics include the following.

Average Thresholds of All Workers

Visual examination of such data can indicate any aberrant shifts that may not be related to noise exposure but may be due to other factors such as the installment of a new audiometer for testing.

List of Workers Showing Occupational Safety and Health Administration Standard Threshold Shifts

This will allow examination of the percentage of workers who show STSs on the initial and retest annual/monitoring audiograms.

List of Workers Showing Occupational Safety and Health Administration Recordable Hearing Loss (29CFR1904.10 eff. Jan. 2003)

This will allow examination of new workers suffering from hearing loss in the presence of an HCP.

List of Workers with Missing or Invalid Audiometric Data

Such a list can be used to examine overall compliance with audiometric testing.

◆ Evaluation of Each Component of the Hearing Conservation Program

A comprehensive evaluation of the effectiveness of an HCP should ideally include measures for each of the components of the HCP (**Table 8.6**). Such a comprehensive evaluation is likely to show which component or components are not properly implemented or are ineffective.

◆ Current Effectiveness of Some Hearing Conservation Programs

Industries with Relatively High Rates of Workers' Compensation Claims

Daniell and colleagues (2006) evaluated noise exposure and hearing loss prevention efforts in industries with a relatively high rate of workers' compensation claims (from 1992 to 1998). The percentage of workers with hazardous noise exposure was 1.5 to 3 times higher using a 3-dB exchange rate instead of the 5-dB exchange rate specified by OSHA. Most companies gave minimal or no attention to noise controls and relied primarily on hearing protection to prevent hearing loss. Recordkeeping of noise measures was poor. Hearing protectors were not used routinely by approximately 38% of the employees. Each industry studied included companies where HCP practices were incomplete.

Canadian Lumber Mill Workers

Davies, Marion, and Teschke (2008) evaluated the effect of HCP on Canadian lumber mill workers using annual audiograms obtained from the Workers' Compensation Board of British Columbia for the period 1979 to 1996. Use of HPDs was associated with a 30% decrease in STS risk, and enrollment in the HCP after 1988 was associated with an additional 30% reduction, suggesting that the introduction of HCPs halved the risk of STS during the study period. However, those with the highest noise exposure were at a 6.6 times greater risk for having hearing loss. Thus, noise control is a critical component of the HCP, and every attempt should be made to reduce noise exposures.

U.S. Coal Mines

Joy and Middendorf (2007) examined the data collected by MSHA inspectors at U.S. coal mines during a period (1987 to 2004) when MSHA issued its new noise regulations, which became effective in 2000. There was a reduction

Table 8.6　Examples of Measures for Evaluating the Effectiveness of Each Component of the HCP

HCP component	Compliance	Effectiveness
Noise measurement	Checklists, examination of records	Evaluate employee knowledge about noise levels in their areas
Engineering noise control	Checklists, records (e.g., if any new machines were purchased, were they designed to be quiet?), maintenance schedules for machines, and noise controls	Evaluate employee and management knowledge about engineering noise controls and what is required to maintain noise controls on equipment and in work areas
Audiometric testing	Checklists, records	Evaluate employee knowledge about the results of their own testing; determine variability in audiometric data. Determine STS rates
Hearing protection	Determine the different types of protectors available; observe workers in areas where protection is required	Evaluate the expected effectiveness of protection using noise measures and individual fit testing of randomly selected workers. Ask workers/supervisors/managers to demonstrate proper insertion techniques
Education and training	Checklists and records	Give quizzes/tests/examinations to employees/supervisors/managers at the beginning and end of each training session
Overall effectiveness	Checklists, records, employee feedback	Examine worker compensation claims and other surveillance statistics

HCP, health conservation program; STS, standard threshold shift.

in the overall annual median noise dose for both surface and underground coal mining, and the reduction accelerated after promulgation of the new noise rule, suggesting effective implementation of the noise control component of HCP. However, increase in shift duration may have counteracted the effect of noise controls to some degree. There was also an increase in the number of workers enrolled in HCPs, use of HPDs, and medical surveillance. However, the authors of the study caution that the reported estimates may be higher than actual rates because the estimates are based on miners who reported being enrolled in an HCP and using HPDs during a compliance inspection. In the presence of a compliance inspector, the compliance may be made to appear better than the actual HCP compliance. Also in 2004 (end of the period examined), 13% of underground miners and 9% of surface miners exposed to a greater than 100% noise dose did not use HPDs, suggesting scope for improvement in the HPD component of the HCPs.

Effectiveness of a Hearing Conservation Program at a Large Surface Gold Mining Company in Ghana

Amedofu (2007) performed a retrospective review of audiograms from 1999 to 2003 to determine the effectiveness of an HCP in a surface gold mining company in Ghana. OSHA STS (without age correction) was apparent in 5.5% of the workers.

Overall, these studies suggest that it is useful to assess the effectiveness of HCPs; generally, there appears to be scope for improving current programs.

◆ Review Questions

1. Why is it necessary to evaluate the effectiveness of HCPs?
2. How frequently should HCPs be evaluated?
3. Discuss the advantages and limitations of checklist audits in evaluating compliance of an HCP with applicable regulations.

4. Review the procedures that can be used for gaining employee feedback about the effectiveness of an HCP. What are the potential advantages and limitations to using employee feedback for evaluating the HCP?
5. Discuss the usefulness of task-based statistics in evaluating compliance of an HCP with applicable regulations.
6. Discuss the usefulness of noise-exposure statistics in evaluating the effectiveness of an HCP.

7. How can audiometric data be used for evaluating the effectiveness of an HCP? What are the potential limitations of this approach?
8. What is the PI, and how is it related to HCP effectiveness?
9. What are the potential advantages of a component-specific approach to evaluating the effectiveness of HCPs?
10. Discuss the usefulness of database software in evaluating the effectiveness of an HCP.

References

Agrawal Y, Niparko JK, Dobie RA. (2010). Estimating the effect of occupational noise exposure on hearing thresholds: the importance of adjusting for confounding variables. *Ear Hear.* 31(2):234–237.

Amedofu GK. (2007). Effectiveness of hearing conservation program at a large surface gold mining company in Ghana. *Afr J Health Sci.* 14:49–53.

American National Standards Institute. (1996). ANSI S3.44-1996. *American National Standard Determination of Occupational Noise Exposure and Estimation of Noise Induced Impairment.* New York: American National Standards Institute.

American National Standards Institute. (2002). *ANSI Technical Report: Evaluating the Effectiveness of Hearing Conservation Programs Through Audiometric Data Base Analysis.* New York: American National Standards Institute.

Amos NE, Simpson TH. (1995). Effects of pre-existing hearing loss and gender on proposed ANSI S12.13 outcomes for characterizing hearing conservation program effectiveness: preliminary investigation. *J Am Acad Audiol.* 6(6):407–413.

Daniell WE, Swan SS, McDaniel MM, Camp JE, Cohen MA, Stebbins JG. (2006). Noise exposure and hearing loss prevention programmes after 20 years of regulations in the United States. *Occup Environ Med.* 63(5):343–351.

Daniell WE, Swan SS, McDaniel MM, Stebbins JG, Seixas NS, Morgan MS. (2002). Noise exposure and hearing conservation practices in an industry with high incidence of workers' compensation claims for hearing loss. *Am J Ind Med.* 42(4):309–317.

Davies H, Marion S, Teschke K. (2008). The impact of hearing conservation programs on incidence of noise-induced hearing loss in Canadian workers. *Am J Ind Med.* 51(12):923–931.

Franks JR, Davis RR, Kreig EF Jr. (1989). Analysis of a hearing conservation program data base: factors other than workplace noise. *Ear Hear,* 10(5):273–280.

Franks JR, Stephenson MR, Merry CJ. (1996). *Preventing Occupational Hearing Loss. A Practical Guide.* DHHS (NIOSH) Publication No. 96–110. Washington, DC: U.S. Department of Health and Human Services, Public Health Service, Centers for Disease Control and Prevention, and National Institute for Occupational Safety and Health.

International Organization for Standardization. (1990). *ISO-1999. Acoustics: Determination of Occupational Noise Exposure and Estimation of Noise-Induced Hearing*

Impairment. Geneva, Switzerland: International Organization for Standardization.

Joy GJ, Middendorf PJ. (2007). Noise exposure and hearing conservation in U.S. coal mines—a surveillance report. *J Occup Environ Hyg.* 4(1):26–35.

Kock S, Andersen T, Kolstad HA, Kofoed-Nielsen B, Wiesler F, Bonde JP. (2004). Surveillance of noise exposure in the Danish workplace: a baseline survey. *Occup Environ Med.* 61(10):838–843.

Kuronen P, Toppila E, Starck J, Pääkkönen R, Sorri MJ. (2004). Modelling the risk of noise-induced hearing loss among military pilots. *Int J Audiol.* 43(2):79–84.

Middendorf PJ. (2004). Surveillance of occupational noise exposures using OSHA's Integrated Management Information System. *Am J Ind Med.* 46(5):492–504.

Morrill JC, Sterrett ML. (1981). Quality controls for audiometric testing. *Occup Health Saf.* 50(8):26–33.

National Institute for Occupational Safety and Health. (1998). *Criteria for a Recommended Standard: Occupational Noise Exposure- Revised Criteria 1998* (Publication No, 98–126). Cincinnati, OH: National Institute for Occupational Safety and Health.

Occupational Safety and Health Administration. (1983). *Guidelines for Noise Enforcement; Appendix A.* OSHA Directive CPL 2-2.35A-29 CFR 1910.95(b)(1). Washington, D.C.: U.S. Department of Labor, Occupational Safety and Health Administration.

Prince MM, Colligan MJ, Stephenson CM, Bischoff BJ. (2004). The contribution of focus groups in the evaluation of hearing conservation program (HCP) effectiveness. *J Safety Res.* 35(1):91–106.

Pyykkö IV, Toppila EM, Starck JP, Juhola M, Auramo Y. (2000). Database for a hearing conservation program. *Scand Audiol.* 29(1):52–58.

Reilly MJ, Rosenman KD, Kalinowski DJ. (1998). Occupational noise-induced hearing loss surveillance in Michigan. *J Occup Environ Med.* 40(8):667–674.

Silverstein B. (2010). Safety & Health Assessment and Research for Prevention (SHARP) program. In Utterback DF, Schnorr TM, eds. *Use of Workers' Compensation Data for Occupational Injury & Illness Prevention Proceedings from September 2009 Workshop* (pp. 5–10). DHHS (NIOSH) Publication No. 2010-152. Washington, DC: Department of Health and Human Services, Centers for Disease Control and Prevention, National Institute for Occupational Safety and Health, Department of Labor, Bureau of Labor Statistics.

Silverstein B, Viikari-Juntura E, Kalat J. (2002). Use of a prevention index to identify industries at high risk for work-related musculoskeletal disorders of the neck, back, and upper extremity in Washington state, 1990–1998. *Am J Ind Med*. 41(3):149–169.

Simpson TH, Stewart M, Kaltenbach JA. (1994). Early indicators of hearing conservation program performance. *J Am Acad Audiol*. 5(5):300–306.

Toppila E, Pyykkö I, Starck J. (2001). Age and noise-induced hearing loss. *Scand Audiol*. 30(4):236–244.

Toppila E, Pyykkö I, Starck J, Kaksonen R, Ishizaki H. (2000). Individuals risk factors in the development of noise induced hearing loss. *Noise Health*. 8(2):59–70.

U.S. Navy and Marine Corps Public Health Center. (2008). *Navy Medical Department Hearing Conservation Program Procedures* (NMCPHC – TM 6260.51.99–2). Portsmouth, VA: U.S. Navy and Marine Corps Public Health Center.

Wolgemuth KS, Luttrell WE, Kamhi AG, Wark DJ. (1995). The effectiveness of the Navy's Hearing Conservation Program. *Mil Med*. 160(5):219–222.Review Questions

Chapter 9

Conservation and Management of Hearing Loss in Musicians

The possibility of the risk of hearing loss in professional musicians has been considered for the last 50 years (Arnold & Miskolczy-Fodor, 1960). Hearing conservation is highly critical for musicians because their livelihood depends on fine hearing abilities. This chapter provides a review of literature related to hearing loss in musicians. In addition, it includes strategies for hearing conservation, information about hearing protection devices (HPDs) and hearing aids, and other coping strategies for musicians with hearing loss.

◆ Applicable Hearing Safety Regulations

Some hearing safety regulations could apply to those musicians who are exposed to hazardous levels of music. Four examples of hearing regulations that could apply to musicians are presented below.

United States

In the United States, facilities with high sound level exposures are regulated by the Occupational Safety and Health Administration (OSHA; 1983). Although musicians are not specifically addressed, the regulation requires action in terms of implementation of a hearing conservation program and recommendation of the use of HPDs when the daily 8-hour time weighted average (TWA) level is equal to or greater than 85 dBA (action value). When the TWA exceeds 90 dBA, HPD use is required, and the exchange rate is 5 dB. Thus if the musician plays on a daily basis only for 4, 2, or 1 hours, then exposures of 90, 95, or 100 dBA

will be allowed. Exposure to impulsive or impact noises (e.g., steel pans) greater than 140 dB sound pressure level (SPL) is not allowed.

European Union

The European Union Directive 2003/10/EC (2003) is directed to all workers including musicians. This directive includes exposure limits of 87 dBA for peak and daily exposures. The upper exposure action values are 85 dBA.

United Kingdom

In the United Kingdom, health and safety law applies to all musicians including self-employed freelancers (Noise at Work Regulations, 2005). According to this law, the lower exposure level where action is required is 80 dBA of daily noise exposure and peak SPL of 135 dBC. At this level, the employer is required to assess the risks, control the risks, make HPDs available for voluntary use, and provide employees with information, instruction, and training. At the upper exposure action value of 85 dBA daily noise exposure or peak exposure of 137 dBC, the employer is required to put more effort into reducing exposures. If exposures are still above the upper level, the employer is required to ensure that the employees use personal HPDs effectively. The noise reaching the ear must not exceed a daily personal noise exposure of 87 dBA or a peak exposure of 140 dBC. In the presence of marked variations in daily exposures, weekly personal noise exposure values can be used to ensure compliance with the regulation. Some musicians may suggest that they are willing to sign a release form wishing not to be protected.

Reid and Holland (2008) pointed out that besides this being an unwise decision, employees cannot consent to be harmed at work. They further emphasized that U.K. health and safety law requires cooperation of employees with their employers in carrying out legal duties.

Sweden

The Swedish National Board of Health and Welfare considers 100 dB L_{Aeq} as a safe limit for a duration of 1 hour/day (5 hours/week) and has recommended a maximum value of 115 dBA during musical performances for adults. LAeq is a constant level of noise that delivers the same amount of energy content as the music being measured. The A represents use of A-weighing, and the eq indicates the use of equivalent level of continuous noise (Chapter 10). The limits are 97 dB L_{Aeq} and 110 dBA at venues where children under 13 years of age have access. For venues that are specifically designed for children, the safety limit is 95 dB L_{Aeq} (Swedish National Board of Health and Welfare, 2005).

Some musicians may practice for 2 to 4 hours daily and increase their practice substantially before performing or preparing for juries or solo concerts (Pascarelli & Hsu, 2001). In addition, some contracts specify the amount of playing that is required; it is 300 hours/year in some cases including performances and rehearsals but excluding personal practice. According to Laitinen, Toppila, Olkinuora, and Kuisma (2003), the average professional musician plays an average of 5.5 hours per day. Thus the duration of sound exposure for musicians may be much greater than 1 hour/day or 5 hours/week, which would require reduction of the 100 dB L_{Aeq} safety limit.

◆ Classical Music versus Industrial Noise

The severity of hearing loss in classical musicians is usually less than can be predicted from their exposure levels. Comparisons of temporary thresholds shifts produced by equal energy exposures (91 dBA for 2 hours) to industrial noise and to classical music show lower temporary threshold shifts for classical music (Strasser, Irle, & Legler, 2003). The equal energy exposure principle cannot be applied to very high levels because 125 dB peak equivalent sound pressure level (peSPL) is considered to be just below the critical level

where cochlear structures can suffer mechanical damage (Levine, Hofstetter, Zheng, & Henderson, 1998). Thus a conservative maximum limit of 115 dBA to music may be appropriate.

Classical music may not appear as hazardous to hearing as industrial noise for the following reasons:

◆ There is a substantial variation in sound levels in classical music (Strasser, Irle, & Legler, 2003). It has more quiet or silent periods than typical occupational or industrial noise, allowing more instances for recovery.
◆ The frequent occurrences of silent periods may allow maintenance of acoustic reflex or prevent decay of acoustic reflex (Rawool, 1996) in some individuals, allowing reduction of stimulus levels entering the cochlea.
◆ Music may induce a toughening effect (Miyakita, Hellström, Frimanson, & Axelsson, 1992).
◆ The differences in efferent suppression may provide a possible reason for less hearing loss in musicians versus nonmusicians (Brashears, Morlet, Berlin, & Hood, 2003). Musicians show greater suppression of otoacoustic emissions (OAEs) with contralateral stimulation than nonmusicians, which can protect hearing (Micheyl, Khalfa, Perrot, & Collet, 1997).
◆ Musicians cannot be forced to participate in human research because of the ethical issues. Those who have hearing loss may not participate (Reid & Holland, 2008) because of the stigma or fear of losing employment due to imperfect hearing.

◆ Sound Exposure Levels

Musicians' daily exposures are expected to vary widely and include exposures during group rehearsals, practicing and playing solo, and providing music instructions to others. Cumulative exposure from a variety of additional activities can lead to hearing loss (Rawool, 2008). Variation in exposure levels to musicians can occur as a result of the factors discussed as follows.

The Repertoire

Some symphonies are written for large orchestras of over 100 instruments often playing *fortissimo* (full volume), while others are written for smaller orchestras of less than 30 instruments that are *forte* (loud). Thus the repertoire being played has an influence on sound exposure levels (Boasson, 2002; O'Brien, Wilson, & Bradley, 2008; Westmore & Eversden, 1981). The rehearsal of *La Valse* composed by Ravel can produce peak levels of 112 dB SPL, whereas the rehearsal of *Mother Goose Suite* by the same composer results in peak levels of only 95 dB SPL (McBride, Gill, Proops, Harrington, Gardiner, & Attwell, 1992).

The Instrument

The sound levels generated by different musical instruments vary widely and are displayed in **Table 9.1**. As shown, many of the instruments exceed the 85 dBA limit that is considered safe, whereas the piano played at moderate levels is well within the safety limit. In a classical orchestra, musicians who play the principal trumpet, first and third horns, and principal trombone are at greatest risk of exposure to excessive sustained noise levels, and those who play the percussion and timpani are at greatest risk of exposure to excessive peak noise levels (O'Brien, Wilson, & Bradley, 2008).

Table 9.1 Sound Levels Generated by Different Instruments

Instrument	Average sound level (dBA)
Bass	80.5[1]
Cello	88.6[1]
Clarinet	85.3[1]
Drum rolls	106[2]
Drum set	93.5–94.6[1]
Flute	88.6–95.5[1]
Horn	90.2–98.6[1]
Marimba	91.3–95[1]
Oboe	88.3–93.5[1]
Piano played at moderate level	60–70[3]
Piano played loudly	92–95[4]
Piccolo	96–112[5]
Piccolo (near right ear)	102–118[5]
Sax	88.2–92[1]
Trombone	92.3–98[1]
Trumpet	97.6–98.5[1]
Tuba	87.9[1]
Viola	84.1–92.9[1]
Violin	85.5–87.8[1]

Data from: [1]Phillips and Mace, 2008; [2]Westmore and Eversden, 1981; [3]Sallows, 2001; [4]Hart, Geltman, Schupbach, and Santucci, 1987; [5]Chasin, 2006.

The Type of Music

The sound levels generated by different musical performances such as concerts or chamber music vary widely and are shown in **Table 9.2**. As can be seen, many of these events are capable of producing damaging sound levels, and some peak levels suggest the possibility of mechanical damage to the cochlea even at very brief durations. Heavy metal music is likely to result in threshold shifts that are similar to those caused by industrial noise (Strasser, Irle, & Scholz, 1999). As shown in **Table 9.2**, chamber music results in less exposure levels compared with the levels generated by jazz/rock or steelbands. The steelband is a relatively modern orchestral form and is played year-round in some countries. The steelpan is created by heating the steel base of a steel drum (commonly used for transporting oil) and hammering and demarcating it into different segments with different shapes. The tuners create steel pans of varying tonal characteristics. Based on their fundamental frequencies, the pans are designated as tenor, cello, bass, guitar, and double second, and can generate very high sound levels in the frequency range of 63 to 1450 Hz (Juman, Karmody, & Simeon, 2004).

The Physical Environment

Performances can occur in concert halls, orchestra pits, town halls, stadiums, and other venues. Rehearsals can occur in a variety of environments, including acoustically treated halls for professional orchestras to basements or garages with highly reflective surfaces for small bands. The presence of reflective surfaces in the room increases the levels. Sound levels generated by instruments are generally higher during performances than during rehearsals (McBride, Gill, Proops, Harrington, Gardiner, & Attwell, 1992).

Setup

An orchestra can be set up in a variety of formats depending on repertoire, venue, orchestra size, the conductor's request, and anticipated noise exposure (O'Brien, Wilson, & Bradley, 2008).

Intramusician Variability

A musician can play the same instrument at differing volumes depending on fatigue, the volume

Table 9.2   Sound Levels Generated by Different Musical Events

Sound source	Sound level	Peak levels
Chamber music in a small auditorium (Sallows, 2001)	75–85 dBA	–
Jazz club with dosimeter on drummer (Kähärit, Zachau, Eklöf, Sandsjö, & Möller, 2003)	100.8 L_{Aeq}, Max:123.9 dBA	141.4 dBC
Orchestra in an acoustically treated rehearsal room with dosimeter within 60 cm of musicians playing various instruments (O'Brien, Wilson, & Bradley, 2008)	77.4 to 95.9 dB L_{Aeq}	103.7 to 144.1 dBC
Orchestra in a concert hall with dosimeter within 60 cm of musicians playing various instruments (O'Brien, Wilson, & Bradley, 2008)	76.1 to 96.3 dB L_{Aeq}	106.9 to 146.9 dBC
Punk jazz/jazz club with dosimeter on drummer (Kähärit, Zachau, Eklöf, Sandsjö, & Möller, 2003)	108.9 L_{Aeq}, Max:108.9 dBA	148.9 dBC
Rock, small stage in a small-sized discotheque with dosimeter on bassist (Kähärit, Zachau, Eklöf, Sandsjö, & Möller, 2003)	115 L_{Aeq}, Max:129.4 dBA	142.8 dBC
Rock, large stage in a discotheque with dosimeter on bassist (Kähärit, Zachau, Eklöf, Sandsjö, & Möller, 2003)	106 L_{Aeq}, Max:120 dBA	133.5 dBC
Steelband, central rhythm section (Juman, Karmody, & Simeon, 2004)	106.5 to 110.7 dBA	-

of music played surrounding musicians, and the request from the conductor to play it louder or softer (O'Brien, Wilson, & Bradley, 2008).

Intermusician Variability

Some musicians play the same part significantly louder than their colleagues either because of differences in instruments, differences in techniques used to play the instrument, or a different interpretation of the piece (O'Brien, Wilson, & Bradley, 2008). Hyperacusis and/or hearing loss in some musicians might also lead to intermusician variability.

◆ Auditory Effects of High Music Levels

The hearing disorders experienced by musicians include hearing loss, tinnitus, hyperacusis, diplacusis, distortion, and difficulty in differentiating a signal of interest from background sounds. If most of these disorders are considered, 68 to 74% of the pop/rock/jazz musicians have hearing

disorders (Axelsson, Eliasson, & Israelsson, 1995; Kähärit, Eklöf, Sandsjö, Zachau, & Möller, 2003).

Hearing Loss

Musicians who do not use hearing protection suffer from sensorineural hearing loss (Juman, Karmody, & Simeon, 2004; Kähärit, Eklöf, Sandsjö, Zachau, & Möller, 2003; Schmuziger, Patscheke, & Probst, 2006). Over 50% of professional musicians can suffer from hearing loss (Emmerich, Rudel, & Richter, 2008), with a significant hearing loss at 6 kHz (Jansen, Helleman, Dreschler, & de Laat, 2009). In choir singers, the hearing loss may occur at lower frequencies (Steurer, Simak, Denk, & Kautzky, 1998). Example of a hearing loss in a pianist who has been playing the piano without hearing protection is shown in **Fig. 9.1**.

Age of Onset

Music-induced hearing loss can begin early in the career. About 44% of college music students have a hearing loss with a notch apparent at

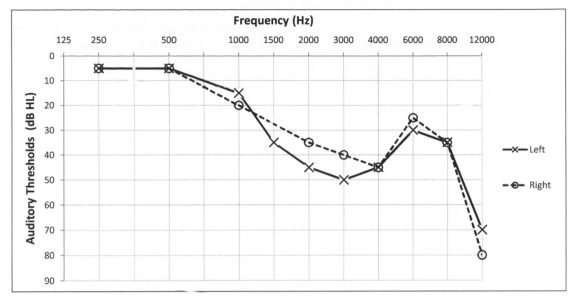

Fig. 9.1 The auditory thresholds of a 61-year-old piano player.

6 kHz. A bilateral hearing loss is apparent in approximately 11.5% of students (Phillips, Henrich, & Mace, 2010).

Ear Asymmetry

Significantly poorer hearing thresholds in the left ear have been reported in male rock/jazz musicians who mostly play in amplified sound environments and may move around on the stage with no fixed location (Kähärit, Eklöf, Sandsjö, Zachau, & Möller, 2003). Among classical orchestral musicians, violinists (Emmerich, Rudel, & Richter, 2008; Ostri, Eller, Dahlin, & Skylv, 1989), violists, and drummers may have worse hearing in the left ear. Flute (Ostri, Eller, Dahlin, & Skylv, 1989) and piccolo players have worse hearing in the right ear. However, a flutist can have a poorer left ear due to the location of a trumpet player on his left side (Chasin, 1998).

Hyperacusis

Hyperacusis is a discomfort or annoyance associated with sound levels that are not considered uncomfortable by individuals with normal hearing. It is often associated with hearing loss. The most common cause of hyperacusis appears to be exposure to loud sounds and more specifically exposure to loud music (Anari, Axelsson,

Eliasson, & Magnusson, 1999). Male musicians with hyperacusis are likely to have poorer auditory thresholds than those without hyperacusis (Kähärit, Zachau, Eklöf, Sandsjö, & Möller, 2003). Approximately 39 to 79% of the musicians report hyperacusis (Anari, Axelsson, Eliasson, & Magnusson, 1999; Jansen, Helleman, Dreschler, & de Laat, 2009; Kähärit, Zachau, Eklöf, Sandsjö, & Möller, 2003; Mendes, Morata, & Marques, 2007), whereas in the general population the incidence may be around 15% (Fabijanska, Rogowski, Bartnik, & Skarzynski, 1999). Among rock/jazz musicians, women report hyperacusis more frequently than men (Kähärit, Zachau, Eklöf, Sandsjö, & Möller, 2003).

Diplacusis

When a single-frequency tone produces noticeably different perception of pitch in the two ears, it is referred to as diplacusis. It is usually associated with sensorineural hearing loss. Diplacusis can cause the musician to play out of tune. Approximately 7% of musicians report diplacusis, and it can be documented through measurements in 18% of musicians. Musicians with diplacusis have increased average threshold levels regardless of age, suggesting that it is likely to be associated with music-induced hearing loss (Jansen, Helleman, Dreschler, & de Laat, 2009).

Tinnitus

The risk of tinnitus is twice as great in musicians than in the general population (Ostri, Eller, Dahlin, & Skylv, 1989). More than 50% of professional musicians report tinnitus (Emmerich, Rudel, & Richter, 2008; Griffiths & Samaroo, 1995; Jansen, Helleman, Dreschler, & de Laat, 2009). Approximately 54% of the percussionists report tinnitus, and professionals are more likely to have tinnitus (57.6%) than amateurs (44.2%) (Cunningham, Curk, Hoffman, & Pride, 2006). More than 60% of violinists suffer from unilateral tinnitus (Emmerich, Rudel, & Richter, 2008). Tinnitus is less likely in low string (cello, double bass) players and is more likely in brass (trumpet, trombone, horn) and high string (violin, viola) players (Jansen, Helleman, Dreschler, & de Laat, 2009). About 30% of orchestral musicians find their tinnitus bothersome, and 6% find it highly bothersome (Reid & Holland, 2008).

Distortion of Tones

Distortion can be defined as pure tones, overtones, and/or harmonics that are not perceived in their original form but as distorted, unclear, fuzzy, and/or out of tune (Kähärit, Zachau, Eklöf, Sandsjö, & Möller, 2003). Up to 24% of musicians report distortion of tones (Jansen, Helleman, Dreschler, & de Laat, 2009).

Impaired Figure-ground Perception

This refers to difficulty in distinguishing a sound of interest in the background of other sounds and is often associated with sensorineural hearing loss. Because of impaired figure-ground perception, the musician may have difficulty hearing conversations on the stage with all other noise in the performance venue. In addition, the musician may not be able to distinguish a particular instrument among the sounds created by other instruments (Reid & Holland, 2008).

Risk Factors for Hearing Symptoms

The number of hearing symptoms and the severity of hearing symptoms experienced by musicians depends on the following factors:

- *Overall sound exposure levels:* Musicians who are exposed to levels under 95 dBA may not suffer from hearing loss (Obeling & Poulsen,

1999) or may show minimal hearing loss (Emmerich, Rudel, & Richter, 2008).
- *Amount of weekly exposure:* Greater weekly exposures increase the risk of hearing loss (Axelsson & Lindgren, 1981; Westmore & Eversden, 1981).
- *Type of instrument:* Musicians who play the French horn, trumpet, trombone, bassoon, and brass are at a higher risk for hearing loss (Axelsson & Lindgren, 1981). Percussionists (Axelsson, Eliasson, & Israelsson, 1995; Behroozi & Luz, 1997; Ostri, Eller, Dahlin, & Skylv, 1989) and brass players (Reid & Holland, 2008) seem to have the worst hearing thresholds of all musicians.
- *Location of the musician:* The noise produced by surrounding instruments can potentially be more harmful than the sound produced by the musician's own instrument (Ostri, Eller, Dahlin, & Skylv, 1989) depending on the location and the closeness of the musician to other musicians. For example, violinists who are seated close to the woodwind players can be exposed to highly intense sounds from behind in addition to the sounds of their own instruments (Emmerich, Rudel, & Richter, 2008).
- *Period as a professional:* Individuals with a greater number of years as a musician are more likely to have hearing loss (Emmerich, Rudel, & Richter, 2008; Juman, Karmody, & Simeon, 2004).
- *Type of music:* Heavy rock metal music is likely to be as hazardous to hearing as industrial noise, while classical music may be less hazardous (Drake-Lee, 1992; Strasser, Irle, & Scholz, 1999).
- *Use of HPDs:* Musicians who use HPDs are less likely to have a hearing loss than are those who do not. Percussionists who wear HPDs have significantly better OAEs than those who do not (Cunningham, Curk, Hoffman, & Pride, 2006).
- *Gender:* Hearing loss tends to be greater in male musicians than in female musicians (Axelsson & Lindgren, 1981; Kähärit, Zachau, Eklöf, Sandsjö, & Möller, 2003; Steurer, Simak, Denk, & Kautzky, 1998), and a higher percentage of men have a hearing loss compared with women (Ostri, Eller, Dahlin, & Skylv, 1989). Men may play instruments louder than women, or hormonal differences may contribute to the variation.
- *Positive emotional associations:* Sometimes, professional musicians are required to

perform music that they do not like. Approximately 10% of orchestral players spend about half of their time playing music they strongly dislike (Reid & Holland, 2008). Temporary thresholds shifts are less in individuals who like a particular type of music compared with individuals who do not like the music (Swanson, Dengerink, Kondrick, & Miller, 1987).

- *Stress:* Self-reported hearing problems are associated with perceived poorer psychosocial environment, mental health symptoms, and long-term stress. A poorer ability to "unwind" from stress is related to increased occurrence of self-reported hearing difficulties (Hasson, Theorell, Liljeholm-Johansson, & Canlon, 2009). Orchestra musicians are exposed to various forms of stress (Liljeholm-Johansson & Theorell, 2003) in addition to high sound levels. Among orchestral players, 16% suffer from performance stress that affects their performance more than once a week, and only 10% do not experience physical effects of stress while playing (Reid & Holland, 2008). In addition, the presence of uncorrected hearing loss can increase stress resulting from the higher effort required in listening to speech.
- *Genetic predisposition:* There is an association between specific genetic variants and the prevalence and severity of noise-induced hearing loss (Konings, Van Laer, Wiktorek-Smagur, et al., 2009; Lin, Wu, Shih, Tsai, Sun, & Guo, 2009; Sliwinska-Kowalska, Noben-Trauth, Pawelczyk, & Kowalski, 2008).

◆ Nonauditory Effects of High Music Levels

Musicians with auditory symptoms can have difficulty in continuing to work with and practice music (Anari, Axelsson, Eliasson, & Magnusson, 1999; Axelsson, Eliasson, & Israelsson, 1995; Behroozi & Luz, 1997). Greater than 50% of the classical musicians feel that the high sound levels affect their performance, concentration, and morale (Holland-Mortiz, 1985). About 86% of orchestral players report that loud music interferes with their performance, and 23% report that this happens frequently. Furthermore, 79% experience pain

because of loud music; in 14% of those cases, this is a frequent occurrence (Reid & Holland, 2008).

Hyperacusis can make it difficult for the musician to perform because of exposure to loud sounds during performances and can often be accompanied by fear and/or depression (Zöger, Svedlund, & Holgers, 2001). It can trigger the fight/flight mechanism, increasing muscle tension and causing the musician to shake with excessive adrenaline (Reid & Holland, 2008). Hyperacusis is associated with higher psychological demands, greater difficulty in relaxing after work, higher stress during individual rehearsals, and insufficient sleep in male musicians (Kähärit, Eklöf, Sandsjö, Zachau, & Möller, 2003).

Tinnitus is associated with greater difficulty in relaxing after work and less energy during musical performances in female musicians (Kähärit, Zachau, Eklöf, Sandsjö, & Möller, 2003). Difficulties in pitch perception or discrimination can have a negative impact on a music career.

◆ Strategies for Prevention of Hearing Loss

Several strategies can be used to minimize the occurrence of hearing loss in musicians. These include controlling sound levels at the source, controlling the propagation of sound toward the musician, and controlling the flow of sound to the musician's eardrum. A combination of these strategies can be effective in preventing hearing loss in musicians. To achieve these goals, knowledge of the generated sound levels can be helpful. Simple devices can inform musicians and conductors about the generated noise levels.

Devices for Indicating Exposure Levels or Noise Dose

dB Check

The dB Check device from Sensaphonics (Chicago, IL; **Fig. 9.2**) provides a reading of ongoing room dBA levels when used in the microphone mode. The device also allows averaging of the dBA levels over a duration of 1 to 120 minutes and shows the average level when the selected duration expires. As an example, the first line in the display in **Fig. 9.2** shows the average dBA level (92 dB) at the end of the selected duration for measurement. The second line shows the maximum duration for

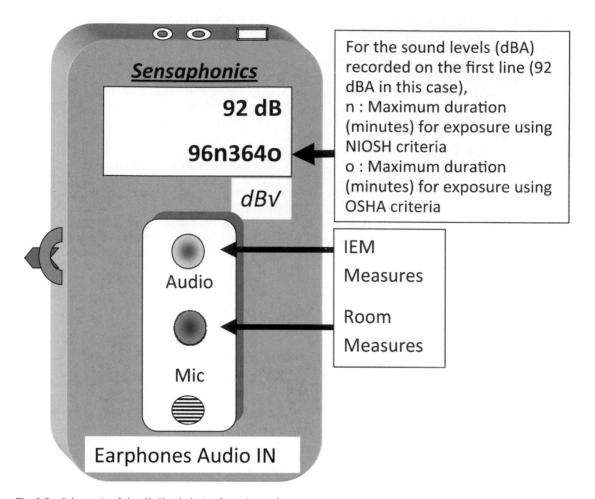

Fig. 9.2 Schematic of the dB Check device from Sensaphonics.

exposure for the measured SPL of 92 dBA recommended by the National Institute of Occupational Safety and Health (NIOSH; 96n; 96 minutes; n indicates use of NIOSH criteria) and the maximum duration using the OSHA (364o; 364 minutes; o indicates use of OSHA criteria) criteria.

SoundCheck

The SoundCheck (**Fig. 9.3**) device from Sensorcom (Annapolis, MD) uses three indicator light-emitting diodes (LEDs) to give an idea of noise levels with the following interpretations:

- Green: flickering = 55 dBA
- Green: on continuously = 60 dBA
- Yellow: flickering = 75 dBA

- Yellow: on continuously = 80 dBA (this is the first action level specified by the Noise at Work Regulations [2005]).
- Red: pulsing slowly = 100 dBA (beyond the second action level)
- Red: pulsing rapidly = greater than 100 dBA (dangerous)
- Red: on continuously = greater than 105 dBA (very dangerous)

Personal Noise Dosimeter

The Personal Noise Dosimeter (**Fig. 9.4**) from Etymotic Research Inc. (ER; Elk Grove Village, IL) uses LED indicators and arrows to show the percent noise dose calculated by taking into consideration the noise level and duration of noise exposure

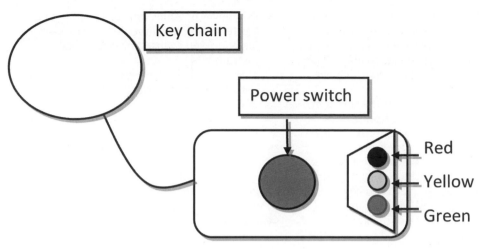

Fig. 9.3 Schematic of the SoundCheck device from Sensorcom.

using the OSHA (1983) criteria. In the normal mode, the noise dose is indicated as follows:

- Green (slow flash) = less than 25% dose; no risk of hearing loss
- Green (fast flash) = 25% daily dose; no risk of hearing loss
- Green 50% = half daily dose reached; no risk of hearing loss
- Yellow = 100% dose; limit of permissible exposure (risk of hearing loss begins)
- Red = 200% dose
- Red = 400% dose
- Red = 800%, 1600%, and 3200% dose

As shown in **Fig. 9.4**, the red indicators are separate for 200%, 400%, and greater than 800% doses.

Control of Sound Levels at the Source

The best way to protect hearing is to control or reduce the sound levels generated by the instruments. The following strategies can be used to achieve this goal (Reid & Holland, 2008):

- Involve composers/conductors in the hearing conservation program. Inform them about the importance of controlling noise below certain levels to prevent hearing loss and encourage them to guide the performers to play less loudly.
- Disperse some quiet pieces among the loud pieces within the program or schedule to reduce the overall noise dose and permit recovery.
- Encourage musicians to use practice mutes or practice pads during individual rehearsals to control the noise dose.
- Different brass instruments have different powers, and the advantage of high-powered instruments is that they require less force to play. Conscious attempts should be made to not play these types of instruments with too much force or too loudly.

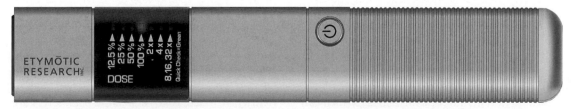

Fig. 9.4 Personal noise dosimeter from Etymotic Research Inc. (© Etymotic Research Inc. Used with permission.)

- Improve propagation of the music toward the audience, which can maintain enjoyment of the music by the audience without having to play too loudly or with too much effort. The following strategies can be used to achieve this goal:
  - ◇ Minimize the absorption of the sound by the listeners seated in the front row by using high risers that are approximately 2 feet above the row in the front.
  - ◇ When risers are not available, musicians can stand up during the performance of loud passages or can play with bells up. Such marking of loud passages may also enhance the elicitation of the acoustic reflex and reduce the sound reaching the inner ear of the musicians.
  - ◇ Spread out the players to allow clear sound paths toward the audience, especially for louder instruments. The increased distance between musicians also minimizes the exposure of sounds to the musicians from other instruments.
  - ◇ Set the orchestra/band back from the edge of the stage to allow the high-frequency sounds reflected off the stage floor to better reach the audience (Chasin, 2009a).

Control of Exposure to the Musician

Many of the strategies listed previously for improving propagation of music toward the audience can also minimize the amount of sound flow toward the musician. In addition, the following strategies can also be used:

- Treat orchestra pits and rehearsal rooms with acoustic paneling and carpeting to reduce reverberation, which increases sound levels. When possible, rehearsal rooms should be treated with acoustic tiles. Renovation of small teaching facilities may not necessarily decrease the noise exposure of the instructors. The best strategy may be to specify the requirements for any rehearsal or music instruction rooms during the designing stage for their intended use (Koskinen, Toppila, & Olkinuora, 2010).
- Place instruments that generate louder overall or peak sound levels such as percussion and brass instruments on risers to allow music to flow over the head of other performers located downwind (Chasin, 2009a), which can cause a slight reduction in sound exposure.

- Whenever possible, musicians should be located out of the direct line of vocalists (e.g., soprano soloists) or directional instruments.
  - ◇ Seat brass players near the front of the pit to minimize exposure of other musicians to loud, highly directional sound coming from the brass instruments (Sallows, 2001).
  - ◇ Stand the conductor on a riser above the brass section to protect the conductor's hearing (Sallows, 2001).
- Provide quiet rest facilities at performance venues (Laitinen & Poulsen, 2008).
- Provide appropriate breaks during rehearsals and between performances. A noise-free interval of 12 hours is recommended between rehearsals and performances (Ostri, Eller, Dahlin, & Skylv, 1989).
- Remind musicians about the risks of high exposure levels and the benefits of the use of preventative strategies. Prior to performances, reminders about risks and HPDs can be e-mailed to musicians. During the performance, reminders can be announced at the beginning of the performance, and written reminders can be placed on stage or music stands. Such reminders are important because young adults may believe that they will not lose their hearing until they become much older (Rawool & Colligon-Wayne, 2008).

Control of Sound Levels Reaching the Musician's Eardrum

The sound levels reaching the musician's ears can be decreased by using either HPDs or sound attenuating in-the-ear monitors (IEMs), also called personal monitors. Such devices should be considered only as a last resort, as they are subject to many problems. Musicians do not always use HPDs and many use them in only one ear. Getting used to HPDs is considered time-consuming by many musicians and thus one-third may give up and stop using HPDs (Laitinen & Poulsen, 2008).

When exposure levels to classical music are under 95 dBA, no or minimal hearing loss is apparent (Emmerich, Rudel, & Richter, 2008; Obeling & Poulsen, 1999). However, music-induced hearing loss can begin early in the career (Phillips, Henrich, & Mace, 2010) and some peak levels are hazardous. Therefore, rather than relying on daily noise doses or exposures to determine if HPD use is necessary, a better approach may be to use HPDs when exposure levels exceed 92 dBA. For musicians who play heavy rock/metal or steelband music, which is likely to be as damaging as industrial noise (Strasser, Irle, & Scholz, 1999), HPD use should be recommended when exposure levels exceed 85 dBA. Different types of HPDs are used by musicians as described subsequently.

Custom-fitted Hearing Protection Devices for Musicians

The ER earplug developed by Elmer Carlson is an example of this type of earplug. It is designed to maintain the natural frequency response of an open ear canal, including the resonance peak at 2.7 kHz, while providing attenuation across frequencies. The earmold contains a sound channel, which acts as an acoustic mass, and a flexible plastic diaphragm, which provides compliance in combination with the compliance of the ear canal volume allowing the formation of

a Helmholtz resonator. A proper manipulation of the diameter and length of the sound channel allows the resonance of the Helmholtz resonator to be at 2.7 kHz (Killion, DeVilbiss, & Stewart, 1988). All earmold laboratories use the same basic principles to determine the accurate diameter and length of the sound channel (bore), and ER and its European affiliate perform regular site visits to ensure uniform practices across laboratories. ER makes "filter buttons" with 9-, 15-, and 25-dB attenuations that fit into the custom-made earmolds. Therefore, it is easy to replace a button for a different amount of attenuation depending on the setting and instrument. The attenuation characteristics of these earplugs are presented in **Fig. 9.5**. The actual attenuation and the uniformity of the attenuation are likely to depend on the quality of the ear impression (good seal and longer ear canal portion) and shape and size of the individual ear canal. In narrow ear canals, when the ear impressions are made beyond the second bend, the bore is not sufficiently wide to achieve the desired resonance around 2.7 kHz.

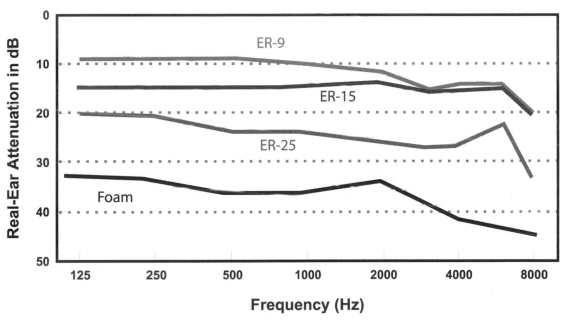

Average sound reduction of Musicians Earplugs and foam earplugs

Fig. 9.5 Attenuation characteristics of the ER earplugs with three different filters and of the foam earplugs. (© Etymotic Research Inc. Used with permission.)

The only solution is to make the earmold canal portion shorter, which increases the occlusion effect (Niquette, 2006).

Preformed Hearing Protection Devices with Relatively Uniform Attenuation

ER-20 is a preformed, low-cost HPD that provides more uniform attenuation than the foam earplug. It is available in regular and junior (Baby Blue) sizes (**Fig. 9.6**). The attenuation characteristics of the ER-20 earplugs are shown in **Fig. 9.7** in both the standard (ETY) and junior (Baby Blues) sizes. The noise reduction rating of ER-20 is 12 dB. About 44% of the musicians may accept and use such hearing protectors (Mendes, Morata, & Marques, 2007).

Foam Hearing Protection Devices

The attenuation characteristic of the foam earplugs are presented in **Fig. 9.5**. These types of HPDs are used commonly (Jansen, Helleman, Dreschler, & de Laat, 2009) and may be effective in minimizing hearing loss. Percussionists who use these types of HPDs have significantly better hearing thresholds than those who do not use foam HPDs (Cunningham, Curk, Hoffman, & Pride, 2006).

Level-dependent Hearing Protection Devices

The Combat Arms Earplug (Aearo Technologies, Indianapolis, IN) is an example of this type of HPD, and it is described in Chapter 6. When the

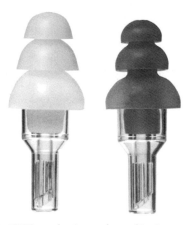

Fig. 9.6   ER-20 earplug in regular and junior (Baby Blue) sizes.

selector dial on the earplug is pointed toward the plug, the plug provides level-dependent protection. The amount of attenuation increases with increases in peak pressure levels. Musicians who play the percussion and timpani are at greatest risk of exposure to excessive peak noise levels (O'Brien, Wilson, & Bradley, 2008). Thus, level-dependent earplugs may be an option for those who play percussion and timpani and may also be suitable for brass and some woodwind instruments. The level-dependent option is available in several off-the-shelf earplugs and earmuffs (Reid & Holland, 2008). Musicians who play percussion and timpani may accept such protection more easily because no attenuation is provided at lower levels, allowing ease in hearing quiet passages in the repertoire and speech.

Use and Acceptance of Hearing Protection Devices

Only one-sixth to half of the musicians in orchestras use hearing protectors, although most are knowledgeable about HPDs (Emmerich, Rudel, & Richter, 2008; Jansen, Helleman, Dreschler, & de Laat, 2009; Laitinen & Poulsen, 2008; Mendes, Morata, & Marques, 2007; Zander, Spahn, & Richter, 2008). The most common type of HPDs used are either the individually fitted HPDs (Zander, Spahn, & Richter, 2008) or disposable foam earplugs or cotton (Jansen, Helleman, Dreschler, & de Laat, 2009; Laitinen & Poulsen, 2008). About 40% of HPD users may switch from the use of one type of protector to another type (Laitinen & Poulsen, 2008).

The frequency of HPD use is higher among musicians who play louder, who have hyperacusis, and who experience tinnitus or fatigue (Laitinen & Poulsen, 2008; Zander, Spahn, & Richter, 2008). Reasons for acceptance of the ER-20 earplug with relatively uniform attenuation characteristics by 44% of the musicians include perception of smoother and more pleasant sound, protection and better sensitivity to singing, lack of tinnitus at the end of the performance, and less bothersome sound (Mendes, Morata, & Marques, 2007). Custom-molded HPDs also can be accepted for frequency-independent attenuation, better fit, and better protection (Laitinen & Poulsen, 2008). The most important consideration for musicians in accepting HPDs appears to be maintenance of the sonority of their musical instrument (Zander, Spahn, & Richter, 2008).

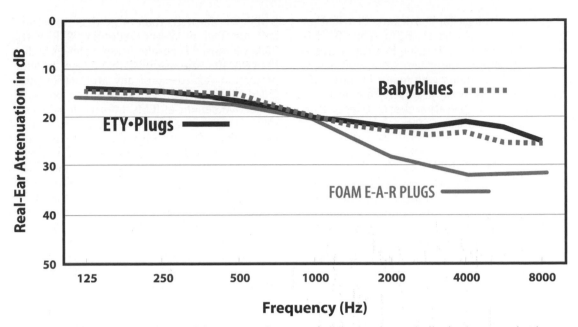

Fig. 9.7 Attenuation characteristics of the ER-20 earplug in standard (ETY) and junior (Baby Blues) compared with a foam plug. (© Etymotic Research Inc. Used with permission.)

Reasons for Lack of Hearing Protection Device Use

In some cases, musicians are concerned about their peers or their audience perceiving them as having less-than-perfect hearing (Ostri, Eller, Dahlin, & Skylv, 1989). Disposable earplugs can be rejected for being too visible. Some musicians prefer foam earplugs over custom-fitted HPDs for the following reasons: difficulty in insertion, perception of altered quality of music, feeling of warmth, sweat, and too much attenuation (Laitinen & Poulsen, 2008). Percussionists may not use HPDs following educational intervention due to hassle (33%), sound quality issues (25%), denial of need (22%), cost (15%), and appearance (5%) (Cunningham, Curk, Hoffman, & Pride, 2006).

Reported reasons for lack of use of HPDs with relatively uniform attenuation characteristics include difficulty in hearing and tuning own instrument, inability to hear the natural sound of the instrument, and difficulty in hearing other musicians or other sounds (Mendes, Morata, & Marques, 2007). Musicians who play brass instruments report significantly greater difficulty in playing music with such earplugs than do percussionists (Chesky, Pair, Yoshimura, & Landford, 2009).

The sound from instruments such as the clarinet is transmitted to the inner ear via bone conduction through the upper teeth. The plugging of the ears by occluding HPDs can result in an occlusion effect, leading to the musician hearing an annoying buzz and difficulty in self-monitoring the output of the instrument through air conduction (Hart, Geltman, Schupbach, & Santucci, 1987). The hollow sound quality and changes in sound image caused by the occlusion effect are considered very annoying and can lead half of musicians to discontinue the use of earplugs (Laitinen & Poulsen, 2008). Additional concerns about HPD use include not being able to hear extremely quiet passages and difficulty in understanding the conductor (Reid & Holland, 2008). Other reasons for rejection of HPDs related to the ear canal include a feeling of pressure from the earplugs, tendency of large amount of earwax, ear infections, and pain (Laitinen & Poulsen, 2008).

Effect of Educational Intervention on Hearing Protection Device Use

Brief educational interventions including information about the dangers of music, awareness of special earplugs for musicians, distribution of free pairs of musicians' earplugs, and knowledge about the risk of hearing loss can increase the use of HPDs (Cunningham, Curk, Hoffman, & Pride, 2006). Students who major in music are more likely to respond positively to education-based hearing conservation efforts (Chesky, Pair, Yoshimura, & Landford, 2009).

Effects of Overprotection

The use of industrial-strength earplugs in some cases can lead to overprotection in musicians. For example, if industrial-strength earplugs are used, too much of the cymbal and "rim-shot" sound is attenuated, which leads to harder hitting by drummers. This in turn can increase wrist and arm injuries (Chasin, 1998).

In-the-Ear Monitors

Musicians can have difficulty hearing their own voices or instruments during live performances because of crowd noise, public announcement systems, onstage amplifiers, and bandmates who increase their sound levels in an attempt to hear their own instruments. Directional wedge-shaped loudspeakers can be placed on the stage in front of the musicians at their knees facing them to allow self-monitoring. A monitor engineer creates mixes for the performers by mixing the output of onstage loudspeakers. One drawback of the onstage loudspeakers is that performers are forced to turn up the volume of their own loudspeaker to hear over the competing sound sources, which can from time to time result in loud whistling feedback. The excessive volume of the loudspeakers and the occasional loud feedback can result in performers being exposed to damaging sound exposures (Santucci, 2006).

Wireless IEMs with custom earpieces made of soft materials have the potential to attenuate crowd and other ambient noises by approximately 25 dB while allowing the musician to hear his or her own instrument or voice and to hear other instruments played by bandmates at safer sound levels. The preferred listening levels using ear monitors under simulated conditions are only around 0.6 dB lower than those preferred using floor monitors. However, the minimum acceptable listening levels are approximately 6 dB lower for IEMs than those that are acceptable for floor monitors (Federman & Ricketts, 2008). If musicians prefer listening levels higher than 90 dBA, the use of IEMs will not provide protection regardless of any attenuation provided by them. Thus, to realize any potential protective benefit of IEMs, informational counseling including recognition of signs of overexposure such as temporary threshold shifts and tinnitus should be provided. Musicians can be informed about the availability of an in-ear-sound analyzer (dB Check, see **Fig. 9.2**), which can read the sound levels reaching the musician's ear and provide data in dBA over time when used in the audio mode along with the IEMs from Sensaphonics (Santucci, 2010). Such a device can alert the musician to take steps to reduce sound exposure. Musicians should also be warned against the practice of using only one earpiece. Use of only one earpiece will cause the musician to increase the volume in one ear to compensate for the loss of binaural summation and leave the other ear unprotected. It is also important to avoid venting of the earpieces, which will allow masking stage sounds to enter the ear canal and force the performer to turn up the volume for self-monitoring (Santucci, 2006).

Earmolds for Custom Fit In-the-Ear Monitors and Hearing Protection Devices

Because of increased comfort, custom-molded earpieces are preferred for IEMs; the best isolation and comfort is provided by earpieces made of soft materials such as silicone or soft vinyl, although these materials are not as durable as acrylic. In making ear impressions, every attempt should be made to minimize the occlusion effect by taking long ear canal impressions past the second bend of the ear canal to seal the bony portion. Asking the musicians to play their own instruments (e.g., flute or singing for vocalists) during curing of the impression material has been recommended (Niquette, 2006).

Verification of Hearing Protection Device Effectiveness

Probe microphone or microphone in the real ear (MIRE) measures can be performed using the procedures described in Chapter 6. Such measures can give some idea of the attenuation provided by HPDs in the frequency range above 1 kHz. The difference in sound field thresholds to narrowband noises with and without the HPDs in place can provide a good estimate of the amount of attenuation across frequencies. During verification of the performance, asking the musicians to play their instrument can allow them to see if a bothersome occlusion effect is present. For larger ear canals, this problem can be resolved by remaking the ear impression and ear mold with a longer ear canal. Comparing the musician's performance with and without HPDs can allow the audiologist to check if the musician plays the instrument more loudly while wearing HPDs. If this is the case, less attenuation or proper instruction to the musician may be necessary.

Use and Care of Custom Earmolds or Hearing Protection Devices

It is important to make sure that the musician can easily insert and remove any HPDs. Slow progression in the use of new custom-made HPDs is recommended to allow the ear canal to adapt to the use and to minimize pain, discomfort, or soreness. One recommendation is to begin wearing the earplug 15 to 20 minutes before playing the instruments so that the ears get used to the plugs and the brain gets adjusted to the altered perception. Perseverance in wearing earplugs is very important so that the brain can adjust to the altered perceptions (Cohen, 1990), including any occlusion effects. Detailed information about the use of IEMs is available at manufacturer's websites that sell such monitors (see Appendix B).

With proper care, earmolds and attenuator buttons can last for prolonged periods. However, these should be inspected on a regular basis and replaced as necessary. Earplugs should be wiped clean after each use. A damp cloth can be used if needed. Use of harsh chemicals or alcohol should be avoided. Earplugs should be stored properly in a clean case. Musicians need to be cautious about the use of corded earplugs while playing their instruments to minimize the possibility of the cord getting tangled in other cords to electrical outlets or the musical instrument.

◆ Potential Future Therapies

Although control of sound levels and use of HPDs when necessary are the best strategies for preventing hearing loss, there are practical limitations in the use of these strategies. The prevention of noise-induced hearing loss can perhaps be augmented in the future by using pharmacological agents such as ebselen (Lynch & Kil, 2005), magnesium (Attias, Sapir, Bresloff, Reshef-Haran, & Ising, 2004), or N-acetylcysteine (Kramer, Dreisbach, Lockwood, et al., 2006). More details about such future trends are included in Chapter 14.

◆ Managing Hearing Loss in Musicians

Case History

The case history form presented in the appendix of Chapter 4 can be used but the onset, duration, and characteristics of tinnitus, hyperacusis, diplacusis, distortion, and any figure-ground perception problems should be noted. Additional information that will be important in managing hearing loss in musicians is presented in **Table 9.3**.

Audiometric Evaluations

Annual audiometric monitoring or evaluations should be completed as detailed in Chapters 4 and 5. Detection of hearing loss at an early stage can motivate musicians to take steps to allow the reduction of further progression of hearing loss. In addition, annual audiograms can indicate any need for adjusting HPDs, hearing aids, or assistive devices.

Otoacoustic Emissions

Routine measurements of OAEs may be helpful in detecting early subclinical pathologies (Guthrie, 2001; Hall & Santucci, 1995). For example, among percussionists who have normal hearing, OAEs are frequently absent or reduced in amplitudes when compared with a normal-hearing group with no significant history of noise exposure (Pride & Cunningham, 2005). In addition, percussionists who use HPDs always or sometimes have significantly better OAEs than

Table 9.3   Additional Information to be Included in the Case History for Musicians

History of music exposure:
The number of years playing:
Current average weekly exposure time: Hours:
Types of instruments played:
Past and current location in the band or orchestra:
Surrounding instruments at the current location: Left:___ Right: ___ Back: ___ Front:___
The environments in which rehearsals/instructions occur:
The environments in which the performances occur:
Types of hearing protection previously worn:
Types of current hearing protection:
Use of IEMs; reasons for using IEMs; type of IEM used; type of encasing material:
Any barriers/difficulties associated with the use of previous or current HPD use:

HPD, hearing protection device; IEM, in-the-ear monitor.

those who do not (Cunningham, Curk, Hoffman, & Pride, 2006).

Tinnitus Evaluation and Management

In the presence of bothersome tinnitus, a complete evaluation and management, as detailed in Chapter 5 and 12, is recommended.

Informational Counseling

All results should be explained carefully, including any deterioration in hearing. Denial of the existence of hearing loss can occur in some cases (Rawool & Kiehl, 2008, 2009) and can interfere with auditory rehabilitation efforts. Even in the presence of pure tone thresholds greater than 40 dB hearing level, musicians may deny the diagnosis of hearing loss and may be concerned about other colleagues finding out about hearing loss. The fear of a loss in personal reputation or of being stigmatized as a disabled person appears to be a major cause for such denial (Emmerich, Rudel, & Richter, 2008). In one study, approximately 19% of musicians indicated that they would be ashamed of having a hearing disorder, and some of them were reluctant to talk about hearing problems (Jansen, Helleman, Dreschler, & de Laat, 2009). The results of OAE testing can be helpful in improving the acceptance of test results because of the objective nature of the test.

Selection of Hearing Aids

For those musicians who have a disabling hearing loss, hearing aids should be considered.

Hearing aids that process music well are currently available. A simple listening comparison of aided and unaided high-quality music played on a high-fidelity system can provide sufficient information about the ability of the hearing aid to process music (Killion, 2009). A good hearing aid for music can also be identified by inspecting the specifications of the hearing aid. The ideal characteristics of hearing aids for musicians are as follows.

Wide Frequency Range

The hearing aid should be capable of providing gain across a very wide range of frequencies including very high and very low frequencies.

Significance of High Frequencies

Instruments such as violin, snare drums, and cymbals elicit sounds that include frequencies as high as 15 kHz (Fletcher, 1931). The perceived quality of orchestral music continues to improve with inclusion of frequencies up to 8 kHz, and a full bandwidth is preferred over any limitation of bandwidth (Snow, 1931). Similarly, the highest rating for perceived "naturalness" of music is obtained with the bandwidth up to 16,854 Hz, while a bandwidth of 313 to 3547 Hz results in a very poor perceived quality (Moore & Tan, 2003).

Beck and Olsen (2008) compared a narrower bandwidth with a high-frequency cutoff of 5.5 kHz to a wider bandwidth with a cutoff of 9 kHz. Ten participants with normal hearing and 20 participants with hearing loss evaluated the quality of short segments of music and a movie sample using a "round-robin"–paired comparison technique. As expected, individuals with normal hearing preferred the wider bandwidth. Participants with slopes less than 8 dB/octave preferred the wider bandwidth or had no preference, while those with greater slopes and more significant high-frequency hearing loss preferred a narrower bandwidth. Such findings may differ among musicians depending on the instrument played and the severity of hearing loss.

The highest sound frequency that can be amplified by digital hearing aids is half the sampling frequency. To achieve amplification of frequencies up to 16 kHz, a sampling frequency of 32 kHz is necessary; hearing aid circuits with such high sampling rates are available (Killion, 2009). Limitation of the bandwidth of the receiver can reduce the quality of music that includes higher frequencies. The hearing aid needs to incorporate receivers that can cover the wide bandwidth.

Significance of Low Frequencies

Instruments such as bass tuba, bass violin, and kettle drums produce sounds that have frequencies as low as 40 Hz (Fletcher, 1931). Musicians may complain about the inability to hear certain sounds. For example, the G bass string of the violin, which has a frequency of 196 Hz, may appear too soft or inaudible (Zakis & Fulton, 2009). Low frequencies are very important for good sound quality for many musical instruments (Snow, 1931), and low frequency response is always preferred for listening to music (Franks, 1982).

Many musicians have normal hearing at lower frequencies, and venting in the earmolds can allow the low frequencies to enter naturally through the ear canal and minimize the occlusion effect. However, depending on the type of instrument played, attenuation of sounds may be necessary to prevent further hearing loss, which would require an occluding earmold. Occlusion effect in such cases can be minimized by making a deep ear impression and by manipulating the gain in the lower frequencies.

Some musicians have hearing loss at low frequencies and will need gain in the lower frequencies. In such cases, if a large vent is added to reduce the occlusion effect, frequencies below 750 Hz will be rolled off, some important elements of the music will become inaudible, and the quality of the music will be perceived as poor. It is important to make a deep ear impression and to use an occluding earmold in these cases. The gain in the low frequencies can be slightly lowered to minimize the occlusion effect.

Wide Intensity Range

The hearing aid needs to be able to handle the wide range of music, including soft sounds created by a violin playing very softly or very quiet passages in a piece to the heaviest playing of a full 75-piece orchestra (Fletcher, 1931). Music quality ratings are somewhat better in the wide dynamic range compression mode when compared with peak clipping or compression limiting modes (Davies-Venn, Souza, & Fabry, 2007). Analog-to-digital converters in hearing aid circuits are available that allow sufficient dynamic range (Killion, 2009; Ryan & Tewari, 2009). Use of a 20-bit precision accuracy can give the hearing aid high precision and the ability to handle a range of 120 dB. The hearing aid also needs to have a receiver with a saturation level above the output limits provided in the fitting software across a wide frequency range.

Multichannel with Adjustable Crossover Frequencies

A high number of channels with the bandwidth of each channel similar to the critical bandwidth of the human ear can allow finer gain adjustments in each channel, including low-frequency channels, depending on the hearing loss. With multiple channels, it is easier to manipulate the gain to remove peaks or dips in the frequency response to obtain a smooth frequency response. A smooth frequency response can prevent one or more notes from being louder or being less audible than other notes (Revit, 2009).

Minimal Processing Delays

Processing delays in digital hearing aids can occur as a result of analog-to-digital conversion, digital-to-analog conversion, and the operation of the signal processing algorithms. Processing delays of less than 1 to 2 milliseconds appear to be less disturbing than longer delays when the gains are low or vary significantly across frequencies (Stone, Moore, Meisenbacher, & Derleth,

2008). Smaller delays also lower the total harmonic distortion. Digital signal processors with conversion delays of just under 0.5 milliseconds at 1 kHz are currently available (Ryan & Tewari, 2009).

Hearing Aid Fitting

A basic hearing aid fitting can begin with a prescriptive approach that incorporates a loudness equalization strategy because many musicians need to hear speech as well as music signals during practice and instruction. Following the initial fitting, it is better to adjust the hearing aid to provide best perception of the specific instrument played by the musician. The hearing aid should be programmed to provide good loudness balance across multiple bands. Most real ear measurement systems allow real ear measures of external stimuli with minor adjustments. Real ear measures for soft, medium, and loud levels across the frequency range are recommended. The hearing aid needs to be programmed to provide good audibility of soft sounds while maintaining loud sounds within comfort levels. Appropriate adjustment of maximum output levels can prevent the high peaks in music (**Table 9.2**) from being transmitted to the ear and may be a satisfying hearing protection option for some musicians (Laitinen & Poulsen, 2008) in the presence of an occluding earmold. The noise reduction and active feedback cancellation needs to be disabled while programming the hearing aid for music (Chasin, 2009b). For most musicians, directional microphones may not be beneficial while performing or listening to music.

Most musicians will need additional adjustments after they listen to music in a variety of different acoustic environments, including rehearsal spaces and performance venues, at softer and louder levels. Two musicians with the same audiometric thresholds may have very different needs, as the perception and expectation of each after the music is processed by the hearing aid may be very different (Punch, 1978). Musicians also need to be informed about the fact that their brains may need some time to adapt to the sounds shaped by the hearing aids. This is especially true for those who have waited for a relatively longer period after having hearing loss to seek hearing aids.

Cochlear Implants

In rare cases, a musician may suffer from severe to profound hearing loss for reasons other than music exposure. Although cochlear implants (CIs) cannot provide the same music perception as that provided by ears with normal hearing, several CI users enjoy listening to music.

Looi, McDermott, McKay, and Hickson (2007) compared the postimplant and aided preimplant ratings of musical quality of nine individuals who were on the waiting list to receive CIs. The ratings after CIs were significantly better than those obtained using hearing aids before implantation. Some of these individuals commented that with hearing aids they could only hear the beat of bass sounds, but with implants they could hear more of the higher-pitched melody instruments. Other individuals reported that with CIs they got a "broader picture" of the musical sounds with finer details. In general, adults with CIs report that their hearing aids provided them with basic rhythmic pulses while the CIs offered more information about pitch and timber (Gfeller, Christ, Knutson, Witt, Murray, & Tyler, 2000).

Combined Use of Hearing Aids and Cochlear Implants

Replacing hearing aids with a CI can adversely affect some aspects of music perception (Looi, McDermott, McKay, & Hickson, 2008). Thus, the best way to maximize listening ability is to maximize the use of residual hearing with hearing aids and use CIs to supplement the information provided by hearing aids. Many individuals have better hearing in the lower frequencies, which are represented at the apical end of the cochlea. Insertion of a shorter electrode array leads to preservation of the apical end, allowing low-frequency stimulation through hearing aids. The shorter electrode array can provide electrical stimulation to the auditory fibers located in the basal or high-frequency end of the cochlea. Some attributes of music perception and appraisal can be improved through such simultaneous use of CIs and hearing aids (Gantz, Turner, Gfeller, & Lowder, 2005; Gfeller, Jiang, Oleson, Driscoll, & Knutson, 2010; Gfeller, Oleson, Knutson, Breheny, Driscoll, & Olszewski, 2008; Gfeller, Turner, Oleson, et al., 2007). The best combination for maximizing the use of residual hearing appears to be the use of CI with a shorter electrode array and hearing aid (hybrid) in one ear and a second hearing aid in the other ear (Dunn, Perreau, Gantz, & Tyler, 2010).

Significance of Individualized Processing Strategy and Fine Tuning

Different individuals benefit from different signal processing strategies for speech perception. The same is likely to be true for music perception. Thus, effort should be made in providing individuals with access to the processing strategy that leads to the enjoyment of their preferred music style. In some cases, when CI users have complaints such as that the music sounds too tinny or too hollow, fine tuning of the CI in terms of the amount of current delivered to different electrodes may improve the perception of music.

Training and Listening Experience

Adults with acquired hearing loss need to be informed to not necessarily expect the same kind of "normal" perception from implants that they had prior to losing their hearing (Rawool, 2007). However, music enjoyment through CIs can be enhanced in a quiet background, using moderate to soft music and visual cues. When possible, background sounds can also be eliminated through direct audio input. Although informal practice in listening to music can result in some music appreciation, formal auditory training may be necessary for full benefit. Preliminary results from a study suggest that formal training in the identification of melodic contour can significantly improve the identification, and this improvement can also lead to improvement in the recognition of familiar melodies (Galvin, Fu, & Nogak, 2007). Formal musical training in early years and music listening practice following implantation can contribute to improvement of familiar melody recognition and recognition of melody excerpts, over time, in adults (Gfeller, Jiang, Oleson, Driscoll, & Knutson, 2010).

Review Questions

1. Why is classical music not as hazardous to hearing as industrial noise?
2. Discuss the factors that cause variation in sound exposure levels across musicians.
3. What are the auditory effects of exposure to hazardous music levels?
4. Discuss the nonauditory effects of exposure to hazardous music levels.
5. Which factors increase the risk of auditory symptoms due to music exposure?
6. Outline the strategies that can be used to minimize the occurrence of hearing loss in musicians.
7. What are some possible reasons for lack of HPD use by musicians?
8. Review the audiogram presented in **Fig. 9.1**. Assume that the musician is a music professor who in addition to teaching music gives solo performances. He is interested in protecting his hearing from further deterioration and is interested in improving his ability to hear his students and music. What will be the potential advantages and disadvantages of earplugs with uniform attenuation, foam earplugs, IEMs, and hearing aids for him? What would you recommend?
9. Review the ideal characteristics of hearing aids for musicians.
10. What is the best option for a musician who has acquired a severe to profound hearing loss?

References

Anari M, Axelsson A, Eliasson A, Magnusson L. (1999). Hypersensitivity to sound—questionnaire data, audiometry and classification. *Scand Audiol.* 28(4): 219–230.

Arnold GE, Miskolczy-Fodor F. (1960). Pure-tone thresholds of professional pianists. *AMA Arch Otolaryngol.* 71:938–947.

Attias J, Sapir S, Bresloff I, Reshef-Haran I, Ising H. (2004). Reduction in noise-induced temporary threshold shift in humans following oral magnesium intake. *Clin Otolaryngol Allied Sci.* 29(6):635–641.

Axelsson A, Eliasson A, Israelsson B. (1995). Hearing in pop/rock musicians: a follow-up study. *Ear Hear.* 16(3):245–253.

Axelsson A, Lindgren F. (1981). Hearing in classical musicians. *Acta Otolaryngol Suppl.* 377:3–74.

Beck DL, Olsen J. (2008). Extended bandwidths in hearing aids. *Hearing Review.* 15(11):22–26.

Behroozi KB, Luz J. (1997). Noise related ailments of performing musicians: a review. *Med Problems Performing Artists.* 12(1):19–22.

Boasson MW. (2002). A one year noise survey during rehearsals and performances in the Netherlands Ballet Orchestra. *Proc Inst Acoust.* 24(4):33–34.

Brashears SM, Morlet TG, Berlin CI, Hood LJ. (2003). Olivocochlear efferent suppression in classical musicians. *J Am Acad Audiol.* 14(6):314–324.

Chasin M. (1998). Musicians and the prevention of hearing loss. *Hearing J.* 51(9):10–16.

Chasin, M. (2006). Hearing aids for musicians. *The Hearing Review* 13(3):24–31.

Chasin M. (2009a). Inexpensive environmental modifications. In: Chasin M, ed. *Hearing Loss in Musicians: Prevention and Management.* San Diego: Plural Publishing: 97–105.

Chasin M. (2009b). Hearing aids and music. In: Chasin M, ed. *Hearing Loss in Musicians: Prevention and Management.* San Diego: Plural Publishing: 107–116.

Chesky K, Pair M, Yoshimura E, Landford S. (2009). An evaluation of musician earplugs with college music students. *Int J Audiol.* 48(9):661–670.

Cohen P. (1990). Drumming: How risky is it to your hearing? *Modern Drummer.* 10:1–11.

Cunningham DR, Curk A, Hoffman J, Pride J. (2006). Despite high risk of hearing loss, many percussionists play unprotected. *Hearing J.* 59(6):58–66.

Davies-Venn E, Souza P, Fabry D. (2007). Speech and music quality ratings for linear and nonlinear hearing aid circuitry. *J Am Acad Audiol.* 18(8):688–699.

Drake-Lee AB. (1992). Beyond music: auditory temporary threshold shift in rock musicians after a heavy metal concert. *J R Soc Med.* 85(10):617–619.

Dunn CC, Perreau A, Gantz B, Tyler RS. (2010). Benefits of localization and speech perception with multiple noise sources in listeners with a short-electrode cochlear implant. *J Am Acad Audiol.* 21(1):44–51.

Emmerich E, Rudel L, Richter F. (2008). Is the audiologic status of professional musicians a reflection of the noise exposure in classical orchestral music? *Eur Arch Otorhinolaryngol.* 265(7):753–758.

European Union Directive(2003). Directive 2003/10/EC of the European Parliament and of the Council of February 6th, 2003 on the Minimum Health and Safety Requirements Regarding the Exposure of Workers on the Risks Arising from Physical Agents (Noise). http://eur-lex.europa.eu/LexUriServ/LexUriServ.do?uri=OJ:L:2003:042:0038:0044:EN:PDF. Accessed July 5, 2001.

Fabijanska A, Rogowski M, Bartnik G, Skarzynski H.(1999). Epidemiology of tinnitus and hyperacusis in Poland. In: Hazell JWP, ed. *Proceedings of the Sixth International Tinnitus Seminar.* London: The Tinnitus and Hyperacusis Centre: 569–771.

Federman J, Ricketts T. (2008). Preferred and minimum acceptable listening levels for musicians while using floor and in-ear monitors. *J Speech Lang Hear Res.* 51(1):147–159.

Fletcher H. (1931). Audible frequency ranges of music, speech and noise. *J Acoust Soc Am.* 3(2.2):1–26.

Franks JR. (1982). Judgments of hearing aid processed music. *Ear Hear.* 3(1):18–23.

Galvin JJ 3rd, Fu QJ, Nogak G. (2007). Melodic contour identification by cochlear implant listeners. *Ear Hear.* 28:302–319.

Gantz BJ, Turner C, Gfeller KE, Lowder MW. (2005). Preservation of hearing in cochlear implant surgery: advantages of combined electrical and acoustical speech processing. *Laryngoscope.* 115(5):796–802.

Gfeller K, Christ A, Knutson JF, Witt S, Murray KT, Tyler RS. (2000). Musical backgrounds, listening habits, and aesthetic enjoyment of adult cochlear implant recipients. *J Am Acad Audiol.* 11(7):390–406.

Gfeller K, Jiang D, Oleson JJ, Driscoll V, Knutson JF. (2010). Temporal stability of music perception and appraisal scores of adult cochlear implant recipients. *J Am Acad Audiol.* 21(1):28–34.

Gfeller K, Oleson J, Knutson JF, Breheny P, Driscoll V, Olszewski C. (2008). Multivariate predictors of music perception and appraisal by adult cochlear implant users. *J Am Acad Audiol.* 19(2):120–134.

Gfeller K, Turner C, Oleson J, et al. (2007). Accuracy of cochlear implant recipients on pitch perception, melody recognition, and speech reception in noise. *Ear Hear.* 28(3):412–423.

Griffiths SR, Samaroo AL. (1995). Hearing sensitivity among professional pannists. *Medical Problems of Performing Artists.* 10(1):11–17.

Guthrie OW. (2001). DPOAEs among normal hearing musicians and nonmusicians. *Hear Review.* 6:26–28.

Hall JW, Santucci M. (1995). Protecting the professional ear: Conservation strategies and devices. *Hearing J.* 48(3):37–45.

Hart CW, Geltman CL, Schupbach J, Santucci M. (1987). The musician and occupational sound hazards. *Medical Problems of Performing Artists.* 3:22–25.

Hasson D, Theorell T, Liljeholm-Johansson Y, Canlon B. (2009). Psychosocial and physiological correlates of self-reported hearing problems in male and female musicians in symphony orchestras. *Int J Psychophysiol.* 74(2):93–100.

Holland-Mortiz K. (1985). Preliminary sound level survey report. *Senza Sordino.* 23(5):2–3.

Jansen EJM, Helleman HW, Dreschler WA, de Laat JA. (2009). Noise induced hearing loss and other hearing complaints among musicians of symphony orchestras. *Int Arch Occup Environ Health.* 82(2):153–164.

Juman S, Karmody CS, Simeon D. (2004). Hearing loss in steelband musicians. *Otolaryngol Head Neck Surg.* 131(4):461–465.

Kähärit K, Eklöf M, Sandsjö L, Zachau G, Möller C. (2003). Associations between hearing and psychosocial working conditions in rock/jazz musicians. *Medical Problems of Performing Artists.* 18:98–105.

Kähärit K, Zachau G, Eklöf M, Sandsjö L, Möller C. (2003). Assessment of hearing and hearing disorders in rock/jazz musicians. *Int J Audiol.* 42(5):279–288.

Killion MC. (2009). What special hearing aid properties do performing musicians require? *Hear Review.* 16(2):22–31.

Killion M, DeVilbiss E, Stewart J. (1988). An earplug with uniform 15-dB attenuation. *Hearing J.* 41(5):14–17.

Konings A, Van Laer L, Wiktorek-Smagur A, et al. (2009). Variations in HSP70 genes associated with noise induced hearing loss in two independent populations. *Eur J Hum Genet.* 73:215–224.

Koskinen H, Toppila E, Olkinuora P. (2010). Facilities for music education and their acoustical design. *Int J Occup Saf Ergon.* 16(1):93–104.

Kramer S, Dreisbach L, Lockwood J, et al. (2006). Efficacy of the antioxidant N-acetylcysteine (NAC) in protecting ears exposed to loud music. *J Am Acad Audiol.* 17(4):265–278.

Laitinen H, Poulsen T. (2008). Questionnaire investigation of musicians' use of hearing protectors, self reported hearing disorders, and their experience of their working environment. *Int J Audiol.* 47(4):160–168.

Laitinen HM, Toppila EM, Olkinuora PS, Kuisma K. (2003). Sound exposure among the Finnish National Opera personnel. *Appl Occup Environ Hyg.* 18(3):177–182.

Levine S, Hofstetter P, Zheng XY, Henderson D. (1998). Duration and peak level as co-factors in hearing loss from exposure to impact noise. *Scand Audiol Suppl.* 48:27–36.

Liljeholm-Johansson Y, Theorell T. (2003). Satisfaction with work task quality correlates with employee health. *Medical Problems of Performing Artists.* 18:141–149.

Lin CY, Wu JL, Shih TS, Tsai PJ, Sun YM, Guo YL. (2009). Glutathione S-transferase M1, T1, and P1 polymorphisms as susceptibility factors for noise-induced temporary threshold shift. *Hear Res.* 257(1–2):8–15.

Looi V, McDermott H, McKay C, Hickson L. (2007). Comparisons of quality ratings for music by cochlear implant and hearing aid users. *Ear Hear.* 28(2 Suppl):59S–61S.

Looi V, McDermott H, McKay C, Hickson L. (2008). Music perception of cochlear implant users compared with that of hearing aid users. *Ear Hear.* 29(3):421–434.

Lynch ED, Kil J. (2005). Compounds for the prevention and treatment of noise-induced hearing loss. *Drug Discov Today.* 10(19):1291–1298.

McBride D, Gill F, Proops D, Harrington M, Gardiner K, Attwell C. (1992). Noise and the classical musician. *BMJ.* 305(6868):1561–1563.

Mendes MH, Morata TC, Marques JM. (2007). Acceptance of hearing protection aids in members of an instrumental and voice music band. *Braz J Otorhinolaryngol.* 73(6):785–792.

Micheyl C, Khalfa S, Perrot X, Collet L. (1997). Difference in cochlear efferent activity between musicians and nonmusicians. *Neuroreport.* 8(4):1047–1050.

Miyakita T, Hellström PA, Frimanson E, Axelsson A. (1992). Effect of low level acoustic stimulation on temporary threshold shift in young humans. *Hear Res.* 60(2):149–155.

Moore BC, Tan CT. (2003). Perceived naturalness of spectrally distorted speech and music. *J Acoust Soc Am.* 114(1):408–419.

Niquette P. (2006). Hearing protection for musicians. *Hear Review.* 13(3):52–58.

Noise at Work Regulations. (2005). *The Control of Noise at Work Regulations.* Milton Keynes, UK: The Stationery Office Limited.

O'Brien I, Wilson W, Bradley A. (2008). Nature of orchestral noise. *J Acoust Soc Am.* 124(2):926–939.

Obeling L, Poulsen T. (1999). Hearing ability in Danish symphony orchestra musicians. *Noise Health.* 1(2):43–49.

Occupational Safety and Health Administration. (1983). 29 CFR 1910.95. Occupational noise exposure; hearing conservation amendment; final rule, effective 8 March 1983. *Federal Register.* 48:9738–9785.

Ostri B, Eller N, Dahlin E, Skylv G. (1989). Hearing impairment in orchestral musicians. *Scand Audiol.* 18(4):243–249.

Pascarelli EF, Hsu YP. (2001). Understanding work-related upper extremeity disorders: clinical findings in 485 computer users, musicians, and others. *J Occup Rehabil.* 11(1):1–21.

Phillips SL, Henrich VC, Mace ST. (2010). Prevalence of noise-induced hearing loss in student musicians. *Int J Audiol.* 49(4):309–316.

Phillips SL, Mace ST. (2008). Sound level measurements in music practice rooms. *Music Performance Research.* 2:36–47.

Pride JA, Cunningham DR. (2005). Evidence of early cochlear damage in a large sample of percussionists. *Medical Problems of Performing Artists.* 20(3):135–139.

Punch JL. (1978). Quality judgments of hearing aid-processed speech and music by normal and otopathologic listeners. *J Am Audiol Soc.* 3(4):179–188.

Rawool VW. (1996). Acoustic reflex monitoring during the presentation of 1000 clicks at high repetition rates. *Scand Audiol.* 25(4):239–245.

Rawool VW. (2007). Potential benefits of cochlear implants for individuals who communicate exclusively through sign language. Part II. Access to music. *Hear Review.* 14(11):40–45.

Rawool VW. (2008). Growing up noisy: The sound exposure diary of a hypothetical young adult. *Hear Review.* 15(5):30, 32, 34, 39–40.

Rawool VW, Colligon-Wayne LA. (2008). Auditory lifestyles and beliefs related to hearing loss among college students in the USA. *Noise Health.* 10(38):1–10.

Rawool VW, Kiehl JM. (2008). Perception of hearing status, communication and hearing aids among socially active older individuals. *J Otolaryngol Head Neck Surg.* 37(1):27–42.

Rawool VW, Kiehl JM. (2009). Effectiveness of informational counseling on acceptance of hearing loss among older adults. *Hear Review.* 16(6):14–22.

Reid AW, Holland MW. (2008). *A Sound Ear II: The Control of Noise at Work Regulations 2005 and Their Impact on Orchestras.* London, United Kingdom: Association of British Orchestras.

Revit LR. (2009). What's so special about music? The demands of a performing musician's hearing aids are very different. *Hear Review.* 16(2):12, 16, 18, 19.

Ryan J, Tewari S. (2009). A digital signal processor for musicians and audiophiles. *Hear Review.* 16(2):38–41.

Sallows K. (2001). *Listen While You Work: Hearing Conservation for the Arts.* Vancouver, BC, Canada: Safety and Health in Arts Production and Entertainment.

Santucci M. (2006). Please welcome on stage... Personal in the ear monitoring. *Hear Review.* 13(3):60, 64, 66, 67.

Santucci M. (2010). Saving the music industry from itself. *Hear J.* 63(6):10–14.

Schmuziger N, Patscheke J, Probst R. (2006). Hearing in nonprofessional pop/rock musicians. *Ear Hear.* 27(4):321–330.

Sliwinska-Kowalska M, Noben-Trauth K, Pawelczyk M, Kowalski TJ. (2008). Single nucleotide polymorphisms in the cadherin 23 (CDH23) gene in Polish workers exposed to industrial noise. *Am J Hum Biol.* 20(4):481–483.

Snow WB. (1931). Audible frequency ranges of music, speech and noise. *J Acoust Soc Am.* 3(1.1):155–166.

Steurer M, Simak S, Denk DM, Kautzky M. (1998). Does choir singing cause noise-induced hearing loss? *Audiology.* 37(1):38–51.

Stone MA, Moore BC, Meisenbacher K, Derleth RP. (2008). Tolerable hearing aid delays. V. Estimation of limits for open canal fittings. *Ear Hear.* 29(4):601–617.

Strasser H, Irle H, Legler R. (2003). Temporary hearing threshold shifts and restitution after energy-equivalent exposures to industrial noise and classical music. *Noise Health.* 5(20):75–84.

Chapter 10

Noise Control and Hearing Conservation in Nonoccupational Settings

Over their lifetimes, humans can be exposed to noise and other ototoxins from several sources outside the occupational environment. Some of these sources are described in this chapter along with suggestions for hearing conservation.

◆ Community Noise

Community noise can be defined as noise from all other sources with the exception of those from industries. Community noise is also referred to as environmental or residential noise (Berglund, Lindvall, & Schwela, 2000). Noises created by transportation, construction and other public works, and communities contribute to community noise.

◆ Community Noise Exposures

In the European Union countries, daytime exposure can exceed 55 dBA for approximately 40% of the population, and it can exceed 65 dBA for 20% of the population. The nighttime exposure can exceed 55 dBA for more than 30% of the population. Excessive exposure to noise has a significant negative impact on human health and hearing (European Agency for Safety and Health at Work, 2005).

◆ Effects of Noise

Noise can interfere with communication, cause sleep disturbance and cardiovascular effects, affect mental health, reduce performance, cause

annoyance responses, and can alter social behavior (European Agency for Safety and Health at Work, 2005). A single incidence of intense noise exposure can cause temporary hearing loss and trigger long-lasting tinnitus and hypersensitivity to sounds (Schmuzigert, Fostiropoulos, & Probst, 2006), and in some cases such tinnitus can be highly debilitating (Rawool, 2010).

Interference with Communication

Noise can interfere with easy and spontaneous communication and may cause strain on the vocal mechanism because of the requirement to speak louder.

Sleep Disturbance

Environmental noise may cause sleep interference, which can have negative effects on physiological and mental functioning. The potential negative effects of noise on sleep are (Berglund, Lindvall, & Schwela, 2000):

- Difficulty in falling asleep
- Awakenings and alterations of sleep stages or depth
- Increased blood pressure, heart rate, and finger pulse amplitude
- Vasoconstriction
- Changes in respiration
- Cardiac arrhythmia
- Increased body movements

Cardiovascular Effects

A study was conducted to evaluate any relationship between noise from aircraft or road traffic near airports and the risk of hypertension. The study included a sample of 4861 individuals within the age range of 45 to 70 years who had lived for at least 5 years near any of six major European airports. Their blood pressure was measured and additional data was collected on health, socioeconomic, and lifestyle factors, including diet and physical activity, via questionnaire at home visits. Their noise exposures were assessed using detailed models with a resolution of 1 dB (5 dB for U.K. road traffic noise) and a spatial resolution of 250 × 250 m for aircraft and 10 × 10 m for road traffic noise. The results showed excess risks of hypertension related to long-term noise exposures, mainly from nighttime aircraft noise and daily average road traffic noise (Jarup, Babisch, Houthuijs, et al., 2008). Another study showed that road traffic noise at home is a stressor that could affect children's blood pressure (Babisch, Neuhauser, Thamm, & Seiwert, 2009). A meta-analysis of 21 epidemiologic studies on exposure to road traffic noise and cardiovascular risk showed an increase in risk of myocardial infarction with increasing noise levels above 60 dBA during the day (Babisch, 2008).

◆ Measurement of Community Noise

Sound levels for community noise measurements are generally A-weighted. For impulsive noise, C-weighted sound levels can be used. A 3-dB exchange rate is used for time average sound levels. Sound quality can be evaluated using octave or one-third octave band levels. The following measures can be used in documenting community noise.

Continuous Equivalent Sound Pressure Level ($L_{Aeq, T}$ dBA)

This is continuous or a constant level of noise that delivers the same amount of energy content as the varying acoustic signal being measured. It is assumed to represent the same potential to damage hearing as the varying signal. The A represents use of A-weighting, and the eq indicates the use of equivalent level of continuous noise. This is a simple way of representing time-varying environmental noises such as those produced by railways and aircrafts. If the sound is recorded as $L_{eq, T}$ dB or $L_{Leq, T}$ dB, it is assumed that the measurements were made without using the A weighting.

Sound Pressure Percentile Level ($L_{AN,T}$)

The measured noise level in dBA is exceeded N% of time, T. For example, $L_{A10,18 \text{ hour}}$, which has been used as an index of traffic noise from 6 AM to midnight for the purposes of noise insulation, indicates the level that was exceeded 10% of the time over a period of 18 hours. The level exceeded 90% of the time is often used as a measure of the background sound present without transient or intermittent sounds. The number of samples measured should be at least 10 times the difference in decibels between the highest and lowest levels to yield reliable measures.

Lday

Lday is the A-weighted long-term average sound level measured over all day periods (usually 12 hours long) of a year and is used as a noise indicator for annoyance during the daytime.

Levening

This is the A-weighted long-term average sound level measured over all the evening periods (usually 4 hours long) of a year and is used as a indicator for annoyance during evenings.

Lnight

This is the A-weighted long-term average sound level measured over all the night periods (usually 8 hours) of a year and serves as an indicator for sleep disturbances during nights.

Ldn, Day–Night Average Sound Level System

This is the 24-hour average sound level, expressed in decibels, with a 10 dB penalty for sound levels measured between 10 PM and 7 AM. The reason for the nighttime penalty is that people are much more annoyed by noise at night than at any other times.

Sound Exposure Level (L$_{AE}$ dBA)

This is the A-weighted sound pressure level, which (over 1 second) contains the same amount of A-weighted energy as a specified single event. This is a way of representing short-duration events such as a passing train or aircraft. It allows comparison of different events: for each event, the energy content is described over a period of 1 second regardless of the actual duration of the original noise.

◆ Community Noise Standards and Guidelines

Community Noise Levels

The U.S. Department of Housing and Urban Development (1991) has specified day–night average sound levels (DNLs) of up to 65 dBA as acceptable for areas where it funds or finances housing. This criterion is based on surveys of people who reported high annoyance related to existing noise in their residential areas. Sound levels between DNLs of 65 and 75 dBA are considered unacceptable unless steps are taken to reduce the noise reaching inside the homes. Five decibel greater noise attenuation than that provided by standard construction is required if the DNLs are between 65 and 70 dBA. Ten decibels additional attenuation is required for DNLs between 70 and 75 dBA. For single-family homes, barriers are required to reduce noise over DNLs of 70. DNLs above 75 dBA are unacceptable because the construction cost required to make the noise levels inside buildings acceptable is likely to be too high and the noise levels in the outdoor environment would remain unacceptable.

Noise Emissions from Motor Vehicles

The main sources of noise from motor vehicles are the engine, the frictional contact of the vehicle with air, and the frictional contact of the tires to the road. At speeds higher than about 37 miles/hour, the road contact noise is generally louder than the engine noise. The following factors partially determine the noise levels generated by road traffic (Berglund, Lindvall, & Schwela, 2000):

- The traffic flow rate
- The speed of the vehicles
- The proportion of heavy vehicles
- The nature of the road surface

The Federal Highway Administration (FHA) in the United States uses a 1-hour equivalent time average sound level criterion of 67 dBA. When expected levels exceed this criterion, noise barriers are considered for new highway projects. The cost and benefit of the barrier per protected home is considered before actually building the barriers. Landscaping is not considered a viable noise abatement measure. The following noise abatement measures may be considered (FHA, 2010):

- Construction of noise barriers
- Traffic management measures including reduction or prohibition of certain types of vehicles through traffic control and signs, time-use restrictions for certain types of vehicles, altered speed limits, and restricted lane designations
- Alteration of horizontal and vertical alignments
- Acquisition of real property (mostly unimproved property) to serve as a buffer zone to preempt development that could be adversely impacted by traffic noise
- Noise insulation of areas such as hotels, auditoriums, daycare centers, campgrounds, etc., through proper designs

Noise Emissions from Airplanes

Airplane traffic can generate loud noise levels in the vicinity of both commercial and military airports. During takeoffs, airplanes can produce intense noise, vibration, and rattle. During landings also, airplanes can produce high noise levels in long low-altitude flight corridors. The following factors determine noise generated at and around airports (Berglund, Lindvall, & Schwela, 2000), some of which can be modified or controlled to reduce overall noise levels near airports:

- The number of airplanes arriving and departing (the proportions of takeoffs and landings)
- The types of airplanes (estimated maximum A-weighted sound levels from some aircrafts are shown in **Table 10.1**)
- The flight paths of airplanes
- The atmospheric conditions

Table 10.1   Estimated Maximum A-Weighted Sound Levels during Takeoff (Federal Aviation Administration, 2010)

Manufacturer	Airplane	Engine	Takeoff gross weight 1000 lb	Estimated maximum dBA
Concord	Concord	0593/M-602	400.00	112.9
Boeing	B-747-100	JT9D-7F, JT9D-7FWET,	750.00	100.5
McDonnell Doug	DC-10-30	CF6-50C1	562.00	93.9
Boeing	B-727-200	JT8D-7QN	172.50	88.00
McDonnell Doug	DC-10-10	CF6-6D1	440.00	85.3
Airbus	A-310-221	JT9D-7R4D1	313.05	77.3
Cessna	152	0-235-L2C	1.70	55.0

The Federal Aviation Administration and the U.S. Department of Defense use a DNL of 65 dBA. Aircraft or military activities generating noise below 65 dBA DNL are considered to have no significant impact. Noise levels at many airports exceed the DNLs of 65 dBA, especially during arrival and departure of flights (Falzone, 1999). The levels may continue to rise in the future because of demands for additional flights.

Noise Emissions from Construction Equipment

Building construction and excavation work can generate a significant amount of noise. Some sources of construction noise include noises from cranes, cement mixers, welding, hammering, boring, and other work processes (Berglund, Lindvall, & Schwela, 2000).

With reference to the European Union, permissible noise emission levels are specified within directive 84/532/EEC/ (European Union European Communities Directive, 1984) on the EEC-type examination certificates for construction plants and equipment. This directive has adopted seven daughter directives for different types of equipment. All the seven daughter directives require that the products must have labels indicating the maximum noise levels guaranteed by the manufacturer and also require the description of procedures used for measuring airborne noise. For example, directive 2000/14/EC (European Parliament and the Council of the European Union, 2000) requires manufacturers of 57 types of equipment used for a variety of outdoor tasks ranging from construction to gardening to label each and every machine to indicate the maximum "guaranteed" sound power level generated by the machine. Of the 57 types, noise limits are set for 22 types of equipment.

◆ Overall Management of Community Noise

A collaborative effort of many individuals is necessary in managing community noise including politicians, noise control engineers, acoustics professionals, community interest groups, technology officials, and law enforcement agencies. A legal framework for managing community noise is presented in **Fig. 10.1** (Berglund, Lindvall, & Schwela, 2000). In cases where community noise problems exist, the problem is likely to be in the enforcement of the noise legislation partly because of the limited number of police officers and the transient and hidden nature of many annoying noises.

◆ Local Noise Ordinances

Several states have state or municipal noise ordinances based on either nuisance or a combination of nuisance and sound levels. These ordinances formally address noise that may annoy or disturb the public but is usually not so loud that it can cause a safety hazard. In simple terms, a nuisance ordinance is usually a prohibition of making any unreasonable or excessive noise, and compliance is based on the subjective responses of two or more listeners. Ordinances that specify sound level limits might appear to provide stronger control over undesirable sound levels compared with nuisance ordinances, but they are hard to implement. The required measurements vary considerably, including A-weighted sound level limits at specified locations, sound levels averaged over specified periods, octave or one-third octave measures, and specific criteria for measuring discrete tone noises. In North America,

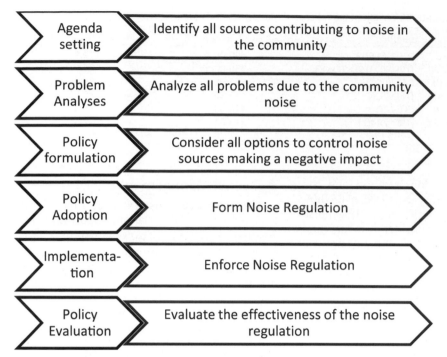

Fig. 10.1   Legal framework for managing community noise.

depending on location and zoning, overall maximum permitted noise levels vary from 45 dBA to 72 dBA (Aaberg, 2008).

As an example of local noise ordinances, the maximum permissible sound levels from stationary sources in Morgantown, WV, are listed in **Table 10.2**. In addition, section 527.03 of this noise ordinance (www.morgantown.com/noiseord.htm) states that, "No person shall make, continue or cause to be made or continued, any loud, unnecessary or unusual noise or any noise which annoys, disturbs, injures or endangers the comfort, repose, health, peace or safety of others, within the city." In reality, annoyances and sleep disturbances at night are experienced routinely by some residents partly due to poorly planned

and highly congested new housing developments without much oversight with reference to sound transmission properties, and partly due to deliberate harassing behaviors of some residents.

In some countries such as India or Pakistan, community noise is often generated by the use of firecrackers or broadcasting of loud music or prayers through loudspeakers during festivals or religious ceremonies. Although local noise ordinances are in place, the execution of the ordinances may not always be effective.

◆ Noise Exposure during a Commute

Of the various forms of mass transit systems (subways, buses, ferries, tramways, and commuter railways) in New York, the highest noise levels are measured in subway cars and at subway platforms (Neitzel, Gershon, Zeltser, Canton, & Akram, 2009). The average noise levels on subway platforms in New York can vary from 82 to 90 dBA, and maximum levels can reach 106 dBA. The maximum levels inside subway cars can reach 112 dBA, while those at bus stops can reach 89 dBA (Gershon, Neitzel, Barrera, &

Table 10.2   Maximum Permissible Sound Levels from Stationary Vehicles in Morgantown, WV

Zoning district	Time of day	Continuous sound (dBA)	Impulsive sound (dBA)
All residential	All	60	80
All business	All	65	90
All industrial	All	70	110

Akram, 2006). The allowable exposure duration for 106 dBA is 3 minutes 45 seconds (National Institute of Occupational Safety and Health [NIOSH], 1998), and 12% of the subway platform levels exceed 100 dBA, which has an allowable exposure duration of 15 minutes. Twenty percent of the maximum noise level readings inside the subway cars show levels over 100 dBA, and more than two-thirds are over 90 dBA with an allowable duration of 2 hours and 35 seconds. Several individuals travel from surrounding cities to New York for work using the mass transit system. Many of them could exceed the allowable durations, especially if they travel over a greater distance and if they are exposed to other noises during the day.

Agencies responsible for operating the subway systems need to make a concerted effort to reduce noise using some of the techniques discussed in Chapter 3, including identification of the noisiest sources, placement of dampening material in noisy sections, and regularly scheduled maintenance of tracks, braking mechanisms, and all other machinery. Individuals who use the mass transit system could benefit from using personal hearing protection (see Chapter 6). Individuals who use personal listening devices need to be especially careful because they are likely to increase the volume of their devices to hazardous levels to overcome the noise levels inside the cars. Williams (2005) measured sound exposure from personal stereo systems under noisy listening conditions. A total of 13 of the 55 personal stereo system users in the study exceeded the 8-hour 85 dBA time weighted average (TWA), and 2 users exceeded 100 dBA TWA. In some cases, the use of noise-cancelling earphones to listen to music may be beneficial.

Noise Exposure from Motorcycles

Motorcyclists can suffer from hearing loss (McCombe & Binnington, 1994; McCombe, Binnington, Davis, & Spencer, 1995). Temporary thresholds shifts and tinnitus can occur after only 1 hour of high-speed riding, and some motorcyclists may suffer from disequilibrium. Earplugs can prevent the temporary thresholds shifts (McCombe, Binnington, & McCombe, 1993) and appear to be relatively safe in terms of detecting important signals while riding (Binnington, McCombe, & Harris, 1993).

◆ Recreational Noise Exposure

Noise exposure can occur during recreational activities including target shooting, hunting, and listening to music.

Recreational Shooting

According to the National Shooting Sports Foundation (NSSF), hunting is a big business in America, and it generates 600,000 jobs in the United States (NSSF, 2011). In 2009, sales of hunting and firearms equipment rose 14% to $5.2 billion from $4.5 billion in 2008 (National Sporting Goods Association, 2010). The noise exposure from gunfire can vary from 134 to 190 dBP (Berger, 2006). Impulse noise exposure above 140 dBP for any amount of time is considered hazardous (NIOSH, 1998). The following precautions can minimize the noise exposure from weapon fire (Schulz, 2006):

- *Practice outdoors, not indoors:* Indoor shooting can increase exposure due to bouncing of sounds off hard surfaces. Outdoor shooting can allow easier dissipation of sound energy.
- *Practice alone:* Shooting at a range with several other shooters leads to exposure to more firing rounds, thus increasing the total exposure.
- *While hunting, add distance between you and other hunters:* With distance, the noise level drops, leading to less exposure.
- *Use smaller caliber weapons:* Larger caliber weapons produce higher intensity exposure; the more the gunpowder, the more hazardous the exposure.
- *Use longer-barreled weapons:* The sound is emitted from the end of the barrel or muzzle. The shorter the barrel, the closer the muzzle is to the ear.
- *Avoid modifying muzzles:* Modifications such as muzzle ports or muzzle breaks increase noise exposure by approximately 10 dBP by sending the noise back to the shooter.
- *Use hearing protection:*
  ◇ Use level-dependent earplugs (see Chapter 6) that provide attenuation for high-level impulse sounds but very little or no attenuation for speech or environmental sounds.

◇ Electronic earplugs or earmuffs can allow softer sounds to be audible but decrease the exposure to hazardous levels produced by weapons.

Music Venues

Young adults spend a significant portion of their social time in venues where loud music is present. For example, in England, Scotland, and Wales, approximately 23% of young adults attend a musical performance once or twice a month or more, 56% of respondents go to a club once or twice a month, and 55% visit a pub or bar where the music is so loud that it is necessary to shout during communication. Of the 55% who go, 76% usually spend 2 to 6 hours in the pub (Bennett, 2006).

The sound levels at discotheques can range from 104 to 112 dBA (Serra, Biassoni, Richter, et al., 2005). The sound levels at concerts can vary with peak levels of up to 153 dBC (**Table 10.3**). Seventy to eighty percent of concert attendees may not be wearing any hearing protection (Bogoch, House, & Kudla, 2005; Widén & Erlandsson, 2004). Ulrich and Pinheiro (1974) reported significant threshold shifts in all participants exposed to pop music with average levels of 110 to 115 dB sound pressure level (SPL), and in one of the participants this threshold shift appeared to be permanent at 5 months following the exposure. Opperman, Reifman, Schlauch, and Levine (2006) requested 29 volunteers to attend three concerts encompassing pop, rock, and heavy metal music in the same concert hall. Average sound levels were 99.8 dBA, and the maximum level was 125.6 dBA. Sixty-four percent (9/14) of the participants without earplugs and twenty-seven percent (4/14) of those using earplugs suffered from significant threshold shifts. Tinnitus is also commonly reported after attending

concerts (Axelsson & Prasher, 2000; Chung, Des Roches, Meunier, & Eavey, 2005). These studies collectively suggest the possibility of cochlear damage after attendance at concerts at least in some individuals.

Strategies for Controlling Levels at Music Venues

Development of Evidence-based Guidelines and Safety Standards

One reported barrier for reducing music levels at different venues such as concerts is the lack of clearly defined levels that are expected to be hazardous for music (Vogel, van der Ploeg, Brug, & Raat, 2009). The Swedish National Board of Health and Welfare considers 100 dB L_{Aeq} as a safe limit for a duration of 1 hour/day (5 hours/week) and has recommended a maximum value of 115 dBA during musical performances for adults. The safe limit and maximum values are 97 dB L_{Aeq} and 110 dBA at venues where children under 13 years have access (Swedish National Board of Health and Welfare, 2005). In 2005, a national project was performed in Sweden to improve environments with high recorded and/or live music levels such as cinemas, concert halls, and restaurants. Out of the 471 establishments that were investigated, 24% exceeded the highest recommended SPLs in Sweden. Out of 171 festival and concert events, 42% exceeded the recommended levels. Therefore, although establishing safety standards is a first step, continuing supervision appears to be necessary for full compliance (Ryberg, 2009).

Acoustic Treatment of Venues

Use of soft furnishings and surround speakers can improve the music experience while allowing lower sound levels (Vogel, van der Ploeg, Brug, & Raat, 2009).

Table 10.3 Sound Levels Generated during Different Music Events (Kähärit, Zachau, Eklöf, Sandsjö, & Möller, 2003)

Sound source	Sound level	dB (A) maximum (fast)	Peak levels
Folk music, restaurant with small stage, dosimeter on listener 1.5 m from loud speaker	91.1 L_{Aeq}	108.8	129.7 dBC
Rock music, medium-sized discotheque with dosimeter on a listener 6 m from the stage	104.3 L_{Aeq}	117.6	150.1 dBC
Rock music, large stage and discotheque with dosimeter on listener 10 m from loudspeaker, 25 m from stage	93.8 L_{Aeq}	114.8	> 140 dBC
Blues/jazz club, on listener 5 m from the stage to the left and the right side	97.4 L_{Aeq}	122.2	153.3 dBC
	98.5 L_{Aeq}	113.8	130.8 dBC

Encouraging Rest Periods

Providing rooms for regeneration breaks at sites such as discotheques may encourage rest periods that allow the ears to recover from loud sound exposure (Weichbold & Zorowka, 2007).

Financial Incentives for Keeping Sound Levels within Safe Limits

Low admission prices may be a strong incentive for attending certain discotheques or musical events (Weichbold & Zorowka, 2007), while softer music levels can lower the attendance with undesired economic consequences (Vogel, van der Ploeg, Brug, & Raat, 2009). Financial subsidies from healthcare insurance providers to event organizers or discotheques may allow them to offer low admission prices, which can improve attendance even in the presence of loud but safe music levels (Weichbold & Zorowka, 2007). Over time, attendees might get used to enjoying music presented at loud but safe levels.

Provision of Earplugs

Provision of earplugs may encourage some of the participants to minimize their music exposure.

Display of Sound Levels in the Venue on a Big Screen

Such displays may encourage everyone involved including disc jockeys to lower music levels.

Demonstration Stations

Individuals who have previously experienced tinnitus are more likely to wear earplugs while conducting noisy activities (Rawool, 2008; Widén, Holmes, Johnson, Bohlin, & Erlandsson, 2009). Therefore, allowing adults to experience simulated tinnitus by presenting either high-frequency pure tones or noises at attractive demonstration stations may encourage them to protect their hearing. Signs showing simple protection strategies such as sitting away from loudspeakers and wearing hearing protection can also be displayed at such stations. Small incentives such as coupons can be provided to approach and experience the activities at such stations.

◆ Reducing Noise at Home

It is important to keep the noise levels at home low. Higher noise levels can interfere with communication and can cause moderate annoyance during daytime and evening hours. During these hours, the levels should be kept below 35 $L_{Aeq, 16}$ dBA. At night, high noise levels can interfere with sleep and lead to poor-quality sleep. The levels inside bedrooms at night should be kept below 30 $L_{Aeq, 8}$ dBA, and the peak levels should not exceed 45 dBA (Berglund, Lindvall, & Schwela, 2000).

Several of the following strategies can be used to reduce noise exposure at home (U.S. Environmental Protection Agency [EPA], 1978), and these strategies are especially useful for hearing aid users:

◆ Windows and doors can allow transmission of outside noises:
  ◇ Keep doors and windows closed.
  ◇ Install storm or soundproof windows.
  ◇ Seal air leaks around the edge of doors or windows with caulking or weather stripping.
  ◇ Use heavy drapery on windows; noise-attenuating drapes are available.
◆ Use techniques that will allow better absorption of sounds and minimize the possibility of sounds bouncing off:
  ◇ Use acoustical tiles on ceilings.
  ◇ Use wall-to-wall and stair carpeting with felt or rubber padding.
◆ Minimize all equipment noise:
  ◇ Buy quiet equipment while purchasing items such as refrigerators, microwaves, hairdryers, air conditioners, heaters, humidifiers, etc.
  ◇ Install exhaust fans on rubber mounts.
  ◇ Put foam pads under small appliances such as blenders and mixers.
  ◇ Use vibration mounts under electrical appliances including washers, dryers, and dishwashers.
◆ Wear earplugs when using equipment that produces sustained loud sounds. For some equipment such as chain saws, use both earplugs and earmuffs.
◆ Buy and use quiet lawnmowers. Electric-powered lawn mowers are generally 10 to 20 dBA quieter than gas (one-half to one-fourth as loud) and also cause less air pollution (Noise Pollution Clearinghouse, 2005).

◆ Minimize noise exposure from entertainment devices: Use of wireless or hardwired surround speakers can allow full experience of the music and other sounds without a loud volume setting. For individuals with hearing loss, use of headphones with volume control or assistive listening devices is recommended. Keep the volume of all entertainment devices such as televisions, mp3 players, stereos, and music playing from cell phones down.

The free field equivalent SPLs from personal stereo systems can vary from 91 to 121 dBA at the highest volume control settings; some peaks in music samples can be as high as 139 dB SPL (Fligor & Cox, 2004), suggesting the possibility of damage to the cochlea for those who listen for long periods and or at high volume levels. Peng, Tao, and Huang (2007) compared the auditory sensitivity of 120 personal listening device users to 30 nonusers. The sensitivity in the region of 3 to 8 kHz and at extended high frequencies was poorer in the group that listened to personal devices. Reported use of personal stereo devices has been associated with a 70% increase in risk for slight to mild hearing loss (Cone, Wake, Tobin, Poulakis, & Rickards, 2010).

◆ Noise Exposure in Children

Children can be exposed to hazardous noise levels from a variety of sources including motor vehicles (including tractors, motorcycles, and automobiles), fireworks, firearms, power tools, amplified music, and farm machinery (Lankford, Mikrut, & Jackson, 1991; Roche, Siervogel, Himes, & Johnson, 1978; Rytzner & Rytzner, 1981). Sound levels from snowmobiles can range from 105 to 136 dBA (Bess & Poynor, 1972, 1974). Tractors may produce sound levels of 95 dBA or greater (Broste, Hansen, Strand, & Stueland, 1989). Approximately 20% of the workforce between the ages of 17 and 25 years entering industries may already have audiometric notches consistent with noise exposure (Rabinowitz, Slade, Galusha, Dixon-Ernst, & Cullen, 2006). Noise exposure at young ages can impair temporal resolution in the auditory cortex (Aizawa & Eggermont, 2006) and can increase the susceptibility to the effects of aging on hearing (Kujawa & Liberman, 2006). Thus, it is necessary to minimize noise exposure at a very early age.

Rawool (2008) identified several ways in which young adults can be exposed to excessively loud sounds, some of which are shown in **Table 10.4** along with some strategies for minimizing the related noise exposure.

Noise Exposure at Daycare Centers

Voss (2005) measured the noise levels at Danish daycare centers (nurseries, kindergartens, and skole og fritidsordning [SFO], which are leisure centers for school children to attend after school). At 95% of the centers, the noise levels exceeded 75 dBA, and the level of 80 dBA was exceeded at 50 to 67% of the centers. The noise levels exceeded 85 dBA TWA at 5% percent of the nurseries, 7% of the kindergartens, and 20% of the SFOs. The noise levels can be expected to vary depending on the number of children at the center, the room acoustics, the type of toys or entertaining items available for children's use, and the social behavior of children and staff. For example, it is important to teach children to express their needs without crying or yelling, and it is important for the staff to keep calm voices while taking any disciplinary actions. In selecting toys, noisy toys should be avoided. Acoustic tiles for ceilings and heavy drapes on windows could reduce reverberation and noise.

Noisy Toys

American Society for Testing and Materials (ASTM; 2007) has issued acoustics standards for toys; these standards are presented in **Table 10.5**. The Consumer Product Safety Improvement Act (Consumer Product Safety Improvement Act, 2008) made the ASTM voluntary standards mandatory. In 2009, many toys on the market exceeded these standards including Secret Saturdays Cryptid Claw manufactured by Mattel (El Segundo, CA) and Kota and Pals Stompers Triceratops manufactured by Playschool (Pawtucket, RI) (Hitchcock, 2009). In addition, many toys may not be used as they are intended to be used (Charbonneau & Goldschmidt, 2004). Unilateral or bilateral hearing loss has been reported in children resulting from the use of toy cap pistols (Segal, Eviatar, Lapinsky, Shlamkovitch, & Kessler, 2003). For example, a handheld toy may be used as though it is a telephone, exposing the child to higher noise levels. The Sight and Hearing Association conducted a noisy toys study in 2009 and

Table 10.4   Participation in Noisy Activities by Young Adults

Activity	Noise level	Strategy for prevention of hearing loss
Music exposure in car	Sound levels in car audio systems can be as high as 154.7 dBA (Gallagher, 1987).	Make it a habit to set the levels just sufficient to hear above the road noise levels; keep car windows closed to allow enjoyable perception of music at lower levels.
Music exposure from personal listening devices	According to a survey, 51% of high school students had experienced at least one of four symptoms of hearing loss. A total of 43% of the students in this survey reported that they listened to their mp3 players at loud volume levels (Zogby International, 2006).	Maximum limits can be set on some personal listening devices such as mp3 players by downloading software via the Internet.
Music exposure from attendance at concerts	At a variety of concerts, the audience can be exposed to hazardous sound levels (see Table 10.3). Eighteen percent of college freshmen prefer to sit near the loudspeaker during concerts, where the sound pressure levels are higher (Rawool & Colligon-Wayne, 2008).	Upper sound exposure limits should be set for concerts. Use of earplugs can reduce the levels of exposure.
Music exposure at night clubs	Gunderson, Moline, and Catalano (1997) measured the sound levels in eight live music clubs in New York. The average sound levels during performances ranged from 94.9 to 106.7 dBA. Fifteen percent of children in the age range of 10 and 17 years may be attending clubs at least once a week (Ising, Babisch, Hanel, Kruppa, & Pilgramm, 1995; Ising, Babisch, & Hanee, 1997).	An upper limit of 95 dBA enforced in clubs may reduce the incidence of hearing loss greater than 10 dB from 10–20% to 1% (Ising, Babisch, Hanel, Kruppa, & Pilgramm, 1995; Ising, Babisch, & Hanee, 1997).
Construction work	Noise exposure for workers in the construction industry can be expected to range from 90 to 130 dBA because of the use of heavy machinery and equipment, transport vehicles, and noise-producing tools (Legris & Poulin, 1998; McClymont & Simpson, 1989). In the United States, among male youths who are 18 years old, construction labor is the second most common occupation during the school year and the most common summer occupation (U.S. Department of Labor, 2003).	Buy quiet equipment; apply noise-reducing measures for existing equipment. Use hearing protection devices when the noise exposure during any activity exceeds 85 dBA.
Woodwork	Noise levels from home power tools vary from 65 to 115 dBA depending on the tool. Our measurements in a metal and wood workshop showed peak measurements as high as 128 dBA from a power-activated nailer. Individuals who do woodwork are 30% more likely to have a hearing loss than those who never do such work (Dalton, Cruickshanks, Wiley, Klein, Klein, & Tweed, 2001).	Buy quiet tools, cover shop/ garage walls with sound-absorbing materials, and use hearing protection devices.
Attendance at sports events	Stadiums have very high noise levels, and the levels can be higher in domed stadiums and near the cheerleading sections. Hodgetts and Liu (2006) measured noise levels at three hockey games. The average levels ranged from 100 to 103 dBA with peaks measured at 120 dBA. Our own measurements at a football game showed levels ranging from 68.3 to 124.8 dBA with peak levels recorded at 138.6 dB SPL (see details in Chapter 13).	Use quieter cheering techniques, overall better social behaviors, and hearing protection devices.
Playing games at arcades	Noise levels of 88 to 90 dBA have been reported in arcade game centers. With less than 1-hour exposure, such levels have the potential to cause a 4 to 8 dB temporary threshold shift at 4 kHz in some individuals (Mirbod, Inaba, Yoshida, Nagata, Komura, & Iwata, 1992)	Limit play time and use hearing protection devices.

Table 10.5   Acoustic Standards for Toys (American Society for Testing and Materials, 2007)

Toy classification	Level limit
Handheld, table-top, floor, and crib toys	Should not exceed 85 dB L_{Aeq} (A-weighted equivalent sound pressure level) when measured from 25 cm
Close-to-the-ear toys	Continuous sound levels should not exceed 65 dB L_{Aeq} when measured from 25 cm; peak levels of impulsive sounds should not exceed 95 dBC
Toys with all impact-type impulsive sounds including recorded sounds such as those on video games	Peak levels should not exceed 115 dBC when measured from 25 cm
Toys with explosive-type impulsive sounds except percussion caps	Peak levels should not exceed 125 dBC when measured from 25 cm

has published a list of noisy toys that can be accessed at their website (www.sightandhearing. org). If a family member suspects that the toy is too loud, it is probably too loud. Under such circumstances, the toy should be left in the off position or the batteries should be removed.

◆ Noise Exposure in Healthcare Settings

Neonatal Intensive Care Unit

A study conducted at a neonatal intensive care unit (ICU) at a major research hospital in western Sweden revealed LA_{eq} values of 53 to 58 dB. The LAF_{Max} levels exceeded 50 dB and LC_{Peak} exceeded 70 dB 90% of the time. Personnel working in the ICU perceived the noise as contributing to stress symptoms (Ryherd, Waye, & Ljungkvist, 2008). A study in Australia found admission to the neonatal ICU or special care nursery to be a significant risk factor for the occurrence of slight to mild sensorineural hearing loss among elementary school children (Cone, Wake, Tobin, Poulakis, & Rickards, 2010). Natus (San Carlos, CA) has developed Mini-Muffs to provide noise attenuation for babies with a reported attenuation of at least 7 dB. The Mini-Muff is reportedly designed to fit comfortably around the baby's ears with a soft foam oval-shaped design and gentle hydrogel adhesive.

Preterm infants can be exposed to noise during various procedures including nasal continuous positive airway pressure (Karam, Donatiello, Van Lancker, Chritin, Pfister, & Rimensberger, 2008). The level of noise exposure is related to the flow rate through the system (Trevisanuto, Camiletti, Udilano, Doglioni, & Zanardo, 2008).

Aural Microsuction

Aural microsuction is a routine procedure used to remove excessive earwax and other debris from ear canals by placing instruments with varying shapes and sizes at different positions in the ear canal. Aural suctioning has been a routine procedure used for decades without regard to noise-induced hearing loss. Noise levels produced during the procedure can vary based on the physical characteristic of the equipment, the size of the suction tip (e.g., #3, #5 and #7, representing 1.0-, 1.5-, and 2.0-mm bore openings), how close the suction tip is to the eardrum, suction pressure (e.g., 9, 35, and 62 mm Hg) and turbulence created by suction noise including shearing and whistling. The levels can vary between 74 to 117 dBA with peaks as high as 140 to 150 dB SPL (Katzke & Sesterhenn, 1982; Mendrygal & Roeser, 2008; Wetmore, Henry, & Konkle, 1993). As expected from the high exposure levels, hearing loss can occur from aural microsuction (Katzke & Sesterhenn, 1982). Limiting the suction tip size to 1.0 mm and using lower suction pressure can reduce the noise exposure levels (Ross, 2009) and minimize the risk of hearing loss.

Exposure to Ototoxic Medications

As noted in Chapter 1, some medications can cause hearing loss (European Agency for Safety and Health at Work, 2009) and ingestion of multiple ototoxic medications can lead to more severe hearing loss due to damage to multiple structures in the cochlea.

Aminoglycosides

Aminoglycosides are narrow-spectrum antibiotics that can counteract aerobic Gram-negative bacilli and are considered effective in treating severe infections like septicemia. Aminoglycosides such as gentamicin, kanamycin, streptomycin, amikacin, tobramycin, and neomycin can damage the cochlea and specifically the outer hair cells (Forge & Schacht, 2000; Govaerts, Claes, van de Heyning, Jorens, Marquet, & De Broe, 1990; Hashino, Shero, & Salvi, 1997). They seem to invade the cochlea through the stria vascularis (Govaerts, Claes, van de Heyning, Jorens, Marquet, & De Broe, 1990; Tran Ba Huy, Meulemans, Wassef, Manuel, Sterkers, & Amiel, 1983). Hearing loss occurs in approximately 20 to 30% of patients receiving aminoglycosides (Fausti, Henry, Helt, et al., 1999; Fee, 1980; Lerner, Schmitt, Seligsohn, & Matz, 1986; Moore, Smith, & Lietman, 1984). The dose and duration of treatment determine the presence and degree of hearing loss, but genetic predisposition can also be a factor. Sequence analysis of the mitochondrial genome has implicated mutations at the 961, 1494, and 1555 loci in the *12SrRNA* gene that can make individuals susceptible to aminoglycoside ototoxicity (Guan, Fischel-Ghodsian, & Attardi, 2000; Li, Greinwald, Yang, Choo, Wenstrup, & Guan, 2004; Wang, Li, Han, et al., 2006; Zhao, Li, Wang, Yan, Deng, Han, et al., 2004). For example, some individuals have a genetic predisposition to hearing loss from aminoglycosides because of a substitution of guanosine at position 1555 in the mitochondrial ribosomal ribonucleic acid by an adenosine (Prezant, Agapian, Bohlman, et al., 1993). As a preventative measure, a quick screening for the existence of this mutation is possible (Usami, Abe, Shinkawa, Inoue, & Yamaguchi, 1999). Approximately 10 to 20% of individuals with aminoglycoside-induced ototoxicity may show a mutation in the *12S rRNA* gene (Fischel-Ghodsian, 1999).

Other factors that increase the risk of hearing loss are preexisting disorders of hearing, older age, use of other medications including loop diuretics, and noise exposure. Auditory threshold shifts are worse when aminoglycoside exposure occurs along with noise exposure or after noise exposure. Soldiers with blast and gunshot wounds often receive aminoglycosides during and after evacuation from warzones in noisy armored personnel carriers or aircrafts. Exposure to moderate or intense noise during combat injuries and medical evacuation and consequent aminoglycoside treatment

can lead to noise-augmented aminoglycoside-induced hearing loss. In such cases, the possibility of hearing loss can be minimized by using nonototoxic drugs and/or reducing the noise dose (Li & Steyger, 2009) to the best possible extent. Another protective measure is to administer aspirin, if possible, along with aminoglycosides; aspirin can reduce the incidence of hearing loss by up to 75% (Sha, Qiu, & Schacht, 2006).

Aminoglycoside treatment is sometimes used in neonatal ICUs, where infants are on ventilators, surrounded by various machines that produce noises including alarms. About 600,000 babies pass through neonatal ICUs in the United States annually, and many receive aminoglycosides for suspected bacterial sepsis for 2 days, or until a negative bacteriologic assay is reported (Escobar, 1999; Pillers & Schleiss, 2005). Some studies have reported alteration of auditory brainstem responses (ABRs) of neonates who receive aminoglycosides (Bernard, 1981). However, a meta-analysis of studies published between 1991 and 2003 found that aminoglycoside toxicity based on auditory testing is 2.3% (10 of 436 cases) in children receiving one strong daily dose and 2.0% (8 of 406 cases) in children receiving multiple daily doses (Contopoulos-Ioannidis, Giotis, Baliatsa, & Ioannidis, 2004). The prevalence of *12S rRNA* mutations related to aminoglycoside ototoxicity is 1%, and many infants with this mutation and aminoglycoside exposure may not suffer from hearing loss. The proportion of infants who fail a repeat ABR screening is similar among those who are exposed to gentamicin and those who are not. In addition, the ABR screening pass rate is similar among babies who are exposed to gentamicin for 2 or fewer days and those who are exposed for more than 2 days (Johnson, Cohen, Guo, Schibler, & Greinwald, 2010).

Anticarcinogenic Drugs

Cisplatin causes hearing loss in humans with a marked loss of hair cells and spiral ganglions and damage to the stria vascularis (Helson, Okonkwo, Anton, & Cvitkovic, 1978; Kopelman, Budnick, Sessions, Kramer, & Wong, 1988; Macdonald, Harrison, Wake, Bliss, & Macdonald, 1994; Nagy, Adelstein, Newman, Rybicki, Rice, & Lavertu, 1999). The reported incidence of cisplatin-induced hearing loss varies from 11 to

97% (Schweitzer, 1993). Cisplatin-induced hearing loss is first apparent at frequencies above 8 kHz (Fausti, Henry, Schaffer, Olson, Frey, & Bagby, 1993), and it can progress after termination of treatment (Bertolini, Lassalle, Mercier, et al., 2004). The ototoxic effects of cisplatin can increase with coexposure to aminoglycosides (Riggs, Brummett, Guitjens, & Matz, 1996), loop diuretics (Komune & Snow, 1981), and hazardous noise exposure (Gratton, Salvi, Kamen, & Saunders, 1990; Laurell, 1992). Potentiation of cisplatin ototoxicity by previous noise exposure has also been reported in clinical cases (Bokemeyer, Berger, Hartmann, et al., 1998).

Carboplatin is another anticarcinogenic drug that may affect hearing, but it is less nephrotoxic than cisplatin. If mannitol is used to disrupt the blood-brain barrier, carboplatin can successfully treat malignant brain tumors, but a high percentage of patients can have hearing loss. However, the hearing loss can be prevented by administering sodium thiosulfate after closing of the blood-brain barrier (Neuwelt, Brummett, Doolittle, et al., 1998).

Loop Diuretics

Ethacrynic acid, furosemide, and bumetanide are loop diuretics that inhibit sodium and chloride ion reabsorption. Loop diuretics are used in the treatment of patients with congestive heart failure or renal failure. These drugs cause excretion of a large volume of water and electrolytes in the urine and reduce fluid overload in the body. They can cause a high-frequency hearing loss through edema and dysfunction of the stria vascularis (Arnold, Nadol, & Weidauer, 1981; Ding, McFadden, Woo, & Salvi, 2002; Forge, 1982; Matz, 1976). In most cases, the hearing loss is temporary, but permanent hearing loss has also been reported in the literature (Gallagher & Jones, 1979). The hearing loss from these loop diuretics can be prevented, when possible, by using the loop diuretic torsemide, which does not appear to be ototoxic (Dunn, Fitton, & Brogden, 1995).

Nonsteroid Analgesics and Anti-inflammatory Drugs

High doses of salicylate (>2.5 g/d) can cause a temporary threshold shift and/or tinnitus (Stypulkowski, 1990), but in some cases permanent hearing loss may occur (Jarvis, 1966; Kapur, 1965). According to the Drug Enforcement Agency of the U.S. Department of Justice, prescriptions for opiate-based drugs have skyrocketed in the past decade. Abuse of opiates can cause a temporary or permanent sensorineural hearing loss in some individuals. In some occupational settings such as military service in areas like Afghanistan where illicit opium is easily available, opiate and noise exposure can occur simultaneously (Rawool & Dluhy, 2010).

Selective Serotonin Reuptake Inhibitors

These drugs, which are administered to chronically depressed individuals, can have negative effects on transient otoacoustic emissions, auditory processing skills, and evoked auditory responses. The enhancement of serotonin (5-HT) through the intake of selective serotonin reuptake inhibitors may be the contributing factor (Gopal, Briley, Goodale, & Hendea, 2005).

◆ Exposure to Other Ototoxins

As mentioned in Chapter 1, ototoxic substances are found in many products used at home, including adhesives, gasoline, nail polish, nail polish remover, cleaning agents, degreasers, and cigarette smoke. Material safety data sheets and the Household Products Database complied by the National Library of Medicine (http://hpd.nlm.nih.gov) can provide information about the ingredients of many household products.

Mercury

Mercury is present in all colors in the QUIKRETE Color-PAK (powder) (Atlanta, GA), except for Charcoal no. 1318, which can be used for coloring cement or concrete. Mercury salts are used in some skin lightening creams, antiseptic creams, and ointments. In water, metallic mercury and mercury are metabolized by bacteria leading to organic or "methyl" mercury, which can build up in fish tissues. As an example, 50% of the fish samples and 17% of hair samples collected from villagers close to a mercury processing plant in KwaZulu-Natal, South Africa, exceeded guidelines of the World Health Organization, possibly because of disposal of mercury waste in the Mngceweni River, located near the plant (Papu-Zamxaka, Mathee, Harpham, et al., 2010). Individuals who consume fish caught in a bay with high mercury content can suffer from severe neurological defects including hearing loss (Mizukoshi, Watanabe, Kobayashi, et al., 1989). Subjects who consume tuna fish regularly have higher levels of mercury in urine and blood than control subjects. In addition, their performance on temporal neurobehavioral tasks involving speed such as color word reaction time, digit symbol reaction time, and finger tapping speed is significantly worse than control subjects (Carta, Flore, Alinovi, et al., 2003). Mercury vapor can also be released from amalgam dental fillings, which is inhaled, transferred to the blood, and gradually accumulated in the nervous (Eggleston & Nylander, 1987) and other systems (Berlin, 2003). The amount of exposure to mercury vapor is dependent on the size and number of amalgam surfaces (Berlin, 2003; Clarkson, Magos, & Myers, 2003). A higher number of amalgam fillings is associated with poorer thresholds at higher frequencies. Use of amalgam for dental fillings should be avoided as much as possible. In addition, during the removal of existing amalgam fillings at the end of their useful life, precautions such as high-volume air extraction can reduce mercury exposure to patients, dentists, and dental assistants (Rothwell & Boyd, 2008). The EPA limit is two parts of mercury per billion parts of drinking water, and the FDA limit is one part of methylmercury in a million parts of seafood.

Lead

Lead is present in the all colors in the Quikrete Color-PAK (powder), except for Charcoal no. 1318, which can be used for coloring cement or concrete. Lead is also present in Mayco Ceramic Clear Glaze (liquid) (Hillard, OH), which is used for arts and crafts. Children can be exposed to lead from consuming lead-based paint chips or playing in polluted soil. A few paints and pigments used as make-up or hair coloring contain lead. It is important to keep such products out of reach from children (Agency for Toxic Substances and Disease Registry, 2007). Blood lead levels greater than 7 μg/dL are significantly associated with hearing loss in adults in the 3 to 8 kHz

range (Hwang, Chiang, Yen-Jean, & Wang, 2009). Intellectual impairment can appear in children with blood lead concentrations below 10 μg/dL (Canfield, Henderson, Cory-Slechta, Cox, Jusko, & Lanphear, 2003). Since August 2009, toys and children's products containing lead in excess of 300 ppm have been banned, and this limit will be lowered to 100 ppm in August 2011 (Consumer Product Safety Improvement Act, 2008). Some of the currently available children's toys and jewelry may contain high levels of lead. Recently, a children's book was found to contain 1900 ppm lead paint, and a piece of jewelry was found to be 71% lead by weight (Hitchcock, 2009). Parents need to be diligent in buying toys, especially when they are bought from small vendors with unknown manufacturers.

Carbon Monoxide

Carbon monoxide (asphyxiant) exposure can occur in homes from faulty stoves, hot water heaters, and furnaces. Razzaq, Dumbala, and Moudgil (2010) presented a case of sudden deafness in a man who had borrowed his friend's generator and used it in a closed space. Fortunately, in this case, at 3 months he reported full recovery of his hearing.

Nicotine

Secondhand smoke exposure is significantly associated with increased risk of hearing loss for low to middle frequencies in nonsmoking adults (Fabry, Davila, Arheart, et al., 2011). Smoking of less than 20 cigarettes/day for 3 years can degrade hearing sensitivity at 12 kHz (Ohgami, Kondo, & Kato, 2011). Smokers also have reduced levels of distortion product otoacoustic emissions compared with nonsmokers, suggesting cochlear dysfunction (Negley, Katbamna, Crumpton, & Lawson, 2007).

Solvent Exposure

Solvent addicts who inhale paint or glue can suffer from auditory brainstem abnormalities or hearing loss (Ehyai & Freemon, 1983; Metrick & Brenner, 1982; Poulsen & Jensen, 1986), which can be expected to be prominent in the 4000 to 16,000 Hz frequency region (Fuente et al., 2009).

Review Questions

1. Define community noise and the potential effects of high levels of community noise.
2. What types of units are used for measuring community noise?
3. Describe the DNL criteria specified by the U.S. Department of Housing and Urban Development for areas where it funds or finances housing.
4. What are the potential sources of noise for road traffic? What noise abatement measures can be used to minimize highway road traffic noise exposures to nearby residents?
5. Which factors determine the noise levels at or around airports due to air traffic?
6. Discuss the potential effects of noise exposure on hearing during a commute via mass transit systems and riding motorcycles.
7. Review the strategies that can be used for reducing hazardous sound exposure during recreational shooting and at music venues.
8. Outline strategies for reducing noise at home.
9. Discuss potential threats to hearing in medical care settings.
10. Review potential exposure to ototoxins in nonoccupational settings.

References

Aaberg D. (2008). Generator set noise solutions. *Pollution Engineering.* 40(3):47–54. Available at: www.pollution-engineering.com. Accessed July 6, 2011.

Agency for Toxic Substances and Disease Registry. (2007). *Toxicological Profile for Lead (Update).* Atlanta, GA: U.S. Department of Public Health and Human Services, Public Health Service.

Aizawa N, Eggermont JJ. (2006). Effects of noise-induced hearing loss at young age on voice onset time and gap-in-noise representations in adult cat primary auditory cortex. *J Assoc Res Otolaryngol.* 7(1):71–81.

American Society for Testing and Materials. (2007). *Standard Consumer Safety Specification for Toy Safety.* ASTM Standard F963-07, Section 4.5. West Conshohocken, PA: American Society of Testing and Materials International.

Arnold W, Nadol JB Jr, Weidauer H. (1981). Ultrastructural histopathology in a case of human ototoxicity due to loop diuretics. *Acta Otolaryngol.* 91(5–6):399–414.

Axelsson A, Prasher D. (2000). Tinnitus induced by occupational and leisure noise. *Noise Health.* 2(8):47–54.

Babisch W. (2008). Road traffic noise and cardiovascular risk. *Noise Health.* 10(38):27–33.

Babisch W, Neuhauser H, Thamm M, Seiwert M. (2009). Blood pressure of 8–14 year old children in relation to traffic noise at home—results of the German Environmental Survey for Children (GerES IV). *Sci Total Environ.* 407(22):5839–5843.

Bennett C. (2006). *Exploring Young People's Attitudes and Behaviors Towards Loud Music.* London, United Kingdom: Royal National Institute for Deaf People.

Berger EH. (2006). *The Noise Navigator™ Database.* Available at: www.e-a-r.com/pdf/hearingcons/Noise_Nav.xls. Accessed December 2010.

Berglund B, Lindvall T, Schwela DH, eds. (2000). *Guidelines for Community Noise.* Geneva: World Health Organization. Available at: www.who.int/docstore/peh/noise/guidelines2.html. Accessed July 6, 2011.

Berlin M. (2003). *Mercury in Dental Fillings: An Updated Risk Analysis in Environmental Medical Terms.* Available at: www.sweden.gov.se/content/1/c6/01/76/11/fb660706.pdf. Accessed November 2010.

Bernard PA. (1981). Freedom from ototoxicity in aminoglycoside treated neonates: a mistaken notion. *Laryngoscope.* 91(12):1985–1994.

Bertolini P, Lassalle M, Mercier G, et al. (2004). Platinum compound-related ototoxicity in children: long-term follow-up reveals continuous worsening of hearing loss. *J Pediatr Hematol Oncol.* 26(10):649–655.

Bess FH, Poynor RE. (1972). Snowmobile engine noise and hearing. *Arch Otolaryngol.* 95(2):164–168.

Bess FH, Poynor RE. (1974). Noise-induced hearing loss and snowmobiles, engine noise, and hearing. *Arch Otolaryngol.* 99(1):45–51.

Binnington JD, McCombe AW, Harris M. (1993). Warning signal detection and the acoustic environment of the motorcyclist. *Br J Audiol.* 27(6):415–422.

Bogoch II, House RA, Kudla I. (2005). Perceptions about hearing protection and noise-induced hearing loss of attendees of rock concerts. *Can J Public Health.* 96(1):69–72.

Bokemeyer C, Berger CC, Hartmann JT, et al. (1998). Analysis of risk factors for cisplatin-induced ototoxicity in patients with testicular cancer. *Br J Cancer.* 77(8):1355–1362.

Broste SK, Hansen DA, Strand RL, Stueland DT. (1989). Hearing loss among high school farm students. *Am J Public Health.* 79(5):619–622.

Canfield RL, Henderson CR Jr, Cory-Slechta DA, Cox C, Jusko TA, Lanphear BP. (2003). Intellectual impairment in children with blood lead concentrations below 10 microg per deciliter. *N Engl J Med.* 348(16):1517–1526.

Carta P, Flore C, Alinovi R, et al. (2003). Sub-clinical neurobehavioral abnormalities associated with low level of mercury exposure through fish consumption. *Neurotoxicology.* 24(4–5):617–623.

Charbonneau D, Goldschmidt C. (2004). *Safety of Noisy Toys: A Current Assessment.* Ontario, Canada: Office of Consumer Affairs, Industry Canada.

Chung JH, Des Roches CM, Meunier J, Eavey RD. (2005). Evaluation of noise-induced hearing loss in young people using a web-based survey technique. *Pediatrics.* 115(4):861–867.

Clarkson TW, Magos L, Myers GJ. (2003). Human exposure to mercury: The three modern dilemmas. *J Trace Elements Experimental Med.* 16(4):321–343.

Cone BK, Wake M, Tobin S, Poulakis Z, Rickards FW. (2010). Slight-mild sensorineural hearing loss in children: audiometric, clinical, and risk factor profiles. *Ear Hear.* 31(2):202–212.

Consumer Product Safety Improvement Act of 2008. (2008). The Consumer Product Safety Improvement Act of 2008, HR 4040. Public Law 110-314-Aug 14, 2008. Title 1, Sec. 106. Mandatory toy safety standards. 122 STAT. 3033–3035. Available at: www.cpsc.gov/cpsia.pdf. Accessed July 6, 2011.

Contopoulos-Ioannidis DG, Giotis ND, Baliatsa DV, Ioannidis JPA. (2004). Extended-interval aminoglycoside administration for children: a meta-analysis. *Pediatrics.* 114(1):e111–e118.

Dalton DS, Cruickshanks KJ, Wiley TL, Klein BE, Klein R, Tweed TS. (2001). Association of leisure-time noise exposure and hearing loss. *Audiology.* 40(1):1–9.

Ding D, McFadden SL, Woo JM, Salvi RJ. (2002). Ethacrynic acid rapidly and selectively abolishes blood flow in vessels supplying the lateral wall of the cochlea. *Hear Res.* 173(1–2):1–9.

Dunn CJ, Fitton A, Brogden RN. (1995). Torasemide. An update of its pharmacological properties and therapeutic efficacy. *Drugs.* 49(1):121–142.

Eggleston DW, Nylander M. (1987). Correlation of dental amalgam with mercury in brain tissue. *J Prosthet Dent.* 58(6):704–707.

Ehyai A, Freemon FR. (1983). Progressive optic neuropathy and sensorineural hearing loss due to chronic glue sniffing. *J Neurol Neurosurg Psychiatry.* 46(4):349–351.

Escobar GJ. (1999). The neonatal "sepsis work-up": personal reflections on the development of an evidence-based approach toward newborn infections in a managed care organization. *Pediatrics.* 103(1 Suppl E):360–373.

European Agency for Safety and Health at Work. (2005). *Noise in Figures.* Luxembourg: Office for Official Publications of the European Communities.

European Agency for Safety and Health at Work. (2009). *Combined Exposure to Noise and Ototoxic Substances.* Luxembourg: Office for Official Publications of the European Communities.

European Union European Communities Directive. (1984). *Council Directive 84/532/EEC of 17 September 1984 on the approximation of the laws of the member states relating to common provisions for construction plant and equipment.* Official Journal L 300, 19/11/1984 P. 0111–0112.

European Parliament and the Council of the European Union (May 8, 2000). Directive 2000/14/EC on the approximation of the laws of the member states relating to the noise emission in the environment by equipment for use outdoors. *Official Journal of European Communities.* 162:1–78.

Fabry DA, Davila EP, Arheart KL, et al. (2011). Secondhand smoke exposure and the risk of hearing loss. *Tob Control.* 20(1):82–85.

Falzone KL. (1999). Airport noise pollution: Is there a solution in sight? *BC Environ Aff Law Rev.* (Summer):769–807.

Fausti SA, Henry JA, Helt WJ, et al. (1999). An individualized, sensitive detection of early detection of ototoxicity. *Ear Hear.* 20(6):497–505.

Fausti SA, Henry JA, Schaffer HI, Olson DJ, Frey RH, Bagby GC Jr. (1993). High-frequency monitoring for early detection of cisplatin ototoxicity. *Arch Otolaryngol Head Neck Surg.* 119(6):661–666.

Federal Aviation Administration. (2010). *Appendix 1. Estimated Maximum A-weighted Sound Levels Measured in Accordance with Part-36 Appendix-C Procedures Takeoff.* Washington, DC: Federal Aviation Administration.

Federal Highway Administration. (2010). *Procedures for Abatement of Highway Traffic Noise and Construction Noise.* FHA 23 CFR Part 772, [FHWA Docket No. 2008-0114] RIN 2125-AF26; FR Doc. 2010-15848. Washington, DC: Federal Highway Administration.

Fee WE Jr. (1980). Aminoglycoside ototoxicity in the human. *Laryngoscope.* 90(10 Pt 2, Suppl 24):1–19.

Fischel-Ghodsian N. (1999). Mitochondrial deafness mutations reviewed. *Hum Mutat.* 13(4):261–270.

Fligor BJ, Cox LC. (2004). Output levels of commercially available portable compact disc players and the potential risk to hearing. *Ear Hear.* 25(6):513–527.

Forge A. (1982). A tubulo-cisternal endoplasmic reticulum system in the potassium transporting marginal cells of the stria vascularis and effects of the ototoxic diuretic ethacrynic acid. *Cell Tissue Res.* 226(2):375–387.

Forge A, Schacht J. (2000). Aminoglycoside antibiotics. *Audiol Neurootol.* 5(1):3–22.

Fuente A, Slade MD, Taylor T, Morata TC, Keith RW, Sparer J, Rabinowitz PM. (2009). Peripheral and central auditory dysfunction induced by occupational exposure to organic solvents. *J Occup Environ Med.* 51(10):1202–1211.

Gallagher G. (1987). Hot music, high noise and hurt ears. *Hear J.* 42:7–11.

Gallagher KL, Jones JK. (1979, Nov). Furosemide-induced ototoxicity. *Ann Intern Med.* 91(5):744–745.

Gershon RRM, Neitzel R, Barrera MA, Akram M. (2006). Pilot survey of subway and bus stop noise levels. *J Urban Health.* 83(5):802–812.

Gopal KV, Briley KA, Goodale ES, Hendea OM. (2005). Selective serotonin reuptake inhibitors treatment effects on auditory measures in depressed female subjects. *E J Pharmacol.* 520(1–3):59–69.

Govaerts PJ, Claes J, van de Heyning PH, Jorens PG, Marquet J, De Broe ME. (1990). Aminoglycoside-induced ototoxicity. *Toxicol Lett.* 52(3):227–251.

Gratton MA, Salvi RJ, Kamen BA, Saunders SS. (1990). Interaction of cisplatin and noise on the peripheral auditory system. *Hear Res.* 50(1–2):211–223.

Guan MX, Fischel-Ghodsian N, Attardi G. (2000). A biochemical basis for the inherited susceptibility to aminoglycoside ototoxicity. *Hum Mol Genet.* 9(12):1787–1793.

Gunderson E, Moline J, Catalano P. (1997). Risks of developing noise-induced hearing loss in employees of urban music clubs. *Am J Ind Med.* 31(1):75–79.

Hashino E, Shero M, Salvi RJ. (1997). Lysosomal targeting and accumulation of aminoglycoside antibiotics in sensory hair cells. *Brain Res.* 777(1–2):75–85.

Helson L, Okonkwo E, Anton L, Cvitkovic E. (1978). cis-Platinum ototoxicity. *Clin Toxicol.* 13(4):469–478.

Hitchcock E. (2009). *Trouble in Toyland: The 24th Annual Survey of Toy Safety.* Washington, DC: U.S. Public Interest Research Group Education Fund.

Hodgetts WE, Liu R. (2006). Can hockey playoffs harm your hearing? *CMAJ.* 175(12):1541–1542.

Hwang YH, Chiang HY, Yen-Jean MC, Wang JD. (2009). The association between low levels of lead in blood and occupational noise-induced hearing loss in steel workers. *Sci Total Environ.* 408(1):43–49.

Ising H, Babisch W, Hanel J, Kruppa B, Pilgramm M. (1995). Empirical studies of music listening habits of adolescents. Optimizing sound threshold limits for cassette players and discoteques [article in German]. *HNO.* 43(4):244–249.

Ising H, Babisch W, Hanee J. (1997). Loud music and hearing risk. *J Audiol Med.* 6:123–133.

Jarup L, Babisch W, Houthuijs D, et al.; HYENA study team. (2008). Hypertension and exposure to noise near airports: the HYENA study. *Environ Health Perspect.* 116(3):329–333.

Jarvis JF. (1966). A case of unilateral permanent deafness following acetylsalicylic acid. *J Laryngol Otol.* 80(3):318–320.

Johnson RF, Cohen AP, Guo Y, Schibler K, Greinwald JH. (2010). Genetic mutations and aminoglycoside-induced ototoxicity in neonates. *Otolaryngol Head Neck Surg.* 142(5):704–707.

Kähärit K, Zachau G, Eklöf M, Sandsjö L, Möller C. (2003). Assessment of hearing and hearing disorders in rock/jazz musicians. *Int J Audiol.* 42(5):279–288.

Kapur YP. (1965). Ototoxicity of acetylsalisylic acid. *Arch Otolaryngol.* 81:134–138.

Karam O, Donatiello C, Van Lancker E, Chritin V, Pfister RE, Rimensberger PC. (2008). Noise levels during nCPAP are flow-dependent but not device-dependent. *Arch Dis Child Fetal Neonatal Ed.* 93(2):F132–F134.

Katzke D, Sesterhenn G. (1982). Suction-generated noise in the external meatus and sensorineural hearing loss. *J Laryngol Otol.* 96(9):857–863.

Komune S, Snow JB Jr. (1981). Potentiating effects of cisplatin and ethacrynic acid in ototoxicity. *Arch Otolaryngol.* 107(10):594–597.

Kopelman J, Budnick AS, Sessions RB, Kramer MB, Wong GY. (1988). Ototoxicity of high-dose cisplatin by bolus administration in patients with advanced cancers and normal hearing. *Laryngoscope.* 98(8 Pt 1):858–864.

Kujawa SG, Liberman MC. (2006). Acceleration of age-related hearing loss by early noise exposure: evidence of a misspent youth. *J Neurosci.* 26(7):2115–2123.

Lankford JE, Mikrut TA, Jackson PL. (1991). A noise-exposure profile of high school students. *Hearing Instruments.* 42:19–24.

Laurell GF. (1992). Combined effects of noise and cisplatin: short- and long-term follow-up. *Ann Otol Rhinol Laryngol.* 101(12):969–976.

Legris M, Poulin P. (1998). Noise exposure profile among heavy equipment operators, associated laborers, and crane operators. *Am Ind Hyg Assoc J.* 59(11):774–778.

Lerner SA, Schmitt BA, Seligsohn R, Matz GJ. (1986). Comparative study of ototoxicity and nephrotoxicity in patients randomly assigned to treatment with amikacin or gentamicin. *Am J Med.* 80(6B):98–104.

Li H, Steyger PS. (2009). Synergistic ototoxicity due to noise exposure and aminoglycoside antibiotics. *Noise Health.* 11(42):26–32.

Li R, Greinwald JH Jr, Yang L, Choo DI, Wenstrup RJ, Guan MX. (2004). Molecular analysis of the mitochondrial 12S rRNA and tRNASer(UCN) genes in paediatric subjects with non-syndromic hearing loss. *J Med Genet.* 41(8):615–620.

Macdonald MR, Harrison RV, Wake M, Bliss B, Macdonald RE. (1994). Ototoxicity of carboplatin: comparing animal and clinical models at the Hospital for Sick Children. *J Otolaryngol.* 23(3):151–159.

Matz GJ. (1976). The ototoxic effects of ethacrynic acid in man and animals. *Laryngoscope.* 86(8):1065–1086.

McClymont LG, Simpson DC. (1989). Noise levels and exposure patterns to do-it-yourself power tools. *J Laryngol Otol.* 103(12):1140–1141.

McCombe AW, Binnington J. (1994). Hearing loss in Grand Prix motorcyclists: occupational hazard or sports injury? *Br J Sports Med.* 28(1):35–37.

McCombe AW, Binnington J, Davis AC, Spencer H. (1995). Hearing loss and motorcyclists. *J Laryngol Otol.* 109(7):599–604.

McCombe AW, Binnington J, McCombe TS. (1993). Hearing protection for motorcyclists. *Clin Otolaryngol Allied Sci.* 18(6):465–469.

Mendrygal M, Roeser RJ. (2008). Ear canal suctioning: a cautionary note for noise-induced hearing loss. *Audiology Today.* 19:35–38.

Metrick SA, Brenner RP. (1982). Abnormal brainstem auditory evoked potentials in chronic paint sniffers. *Ann Neurol.* 12(6):553–556.

Mirbod SM, Inaba R, Yoshida H, Nagata C, Komura Y, Iwata H. (1992). Noise exposure level while operating electronic arcade games as a leisure time activity. *Ind Health.* 30(2):65–76.

Mizukoshi K, Watanabe Y, Kobayashi H, et al. (1989). Neurotological follow-up studies upon Minamata disease. *Acta Otolaryngol Suppl.* 468:353–357.

Moore RD, Smith CR, Lietman PS. (1984). Risk factors for the development of auditory toxicity in patients receiving aminoglycosides. *J Infect Dis.* 149(1):23–30.

Nagy JL, Adelstein DJ, Newman CW, Rybicki LA, Rice TW, Lavertu P. (1999). Cisplatin ototoxicity: the importance of baseline audiometry. *Am J Clin Oncol.* 22(3):305–308.

National Institute for Occupational Safety and Health. (1998). *Criteria for a Recommended Standard: Occupational Noise Exposure- Revised Criteria 1998* (Publication No, 98-126). Cincinnati, OH: National Institute for Occupational Safety and Health.

National Sporting Goods Association (2010). New NSGA Consumer Purchases survey: 2009 sporting goods sales fall 3%. Available at http://www.nsga.org/i4a/pages/index.cfm?pageid=4331. Accessed on July 6, 2011.

National Shooting Sports Foundation (NSSF, 2011). Hunter's pocket fact card. Available at: http://nssf.org/PDF/HunterFactCard.pdf. Accessed July 6, 2011.

Negley C, Katbamna B, Crumpton T, Lawson GD. (2007). Effects of cigarette smoking on distortion product otoacoustic emissions. *J Am Acad Audiol.* 18(8):665–674.

Neitzel R, Gershon RRM, Zeltser M, Canton A, Akram M. (2009). Noise levels associated with New York City's mass transit systems. *Am J Public Health.* 99(8):1393–1399.

Neuwelt EA, Brummett RE, Doolittle ND, et al. (1998). First evidence of otoprotection against carboplatin-induced hearing loss with a two-compartment system in patients with central nervous system malignancy using sodium thiosulfate. *J Pharmacol Exp Ther.* 286(1):77–84.

Noise Emission in the Environment by Equipment for Use Outdoors Directive.(2000). *Directive 2000/14/EC.*

Noise Pollution Clearinghouse. (2005). *Quiet Lawns: Creating the "Perfect" Landscape without Polluting the Soundscape.* Montpelier, VT: Noise Pollution Clearinghouse.

Ohgami N, Kondo T, Kato M. (2011). Effects of light smoking on extra-high-frequency auditory thresholds in young adults. *Toxicol Ind Health.* 27(2):143–147.

Opperman DA, Reifman W, Schlauch R, Levine S. (2006). Incidence of spontaneous hearing threshold shifts during modern concert performances. *Otolaryngol Head Neck Surg.* 134(4):667–673.

Papu-Zamxaka V, Mathee A, Harpham T, et al. (2010). Elevated mercury exposure in communities living alongside the Inanda Dam, South Africa. *J Environ Monit.* 12(2):472–477.

Peng JH, Tao ZZ, Huang ZW. (2007). Risk of damage to hearing from personal listening devices in young adults. *J Otolaryngol.* 36(3):181–185.

Pillers DM, Schleiss MR. (2005). Gentamicin in the clinical setting. *The Volta Review.* 105:205–210.

Poulsen P, Jensen JH. (1986). Brain-stem response audiometry and electronystagmographic findings in chronic toxic encephalopathy (chronic painter's syndrome). *J Laryngol Otol.* 100(2):155–156.

Prezant TR, Agapian JV, Bohlman MC, et al. (1993). Mitochondrial ribosomal RNA mutation associated with both antibiotic-induced and non-syndromic deafness. *Nat Genet.* 4(3):289–294.

Rabinowitz PM, Slade MD, Galusha D, Dixon-Ernst C, Cullen MR. (2006). Trends in the prevalence of hearing loss among young adults entering an industrial workforce 1985 to 2004. *Ear Hearing.* 27(4):369–375.

Rawool VW. (2008). Growing up noisy: The sound exposure diary of a hypothetical young adult. *Hearing Review.* 15(5):30, 32, 34, 39–40.

Rawool VW. (2010). "Debilitating Tinnitus Triggered by a Single Noise Exposure Incidence." Clinical poster presentation at the American Academy of Audiology's annual convention, AudiologyNOW! 2010, San Diego, CA, April 14–17.

Rawool VW, Colligon-Wayne LA. (2008). Auditory lifestyles and beliefs related to hearing loss among college students in the USA. *Noise Health.* 10(38):1–10.

Rawool VW, Dluhy C. (2010). "Can Opiates and Noise Interact in Increasing Hearing Loss?" Podium presentation at the American Academy of Audiology's annual meeting, AudiologyNOW!, San Diego, CA, April 14–17.

Razzaq M, Dumbala S, Moudgil SS. (2010). Neurological picture. Sudden deafness due to carbon monoxide poisoning. *J Neurol Neurosurg Psychiatry.* 81(6):658.

Riggs LC, Brummett RE, Guitjens SK, Matz GJ. (1996). Ototoxicity resulting from combined administration of cisplatin and gentamicin. *Laryngoscope.* 106(4):401–406.

Roche AF, Siervogel RM, Himes JH, Johnson DL. (1978). Longitudinal study of hearing in children: baseline data concerning auditory thresholds, noise exposure, and biological factors. *J Acoust Soc Am.* 64(6):1593–1616.

Ross, JR. (2009). Re: Noise levels generated within the external auditory canal during microsuction aural toilet. *Clin Otolaryngol.* 34(5):494–496, author reply 496.

Rothwell JA, Boyd PJ. (2008). Amalgam dental fillings and hearing loss. *Int J Audiol.* 47(12):770–776.

Ryberg JB. (2009). A national project to evaluate and reduce high sound pressure levels from music. *Noise Health.* 11(43):124–128.

Ryherd EE, Waye KP, Ljungkvist L. (2008). Characterizing noise and perceived work environment in a neurological intensive care unit. *J Acoust Soc Am.* 123(2):747–756.

Rytzner B, Rytzner C. (1981). Schoolchildren and noise. The 4 kHz dip-tone screening in 14391 schoolchildren. *Scand Audiol.* 10(4):213–216.

Schmuzigert N, Fostiropoulos K, Probst R. (2006). Long-term assessment of auditory changes resulting from a single noise exposure associated with non-occupational activities. *Int J Audiol.* 45(1):46–54.

Schulz TY. (2006). Recreational shooting and hearing safety. *CAOHC Update.* 18(3):6–7.

Schweitzer VG. (1993). Cisplatin-induced ototoxicity: the effect of pigmentation and inhibitory agents. *Laryngoscope.* 103(4 Pt 2):1–52.

Segal S, Eviatar E, Lapinsky J, Shlamkovitch N, Kessler A. (2003). Inner ear damage in children due to noise exposure from toy cap pistols and firecrackers: a retrospective review of 53 cases. *Noise Health.* 5(18):13–18.

Serra MR, Biassoni EC, Richter U, et al. (2005). Recreational noise exposure and its effects on the hearing of adolescents. Part I: an interdisciplinary long-term study. *Int J Audiol.* 44(2):65–73.

Sha SH, Qiu JH, Schacht J. (2006). Aspirin to prevent gentamicin-induced hearing loss. *N Engl J Med.* 354(17):1856–1857.

Stypulkowski PH. (1990). Mechanisms of salicylate ototoxicity. *Hear Res.* 46(1–2):113–145.

Swedish National Board of Health and Welfare. (2005). *High Sound Levels. General Recommendations Issued by the Swedish National Board of Health and Welfare SOSFS, 7.* Stockholm: Socialstyrelsens författningssamling.

Tran Ba Huy P, Meulemans A, Wassef M, Manuel C, Sterkers O, Amiel C. (1983). Gentamicin persistence in rat endolymph and perilymph after a two-day constant infusion. *Antimicrob Agents Chemother.* 23(2):344–346.

Trevisanuto D, Camiletti L, Udilano A, Doglioni N, Zanardo V. (2008, Sep). Noise levels during neonatal helmet CPAP. *Arch Dis Child Fetal Neonatal Ed.* 93(5):F396–F397.

Ulrich RF, Pinheiro ML. (1974). Temporary hearing losses in teen-agers attending repeated rock-and-roll sessions. *Acta Otolaryngol.* 77(1):51–55.

U.S. Department of Housing and Urban Development. (1991). *The Noise Guidebook. A Reference Document for Implementing the Department of Housing and Urban Development's Noise Policy.* Washington, DC: The Environment Planning Division, Office of Environment and Energy.

U.S. Department of Labor. (2003). *Employment Experience of Youth During the School Year and Summer.* Washington, DC: U.S. Department of Labor.

U.S. Environmental Protection Agency. (1978). *Is Quiet Possible at the Dudley Home?* Washington, DC: U.S. Environmental Protection Agency, Office of Noise Abatement and Control.

Usami S, Abe S, Shinkawa H, Inoue Y, Yamaguchi T. (1999). Rapid mass screening method and counseling for the 1555A—>G mitochondrial mutation. *J Hum Genet.* 44(5):304–307.

Vogel I, van der Ploeg CP, Brug J, Raat H. (2009). Music venues and hearing loss: Opportunities for and barriers to improving environmental conditions. *Int J Audiol.* 48(8):531–536.

Voss P. (2005). *Noise in Children's Daycare Centers.* Noise at Work. *Magazine of the European Agency for Safety and Health at Work.* 8:23–25. Available at: http://osha.europa.eu/en/publications/magazine/8. Accessed July 6, 2011.

Wang Q, Li QZ, Han D, et al. (2006). Clinical and molecular analysis of a four-generation Chinese family with aminoglycoside-induced and nonsyndromic hearing loss associated with the mitochondrial 12S rRNA C1494T mutation. *Biochem Biophys Res Commun.* 340(2):583–588.

Weichbold V, Zorowka P. (2007). Can a hearing education campaign for adolescents change their music listening behavior? *Int J Audiol.* 46(3):128–133.

Wetmore RF, Henry WJ, Konkle DF. (1993). Acoustical factors of noise created by suctioning middle ear fluid. *Arch Otolaryngol.* 106:92–96.

Widén SE, Erlandsson SI. (2004). The influence of socioeconomic status on adolescent attitude to social noise and hearing protection. *Noise Health.* 7(25):59–70.

Widén SE, Holmes AE, Johnson T, Bohlin M, Erlandsson SI. (2009). Hearing, use of hearing protection, and attitudes towards noise among young American adults. *Int J Audiol.* 48(8):537–545.

Williams W. (2005). Noise exposure levels from personal stereo use. *Int J Audiol.* 44(4):231–236.

Zhao H, Li R, Wang Q, et al. (2004). Maternally inherited aminoglycoside-induced and nonsyndromic deafness is associated with the novel C1494T mutation in the mitochondrial 12S rRNA gene in a large Chinese family. *Am J Hum Genet.* 74(1):139–152.

Zogby International. (2006). *Survey of Teens and Adults about the Use of Personal Electronic Devices and Head Phones.* http://www.asha.org/uploadedFiles/about/news/atitbtot/zogby_survey2006.pdf#search="Survey". Accessed December 2010.

Chapter 11

Workers' Compensation for Noise-Induced Hearing Loss and Forensic Audiology

The concept of compensation for hearing loss is very old. The ancient Roman Empire recognized that the noise of metal could cause hearing loss and that their soldiers were therefore eligible for compensation (Mackenzie, 1997). In ideal cases, implementation of effective hearing conservation programs (HCPs) should prevent hearing loss in workers. However, it is still necessary to have a policy for workers' compensation. According to the Bureau of Labor (Bureau of Labor Statistics, 2009), in 2008 hearing loss was the second most prevalent work-related illness, with approximately 22,000 reported cases. The most prevalent service-connected disability for U.S. veterans receiving compensation at the end of fiscal year 2008 was tinnitus (558,232), followed by hearing loss (519,834). **Figure 11.1** shows the number of veterans receiving benefits for auditory problems at the end of fiscal years 2004 to 2008 (Veterans Benefits Administration, 2008). Noise-induced hearing loss (NIHL) is a worldwide problem. For example, the Accident Compensation Corporation in New Zealand is concerned about the fact that even with implementation of HCPs, new cases of NIHL are still reported (Thorne, Ameratunga, Stewart, et al., 2008).

The workers' compensation system is designed to minimize legal actions between employers and employees. The purpose is to minimize disputes in society without bias or force (Jones, 2007). The principle underlying the workers' compensation system is that the employer is expected to automatically assume responsibility for any work-related injuries and illnesses, and the employee gives up the right to civil suit. Compensation for work-related hearing loss is usually awarded by taking into account a variety of factors such as occupation, duration of work, current earnings, life expectancy, age, tinnitus, etc., and varies according to the jurisdiction, state, or country. Individuals who are working with employees seeking compensation for hearing loss should make themselves familiar with the specific workers' compensation policies in their jurisdictions.

◆ Need for Workers' Compensation Policies

There are several reasons for the need for workers' compensation policies, even in the presence of effective HCPs, including the following:

- The most effective strategy for preventing hearing loss is to control noise exposure levels below 75 dBA. Universal implementation of strategies for such noise control is not yet practical.
- All workers are unlikely to wear hearing protection devices (HPDs) for a variety of reasons, as stated in Chapters 6 and 9.
- When worn in real work settings, HPDs may not offer the expected or desired degree of protection.
- Sounds above 85 dBA with exposures of 8 hours per day can produce permanent hearing loss after many years (National Institutes of Health Consensus Statement, 1990). The 90-dBA criterion level for requiring use of hearing protection can be expected to result in hearing loss in at least some workers because of individual susceptibility.

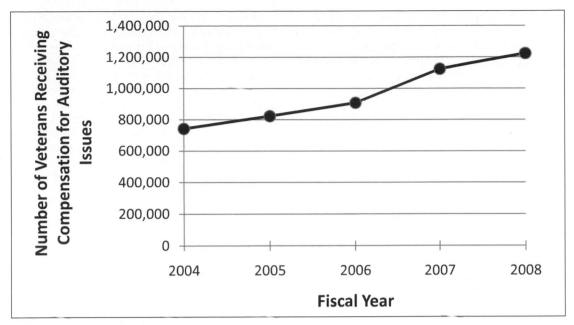

Fig. 11.1 The number of veterans receiving benefits for auditory problems at the end of fiscal years 2004 to 2008 (Veterans Benefits Administration, 2008).

- The Occupational Safety and Health Administration (OSHA) has had difficulty enforcing the 90 dBA standard because of opposition from employers and court decisions finding that engineering controls may not be economically feasible (Ginnold, 1979). Thus, many workers may be exposed to noise levels above 90 dBA.

Impairment and Disability

Previously, a distinction was made between the terms *impairment*, *handicap*, and *disability*. The American Medical Association (AMA) (1979) defined permanent impairment as a change for the worse in the structure or function outside the normal range. Handicap was defined as the disadvantage imposed by the impairment sufficient to affect a person's efficiency in performing daily activities. An actual or presumed inability to remain employed at full wages was considered a disability. The term *handicap* has a negative connotation because it is originated from the phrase *cap in hand*, which may be associated with a beggar (assumed to be handicapped) with a *cap in his hand*. In addition, the terms *disability*, *limitation*, and *restrictions* could also have negative connotations depending on the context, geographical locations, and cultural factors.

The World Health Organization (WHO; 2001) has proposed the terms *impairment, activity limitation*, and *participation restriction* to describe a person's functioning, disability, and health. Impairment is defined as a problem in structure with a significant deviation or loss. Activity limitations are difficulties experienced by individuals in executing activities (tasks or actions) and can be described in terms of the person's capacity to perform tasks. Participant restrictions are problems that individuals have in involving themselves in regular life situations and can be described in terms of the person's performance in such situations. In addition, WHO recommends the assessment of the person's physical, social, and attitudinal environments in terms of barriers and facilitators.

In terms of hearing loss, both activity limitation and participant restriction are difficult to judge based on audiometric thresholds alone, which are often used to determine the award of compensation for hearing loss. From the perspective of WHO's International Classification of Functioning, Disability, and Health (WHO, 2001), an individual's functioning and disability is not just related to the underlying health condition such as hearing loss, but is also related to the society within which the person is expected to function. Currently, attempts are being made to develop reliable, comprehensive, and valid International Classification of Functioning, Disability, and Health core sets for hearing loss (Danermark, Cieza, Gangé, et al., 2010). In this chapter, the broader term *hearing impairment* is used to accommodate for the term *handicap* used in previous literature, guidelines, and regulations.

◆ Determination of Eligibility for Compensation

Before determining compensation for any worker, it is important to determine if the worker is eligible for compensation. Presence of any complicating factors such as nonoccupational noise exposure including use of firearms or other loud recreational activities, head trauma, diseases, or ototoxic medications should be considered.

Waiting Period

Some jurisdictions have waiting periods to allow recovery from any temporary thresholds shifts before a claim can be filed, and these periods can vary from 3 days to 6 months.

Claim Submission Time Limit or Statute of Limitation

Many states in the United States have a statute of limitations on submitting a claim; the claim must be submitted within a specified timeframe after the injury or last exposure. Some states allow the "discovery" rule, which specifies that the time limits imposed on filing do not begin until the worker has become aware of a disability. If this time limit has expired, then the worker is automatically ineligible for compensation. As examples of time limits, in Pennsylvania, the employer needs to be informed about the compensable disability within 21 days, and the parties have to agree on the payable compensation within 16 months after the disability begins. In Arkansas, the claim needs to be filed within 2 years after the worker becomes aware of his hearing loss; the worker does not need to be aware that the loss is work-related. Another example is the Federal Employee Liability Act (1908; 45 U.S.C. §§51–60), which requires that the claim be filed within 3 years of the date the cause of action occurs.

Most jurisdictions consider hearing loss actions to accrue starting at the time when the claimant should have known of his hearing loss, and most entertain the possibility that the hearing loss may be work-related. A definitive diagnosis of hearing loss is not required. A worker who experienced temporary hearing loss and/or tinnitus at the end of a workday may have difficulty claiming that he or she was unaware of the loss or that he or she did not realize that the loss may be work-related. The worker is considered to have an obligation to try to investigate the possible cause of the hearing-related symptoms. In this regard, pretrial statements made by the worker to an audiologist or medical professionals may be considered more valid than any statements made after consulting an attorney and after being aware of problems associated with the statute of limitations (Spence & Spencer, 1994).

A person who has worked in a noisy environment where an HCP is not in place may not necessarily be aware of hearing loss because of the slow progression of hearing loss, or he or she may not be aware that it is work-related or that it is compensable. In addition, psychologically, many individuals have difficulty accepting the presence of hearing loss and may stay in denial (Rawool & Kiehl, 2009) for a variety of reasons, including the stigma associated with hearing loss, which may cause further delays in claiming compensation.

Hazardous Exposure

Some states require a certain noise dose (e.g., 85 dBA or 90 dBA) to prove hazardous noise exposure. For example, in Utah, a professional noise test may be conducted to document the noise exposure of 90 dBA time weighted average (TWA) as evidence of harmful noise exposure. Missouri specifies that only when a worker is exposed to hazardous noise levels for a period of at least 90 days does the employer becomes liable for hearing loss caused by that exposure. Requirements of a record of a specific amount of noise exposure can be problematic for the following reasons:

◆ Although current noise surveys may show noise levels below 90 or 85 dBA, this does not necessarily mean that the employee was previously not exposed to higher noise levels. Improved noise controls may have resulted in reduction of noise levels.
◆ Employer records of previous noise surveys may be incomplete, inaccurate, or self-serving.

Regardless, it is beneficial to determine the amount of noise exposure. If hazardous noise exposure can be recorded in the work environment, it is easy to establish that the hearing loss is at least partially work-related. Conversely, if the exposure levels are below 75 dBA, then it is highly unlikely that the hearing loss is work-related (U.S. Environmental Protection Agency, 1974), unless there is exposure to impulse noise above 140 dB sound pressure level (SPL), which can result in permanent acoustic trauma (National Institutes of Health Consensus Statement, 1990).

◆ **Percentage of Hearing Impairment**

Once it is decided that there is work-related hearing loss, many jurisdictions use a formula to determine the amount of hearing impairment, which can vary from 0% (no impairment) to 100% (complete impairment). Web-based calculators (see www.occupationalhearingloss.com) are available to determine the percentage of hearing impairment using various formulae (Kavanagh, 2001). The most frequently used procedure for determining the percentage of impairment is the one proposed by the American Academy of Otolaryngology and American Council of Otolaryngology (AAO/ACO; 1979). The procedure was published in the *Journal of the American Medical Association* (JAMA) and thus is sometimes referred to as the AAO/AMA procedure. The steps in this procedure, the underlying assumptions for each step, and an example of calculation of hearing impairment are shown in **Table 11.1**.

Table 11.1   Example of Calculation of Hearing Impairment Using the AAO/ACO (1979) Procedure

Hypothetical air conduction thresholds			
Frequency (Hz) 500	1000	2000	3000
Right (dB HL) 10	15	20	20
Left (dB HL) 20	35	55	55

Steps	Assumption	Example of calculations for thresholds displayed above
1. Find the PTA for 0.5, 1, 2, and 3 kHz for each ear, air conduction only.	The average air conduction threshold at 0.5, 1, 2, and 3 kHz is a valid indicator of a person's ability to hear speech in various daily listening conditions.	• Right ear PTA: (10 + 15 + 20 + 20) / 4 = 16.25. • Left ear PTA: (20 + 35 + 55 + 55) / 4 = 41.25
2. Subtract 25 dB from the PTA found in step 1.	Impaired hearing begins when average thresholds (dB HL) at 0.5, 1, 2, and 3 kHz are above 25 dB (the low fence) and is complete at 92 dB (the high fence); there is no disability below 25 dB.	• Right ear: The average threshold is 16.25, which is below the 25 dB fence. Thus, there is 0% disability in the right ear • Left ear: 41.25 − 25 = 16.25
3. Multiply values in step 2 by 1.5% to find percentage of hearing loss for each ear.	The range of hearing loss in step 2 from high fence to low fence (92 − 25 = 67 dB) allows each dB unit to be assigned a value of 1.5% assuming a linear growth (100% / 67 = 1.5%).	• Right ear: 0 × 1.5%/dB = 0% • Left ear: 16.25 × 1.5%/dB = 24.375%
4. Multiply the smaller of the two percentages (better ear) by five and add the percentage impairment for the poorer ear. This creates a total of six values: five from the better ear and one from the worse ear. Thus, the average is calculated by dividing the total by 6, which yields the total percentage of hearing disability.	Better ear sensitivity contributes to binaural audibility by a factor of 5:1.	[(0% × 5) + 24.375] / 6 = 4.0625% binaural hearing loss

AAO, American Academy of Otolaryngology; ACO, American Council of Otolaryngology; HL, hearing level; PTA, pure tone average.

Variations in Procedures Used For Calculating Percentage of Hearing Impairment

The exact procedures used for calculating percentage of hearing impairment vary depending on the jurisdiction as well as on some of the following variations.

Variation in Frequencies Considered in Determining the Impairment

Consideration of the following frequency combinations have been recommended for calculating the percentage of impairment:

- 0.5, 1, and 2 kHz (American Academy of Ophthalmology and Otolaryngology [AAOO], 1959)
- 0.5, 1, 2, and 3 kHz (AAO/ACO, 1979)
- 0.5, 1, 2, 3, and 4 kHz (Hardick, Melnick, Hawes, Pillion, Stephens, & Perlmutter, 1980)
- 1, 2, and 3 kHz (Committee on Hearing, Bioacoustics, and Biomechanics, 1975; King, Coles, Lutman, & Robinson, 1992)
- 1, 2, 3, and 4 kHz (American Speech-Language-Hearing Association [ASHA] Task Force, 1981)
- 1, 2, and 4 kHz (International Organization of Standardization, 1990 [Annex D of ISO-1999])
- 0.5, 1, 2, 3, 4, and 6 kHz (Department of Insurance and Finance of the State of Oregon, 1988)
- 0.5, 1, 1.5, 2, 3, and 4 KHz; 6 and 8 kHz in special circumstances (National Acoustic Laboratories [NAL], 1976; Macrae, 1988)

The inclusion of specific frequencies is related to the importance of those frequencies in understanding speech. The Speech Intelligibility Index is a simple way to predict the contribution of various frequency bands to speech understanding. Frequency bands that contribute equally and independently to speech understanding have been described, and the sum of these bands results in an index of 1.0 or 100% speech intelligibility (American National Standards Institute, 1997; S3.5 [R 2007]). The actual speech recognition ability of a specific person depends on various factors, including the type and level of speech material; background noise; reverberation; distance from the speaker; availability of visual and contextual cues; the cognitive skills and age of the listener; language fluency; the type, degree, and configuration of hearing loss; and any auditory-processing deficits.

Inclusion of 0.5 kHz is likely to reduce the amount of calculated percentage of hearing impairment because most individuals can be expected to have good hearing sensitivity at this frequency and it is least affected by noise exposure or age (International Organization of Standardization, 1990 [Annex D of ISO-1999]).

Consideration of higher frequencies such as 8 KHz may allow for recognition of the impact on quality of life due to reduction of the enjoyment related to listening to several stimuli including bird songs and music and a feeling of security related to being able to hear noises such as footsteps from behind. If frequencies above 5 kHz are filtered out, an appreciable effect on the quality of most musical instruments is apparent. The quality of orchestral music continues to improve with inclusion of frequencies up to 8 kHz, and a full bandwidth is preferred over any limitation of bandwidth. In addition, high frequencies up to approximately 10 or 12 kHz are apparent in noises made by footsteps (Snow, 1931). A need for inclusion of both 6 and 8 kHz has been recommended for workers such as electronic technicians and sonar operators who may have a special need for being able to hear these frequencies (Macrae, 1988).

The advantage of averaging more frequencies is that statistically a larger "N" is expected to result in a more stable mean. Thus, averaging of 0.5, 1, 1.5, 2, 3, 4, and 6 kHz is expected to minimize nonsystematic errors in the measurement of audiometric thresholds compared with the averaging of 1, 2, and 3 kHz (Atherley, 1973). A further advantage is that any dips occurring at midoctave frequencies will be apparent when testing is conducted at those frequencies. One disadvantage of this procedure is that more time is necessary to obtain thresholds and some patients may experience fatigue, which may lead to more unstable thresholds. This is more likely to be true when masking is required during testing in the presence of asymmetric hearing loss.

Frequency Weighting versus Frequency Averaging

Most procedures use a simple pure tone average of auditory thresholds at specific frequencies to determine the percentage loss. In the original procedure described by the AMA (1942), percentage values were assigned to frequencies between 256 and 4096 Hz, and the frequency weighting varied with intensity. Fowler (1942) assigned 15%

weight to 0.5 kHz, 30% to 1 kHz, 40% to 2 kHz, and 15% to 4 kHz.

NAL (1976) recommended a complex procedure for determining percentage loss of hearing. In this procedure, percentage loss is calculated for 0.5, 1, 1.5, 2, 3, and 4 kHz separately after assigning different weights to each frequency. The percentage loss for all six frequencies are then added. For ease of calculation, tables are provided that allow reading of percentage loss based on thresholds ranging from 15 to 95 dB HL in the better and worse ear. The highest weight is assigned to 1 kHz, and the lowest weight is assigned to 4 kHz. The weights for 500 and 1500 Hz are similar.

When a low weight is assigned to 4 kHz, which is a frequency most affected by NIHL, frequency weighting may reduce the percentage of hearing impairment when compared with simple frequency averaging. It appears unlikely that frequency weighting will improve the prediction of speech recognition ability significantly because the actual ability of a specific person depends on a variety of factors, as noted previously.

Variations in the Low Fence

The low fence is the hearing level above which the disability is expected to start. Low fences used or recommended vary from 15 (AAOO, 1959) to 55 dB. For example, the low fence used in West Virginia is 27.5 dB. The AAOO (1959) guidelines noted that if the average hearing level (HL) at 0.5, 1, and 2 kHz is 15 dB HL or less, the ability to hear everyday speech under everyday conditions is usually not impaired. Based on a review of literature related to audiometric thresholds and self-reported disability, Hardick and colleagues (1980) also suggested a low fence of 15 dB average for the frequencies of 0.5, 1, 2, and 3 kHz. Hearing disability can certainly begin at 15 dB HL for older individuals who may have poorer cognitive skills and thus may have difficulty in filling in missing elements especially in noisy or reverberant backgrounds (Rawool, 2007).

With more workers becoming eligible for compensation with a lower fence, selection of a lower low fence can have a significant economic impact. In terms of general clinical experience, most individuals do not seek assistance for hearing loss at 15 dB HL and are more likely to seek assistance after the average loss at 0.5, 1, 2, and 3 kHz is 25 dB HL or worse.

Variations in the High Fence

The high fence is the hearing level at which the disability is considered to be complete. The recommended high fences vary from 70 (Hardick, Melnick, Hawes, Pillion, Stephens, & Perlmutter, 1980) to 105 dB HL. Kryter (1973) proposed a fence of 75 dB using the auditory thresholds at 1, 2, and 3 kHz and the ASHA Task Force (1981) recommended the same fence but for thresholds at 1, 2, 3, and 4 kHz. A high fence of 75 dB assumes that a person with an average loss of 75 dB HL or greater at 1, 2, 3, and 4 kHz will have 100% impairment. ASHA argued that conversations at 75 dB HL would be difficult to sustain because of the requirement of extreme vocal effort. In addition, even at very high levels, speech comprehension for a person with a greater-than-75 dB HL loss would be minimal.

If a higher fence such as 105 dB is used or if it is assumed that the hearing loss is complete at 105 dB HL, then an average loss of 75 dB HL will be considered only partial. Thus, selection of a higher fence such as 105 dB HL is likely to result in reduction in the award for compensation. If both the hearing loss and speech recognition ability is considered in awarding compensation and if hearing aids or cochlear implants and related costs are provided free of charge as part of the award, use of a high fence of 105 dB HL can perhaps be justified. On the other hand, the use of hearing aids and cochlear implants can be considered undue burdens to the worker, and these devices are not likely to correct for poor frequency discrimination or any central auditory deficits such as poor gap detection (see Chapter 5).

Variation in Weight Assignment to Poor and Better Ears

Fowler (1947) recommended a variable ratio that weighted the better ear by 10 and the poorer ear by a factor equal to 0.1 of the loss of the better ear. He also proposed that one totally deaf ear resulted in a handicap of no greater that 10% in the presence of a normal better ear. Most other investigators have recommended fixed ratios, with the weights between better and poor ears varying from 1:1 (Ginnold, 1979) to 8:1 (Sabine, 1942). The amount of calculated percentage impairment decreases slightly with an increase in weight given to the better ear when the ears have fairly similar thresholds. The decrease in percentage binaural impairment with an increase in weight for the better ear is more obvious when the asymmetry between the two ears is high.

Macrae (1974) recommended a fixed weight of 4:1 based on correlations between hearing loss and self-assessed disability. Using a 4:1 weighting for better/poor ear, Macrae obtained a correlation of 0.91 between the binaural impairment and self-assessed disability based on responses to a questionnaire. A variable ratio formula did not provide such high correlation.

In some jurisdictions, a monaural hearing loss is calculated without giving any weight to the better ear; a binaural hearing loss is calculated by giving greater weight to the better ear. Amount of awards differ for monaural and binaural hearing loss. For example, in West Virginia, if the hearing loss is monaural, the percentage of monaural hearing loss is calculated. In cases of binaural hearing loss, the better ear gets a weight of 5. A total and irrecoverable monaural hearing loss is considered a 22.5% disability, and a similar binaural hearing loss is considered a 55% disability; the amounts of awards differ accordingly.

Variations in the Growth Function

The increase in percentage hearing impairment with increase in auditory thresholds can be assumed to be either linear or nonlinear (**Fig. 11.2**).

Linear Growth

In most cases, the calculated percentage of hearing impairment is assumed to be linearly related to auditory thresholds. Such assumptions allow for easier calculation of percentage of hearing impairment. For example, the ASHA Task Force (1981) recommends a low fence of 25 dB and a high fence of 75 dB HL. An assumption of linear growth allows assignment of 2%/dB growth because of the range of 50 dB between 25 and 75 dB HL.

Nonlinear Growth

The prediction of hearing impairment can be based on the difference limen or differential sensitivity for changes in sound intensity. Because the difference limen decreases with increasing intensity, hearing disability can be assumed to grow in a nonlinear manner, with increases in auditory thresholds by some investigators (Sabine, 1942). Other investigators have proposed a curvilinear relationship between hearing disability and hearing threshold levels over the entire range (King, Coles, Lutman, &

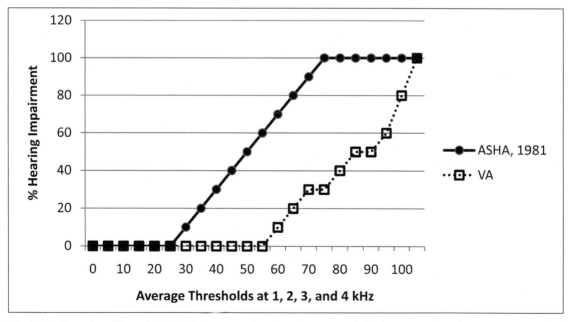

Fig. 11.2 Examples of linear (ASHA Task Force, 1981) and nonlinear growth (Veterans Benefits Administration, 2008) of percentage hearing impairment as a function of auditory thresholds assuming bilateral symmetrical auditory thresholds.

Robinson, 1992). Ontario, Canada, has adopted a nonlinear growth function where a minimum disability of 8% is considered with a 35 dB low fence. Then the growth of disability is 1%/dB up to 55 dB HL, 1.2%/dB from 55 to 65 dB HL, 1.5%/dB from 66 to 75 dB HL, 1.8%/dB from 76 to 89 dB, and 3%/dB for 90 dB and above (Alberti, Morgan, Fria, & LeBlanc, 1976). The NAL (1976) assumed a slow growth for mild losses, a rapid increase through moderate losses, and a tapering off for severe losses.

◆ Determination of the Amount of Compensation

Once the percentage of hearing impairment is determined, the compensation is usually calculated for a specified number of weeks and is a particular percentage of the average weekly wage (AWW) for the previous year. The specified number of weeks can vary from 17 to 425 weeks for a 100% monaural loss and from 77 weeks to a lifetime for a 100% binaural hearing loss. For example, the U.S. Code Compensation For Work Injuries (2008) allows 52 weeks of compensation for 100% monaural hearing loss and 200 weeks of compensation for 100% binaural loss for federal employees. The compensation rate for each week is 66.66% of the weekly wage; for individuals with dependents, the rate is 75% of the weekly wage.

Example of Determination of Amount of Compensation

The following is an example of determination of the amount of compensation using the Division of Longshore and Harbor Worker's Compensation (DLHWC) Procedures. The DLHWC program covers workers in private shipyards. The first step in this calculation is to determine the percentage of hearing impairment. Examples of percentage impairment calculations for monaural and binaural compensable hearing loss are shown in **Tables 11.2** and **11.3**.

After the calculation of percentage impairment, the amount of compensation is determined by using the following steps.

Step 1

Determine the length of entitlement: For 100% monaural loss, it is 52 weeks; for 100% binaural loss, it is 200 weeks. Calculate the number of weeks for the patient's percentage hearing impairment.

Example 1, based on monaural impairment shown in **Table 11.2**:

Length of entitlement = 24.375% monaural loss × 52 weeks = 12.675 weeks (stated differently, if the length of entitlement for 100% impairment is 52 weeks, then for 24.375% impairment, it is 12.675 weeks)

Table 11.2   Example of Calculation of Percentage Monaural Hearing Impairment Using the DLHWC Procedure

Air conduction thresholds			
Frequency (Hz)	500	1000	2000	3000
Right (dB HL)	10	15	20	20
Left (dB HL)	20	35	55	55

Steps in determining percentage hearing impairment	Calculation
1. Determine the average dB HL for 0.5, 1, 2, and 3 kHz for each ear:	1. Right ear average: (10 + 15 + 20 + 20) / 4 = 16.25. 16.25 is below the 25 dB fence which assumes no disability below 25 dB. 2. Left ear average: (20 + 35 + 55 + 55) / 4 = 41.25 Compensable hearing loss is monaural.
2. Subtract the low fence of 25 dB from the average loss in the left ear. (Assumption: No disability below 25 dB.)	41.25 − 25 = 16.25
3. For each dB that the estimated HL exceeds by 25 dB, assign 1.5%/dB monaural loss.	16.25 × 1.5%/dB = 24.375% monaural impairment

DLHWC, Division of Longshore and Harbor Worker's Compensation; HL, hearing level.

Table 11.3 Example of Calculation of Percentage Binaural Hearing Impairment Using the DLHWC Procedure

Air conduction thresholds					
Frequency (Hz)	500	1000	2000	3000	4000
Right (dB HL)	15	20	50	55	55
Left (dB HL)	15	30	50	55	55

Steps in determining percentage hearing impairment	Calculation
1. Determine the average dB HL for 0.5, 1, 2, and 3 kHz for each ear.	1. Right ear average: (15 + 20 + 50 + 55) / 4 = 35 2. Left ear average: (15 + 30 + 50 + 55) / 4 = 37.5 Compensable hearing loss is binaural because both averages are above 25 dB.
2. Subtract the low fence of 25 dB from the average loss in the left ear. (Assumption: No disability below 25 dB.)	Right ear: 35 − 25 = 10 Left ear: 37.5 − 25 = 12.5
3. For each dB that the estimated HL exceeds by 25 dB, assign 1.5%/dB impairment.	Right ear: 10 × 1.5%/dB = 15% Left ear: 12.5 × 1.5%/dB = 18.75%
4. Better (right) ear is given five times the weight assuming that the better ear will reduce the overall impairment considerably.	[(5 × 15%) + 18.75%] / 6 = 15.625% binaural impairment

DLHWC, Division of Longshore and Harbor Worker's Compensation; HL, hearing level.

Example 2, based on binaural impairment shown in **Table 11.3**:

Length of entitlement = 15.625% binaural loss × 200 weeks = 31.25 weeks

Step 2

Determine the average daily wage of the employee. Divide the total earnings for the 12 months immediately preceding the injury (e.g., $15,300) by the number of days actually worked (e.g., 245).

15,300 / 245 = $62.449 average daily wage

Step 3

Determine the average annual earnings of the employee. One of the following procedures can be used for calculating average annual earnings.

Workers Employed For the Entire or Most of the Year

1. For a worker who works 6 days a week, the average annual earning is 300 times the average daily wage.

For a worker who works 5 days a week, the average annual earning is 260 times the average

daily wage. For example, if the average daily wage in step 2 is $62.449, then the average annual earning is $62.449 × 260 = $16,236.74.

Workers Employed For Less Than the Entire Year

Select an employee of the same class, working substantially the whole year, in the same or similar employment, in the same or a neighboring place on the days when similarly employed. Use the average annual earnings of such a worker.

Step 4

Determine the AWW by dividing the average annual earnings by 52. For example, if the average annual earning in step 3 is $16,236.74, then the AWW is $16,236.74 / 52 = $312.245.

Step 5

Determine the amount of compensation: Multiply the length of entitlement in step 1 by the allowed compensation, assuming a compensation rate of two-thirds of the AWW; AWW is shown in step 4.

Example 1: 12.675 weeks × (312.245 × ⅔) = $2638.47

Example 2: 31.25 weeks × (312.245 × ⅔) = $6505.10

Step 6

Recommend the award, taking into consideration any other factors (described later in the chapter) and compensations.

Step 7

Notify the employee, the employer, and the insurance carrier about the recommendations.

Accounting for Age-related Hearing Loss

In some jurisdictions, some of the hearing loss is assumed to be age-related. Because every individual does not necessarily have age-related hearing loss (or presbycusis), age-related corrections give the benefit of doubt about the possibility of age-related hearing loss to the employer. The following procedures can be used for accounting for age-related hearing loss.

Specified Age Corrections

In some cases, age correction is achieved by subtracting a specific amount of hearing loss after a certain age. For example, Missouri deducts a half decibel for each year after the age of 40 years to correct for nonoccupational causes of hearing loss including presbycusis.

Age Corrections Based on Allocation

In some jurisdictions, individuals who are evaluating the medical evidence might apply age-related corrections. Different correction procedures have been suggested (Corso, 1980; Dobie, 1993a, 1993b, 1996). Such corrections often recommend the use of published median data on age-related hearing loss in populations that have not been exposed to any noise or those that may have been exposed to only nonoccupational noise (International Organization of Standardization, 1990 [Annex D of ISO-1999]; Johansson & Arlinger, 2002). Such data are used in combination with the data on expected amount of occupational NIHL for a given amount and duration of exposure (International Organization of Standardization, 1990

[Annex D of ISO-1999]). The datasets are used to estimate the percentage of age-related hearing loss that may have contributed to the total percentage of loss for those who report exposure to only occupational noise and those who report exposure to both occupational and nonoccupational noise. Some investigators have suggested that the notion of dividing any audiogram into several principal segments needs to be discarded, and each audiogram needs to be considered within its own stochastic nature (Hinchcliffe, 2000).

Use of Age Correction Tables Provided by the Occupational Safety and Health Administration (1983)

A simple and conservative way to account for age-related hearing loss is to use the age correction tables provided by OSHA (1983). The ISO-1999 (International Organization of Standardization, 1990) values for 500 Hz and 1000 Hz for the 90th percentiles are within 26 dB up to the age of 60 years for both screened and unscreened populations. When a low fence of 25 dB is used, age correction appears unnecessary at 500 and 1000 Hz. The hearing loss at 2000 and 3000 Hz can be corrected for age using thresholds provided by OSHA (1983). Then the percentage impairment can be calculated using the corrected threshold values.

Reasons for Not Allowing Age Corrections

Many jurisdictions do not allow age-related corrections, thus giving the benefit of doubt to the employee. Not allowing age corrections may be justified for the following reasons:

♦ Among individuals who are 55 to 99 years old, the prevalence of hearing loss is 39.4% (Sindhusake, Mitchell, Smith, et al., 2001). Thus approximately 60% of this population does not have age-related hearing loss. The noise-exposed worker may or may not have an age-related component in the hearing loss.
♦ There is considerable variability in age-related hearing loss (Robinson & Sutton, 1979). It is difficult to predict the severity or degree of any age-related component.
♦ Group results cannot be used to assess or predict the hearing impairment of any specific

individual (International Organization of Standardization, 1990 [Annex D of ISO-1999]).

Use of Age-related Corrections in Special Circumstances

Age-related corrections may be appropriate when someone retires at the age of 65 years and is allowed to apply for workers' compensation at the age of 75 years (Macrae, 1988). It would be unfair for the employer to have to pay for any deterioration in hearing that may have occurred during the period after retirement. Differences in audiometric thresholds at the age of 65 years and those obtained at the age of 75 years will provide a fairly accurate picture of age-related or non-employment–related hearing loss during the 10-year period in such cases.

Consideration of Speech Recognition Scores in the Calculation of Awards

Speech recognition scores (SRS) are not always considered in the calculation of awards, probably because savvy clients can exaggerate their difficulties and yield poor performance on speech recognition tests. However, in some cases such as blast injuries to the head, speech recognition can be much poorer than that predicted based on audiometric thresholds. In such cases, consideration of speech recognition abilities may be important. Different approaches have been used for considering SRS, as described subsequently.

Use of a Combination of Speech Recognition Scores and Audiometric Air Conduction Thresholds

Walsh and Silverman (1946) noted the insufficiency of just pure tone measures of hearing and proposed the Social Adequacy Index as the average of the SRS obtained at faint, average, and loud conversation levels using a phonetically balanced (PB) words lists. Davis (1948) compiled a table to allow clinicians to predict the Social Adequacy Index by using the speech recognition threshold (which is closely related to the pure tone average at 0.5, 1, and 2 kHz) and the maximum SRS for PB word lists. The Department of Veterans Affairs (VA) similarly assigns Roman numerals to each ear from I to XI based on a combination of pure tone hearing loss at 1, 2, 3, and 4 kHz and SRS (**Table 11.4**). The testing has to be conducted by a state-licensed audiologist and speech discrimination scores are determined using the Maryland Consonant-Nucleus-Consonant (CNC) test without hearing aids. The CNC test consists of monosyllabic words that have consonants in the initial and final position and a vowel in the middle. This assignment of numerals is altered under the following special circumstances:

◆ When SRS are unreliable or cannot be determined accurately because of language barriers, only pure tone averages are used to assign numerals to each ear as shown in **Table 11.5**.

Table 11.4   Veterans Affairs Numeric Assignments to Each Ear Using Pure Tone Average and SRS for the Maryland Consonant-Nucleus-Consonant (CNC) Test (Adapted from Table VI, Department of Veterans Affairs, 1999)

% SRS	Average of auditory thresholds (dB HL) at 1, 2, 3, and 4 kHz								
	0–41	42–49	50–57	58–65	66–73	74–81	82–89	90–97	98+
92–100		I			II		III		IV
84–90		II			III			IV	
76–82		III		IV				V	
68–74	IV		V		VI			VII	
60–66	V		VI		VII			VIII	
52–58	VI		VII			VIII			IX
44–50	VII			VIII			IX		X
36–42		VIII			IX			X	
0–34	IX	X			XI				

HL, hearing level; SRS, speech recognition scores.

Table 11.5 Veterans Affairs Numeric Assignments for Hearing Impairment Based on Mean Thresholds (dB Hearing Level) at 1, 2, 3, and 4 kHz (Adapted from Table VI, Department of Veterans Affairs, 1999)

Mean thresholds (dB hearing level) in the following range	Numeric designation	Percentage hearing impairment in the presence of the same numeric designation in both ears
0–41	I	
42–48	II	0
49–55	III	
56–62	IV	10
63–69	V	20
70–76	VI	30
77–83	VII	40
84–90	VIII	50
91–97	IX	60
98–104	X	80
105+	XI	100

- When the thresholds at each of the four frequencies (1, 2, 3, and 4 kHz) exceed 55 dB HL, the higher of the numeral designations found using **Tables 11.4** and **11.5** is used.
- When the thresholds at 1 kHz are 30 dB HL or lower and the thresholds at 2 kHz are 70 dB HL or greater, the higher of the numeral designations found in **Tables 11.4** and **11.5** is first determined and then that numeral is elevated to the next higher level.

After determination of the numerical designations for each ear (better and poor ear), the percentage impairment is decided as shown in **Table 11.6**. An example of calculation of percentage impairment using the VA procedure is shown in **Table 11.7**.

Assignment of Additional Disability Based on Speech Recognition Scores

In some jurisdictions, the percentage disability/impairment is first calculated using audiometric thresholds and then extra percentage disability is added based on the SRS. As an example of this, in West Virginia, a certain percentage is added to permanent partial disability depending on the SRS (**Table 11.8**). For

Table 11.6 Determination of Percentage Hearing Impairment Based on Numeric Designations Obtained from Table 11.4 or Table 11.5 for Each Ear (Adapted from Table VII, Department of Veterans Affairs, 1999)

Better ear		i	ii	iii	iv	v	vi	vii	viii	ix	x	xi
B	xi											100
e	x										80	90
t	ix									60	70	80
t	viii								50	50	60	70
e	vii							40	40	50	60	60
r	vi						30	30	40	40	50	50
e	v					20	20	30	30	40	40	40
a	iv				10	10	20	20	20	30	30	30
r	iii				10	10	10	20	20	20	20	20
	ii	0	0	0	0	10	10	10	10	10	10	10
	i	0	0	0	0	0	0	0	0	0	10	10

Worse ear

Table 11.7 Example of Determination of Percentage Hearing Impairment with the System Used by the VA in the Presence of Unreliable SRS for Hypothetical Air Conduction Thresholds Showing Compensable Hearing Loss in Both Ears

Frequency (Hz)	500	1000	2000	3000	4000	Average of thresholds at 1, 2, 3, and 4 kHz
Right (dB HL)	15	30	50	55	55	47.5 (III)
Left (dB HL)	20	35	55	55	55	50 (III)

As shown in **Table 11.5**, average thresholds between 44 and 50 dB are assigned the numeric designation III; as shown in **Table 11.6**, 0% impairment is assigned when both ears have the designation of III.

SRS, speech recognition scores; VA, Department of Veterans Affairs.

monaural hearing loss, the percentage SRS in the injured ear are used. For binaural hearing loss, the average percentage SRS in the two ears are used. The test to be used in documenting speech discrimination scores is not specified.

Increasing Percentage of Hearing Impairment in the Presence of Abnormally Poor Speech Recognition Scores

The following steps are involved in this procedure (Macrae, 1991):

◆ Determine the SRS using the Central Institute for the Deaf everyday sentence lists (Davis & Silverman, 1978). There are 10 sentences in each list, which are scored based on correct recognition of 50 keywords. The sentences are to be presented at 60 dB SPL in a quiet room. If the claimant scores 0% at this level, the sentences can be presented at 80 dB SPL.
◆ Determine if the claimant's SRS are poorer than what can be predicted from his or her average auditory thresholds; data are provided to determine this (Macrae & Brigden, 1973).
◆ If the scores are abnormally poor, find the expected threshold average corresponding to the client's poor SRS; established data

Table 11.8 SRS and Related Percentage of Permanent Partial Disability in West Virginia

Percentage of speech discrimination	Percentage of permanent partial disability
90–100%	0
80–89%	1%
70–79%	3%
60–69%	4%
0–59%	5%

SRS, speech recognition scores.

are provided to determine this (Macrae & Brigden, 1973).
◆ Instead of using the actual threshold average, use the expected threshold average to decide the percentage of hearing loss; data are provided to determine this (Macrae & Brigden, 1973).

Consideration of Tinnitus in Calculating the Amount of Compensation

It has been well established that exposure to occupational noise can result in tinnitus and approximately 17 to 30% of individuals exposed to noise have chronic tinnitus (Gabriels, Monley, & Guzeleva, 1996; Griest & Bishop, 1996), though prevalence estimates can vary depending on the specific population studied. A variety of procedures are used in awarding compensation for tinnitus.

Wisconsin allows the addition of 5% to the hearing impairment in the presence of work-related tinnitus. The VA assigns a separate 10% disability rating for recurrent tinnitus. In Sweden, a slight NIHL is not compensable by itself, but if the patient spontaneously reports troublesome tinnitus, the slight hearing loss can be considered compensable. Sweden and the United Kingdom allow up to a 20% increase in compensation of NIHL for tinnitus. Australia allows a 5% increase, Denmark allows up to a 5% increase, and Germany allows a 2.5 to 10% increase, while some countries do not compensate for tinnitus (Axelsson & Coles, 1996). Some states like West Virginia in the United States specifically include a declaration stating that no permanent partial disability benefits will be granted for tinnitus. In rare cases, compensation for tinnitus in nonindustrial settings can be quite high. For example, a Hollywood actress claimed that her career was in ruins because of tinnitus caused by a pistol fired from near her head in a Thames television studio. Her claim was supported by three Beverly Hills psychiatrists and was settled for £75,000 (Chuang, 1986).

Allowing compensation for tinnitus only within the calculation of percentage of hearing loss can be problematic because approximately 15 to 35% workers report tinnitus but have no hearing loss (Axelsson, 1996; Gabriels, Monley, & Guzeleva, 1996) and distress from debilitating tinnitus can be "on" all the time. Distress from hearing loss can be temporarily reduced when the person is alone (Axelsson, 1996).

If it is carefully evaluated and documented (see Chapter 5) as being a result of work-related noise exposure (Dejonckere, Coryn, & Lebacq, 2009; Dejonckere & Lebacq, 2005), compensation should be provided for tinnitus separately from hearing loss because it can lead to annoyance, depression, and degraded quality of life. There is some evidence suggesting that tinnitus interferes with speech perception, thus worsening the disability caused by hearing loss. Tinnitus can also be considered as causing "suffering" (Chuang, 1986).

One issue that can be raised about tinnitus is whether or not the tinnitus is permanent. It has been suggested that if tinnitus remains essentially unchanged for 2 years, it can be considered permanent (Vernon, 1996). During these 2 years, the worker should be allowed to try treatment and should be compensated for any treatment-related costs. Another issue is related to the determination of severity of tinnitus, which is based on the patient's self-report. Such self-reports can result in exaggeration of the severity by a few savvy patients for greater compensation. Although a repeated severity grading can offer some information about reliability of the self-report, it may be simpler to offer a set amount of compensation regardless of severity.

Allocation of Hearing Disability to More Than One Employer

Such allocation can be based on the noise exposure level with each employer and the duration of exposure. This data can be used in combination with the ISO-1999 (International Organization of Standardization, 1990) curves, which provide information about expected hearing levels for various exposure levels and durations (Dobie, 1993b).

Evaluation of Disability Based on Self-reports

Medical professionals often ask patients about how much difficulty they are having in hearing speech and other stimuli in quiet and noisy environments. The answers to these questions can be considered part of the medical evidence that is allowed in many jurisdictions. Railroads sometimes employ questionnaires sent to employee/claimants in an effort to resolve potential claims for hearing loss and to minimize litigations (Spence & Spencer, 1994). More formal, detailed interviews and questionnaires have also been developed to provide estimates of hearing disability (Giolas, Owens, Lamb, & Schubert, 1979). However, such self-reports can be affected by exaggeration of hearing loss due to neurotic tendencies (Gatehouse, 1990) or for gaining maximum compensation. On the other hand, some patient may underestimate the disability because of psychological denial of disability (Rawool & Kiehl, 2009), adaptation to the gradual or slowly progressing hearing loss, or lack of awareness of the presence of inaudible sounds (Kryter, 1998).

Consideration of Nonoccupational Noise Exposure and Other Factors

The case history form discussed in Chapter 4 can point to possible sources of nonoccupational noise exposure. Use of loud recreational or other activities (Rawool, 2008; Rawool & Colligon-Wayne, 2008) without the use of hearing protection can contribute to the overall hearing loss of the worker and weaken the claim for compensation depending on the severity of loss. The data from ISO-1999 (International Organization of Standardization, 1990) shows the difference in average thresholds between screened and unscreened populations. The unscreened population gives some indication of the impact of nonoccupational noise exposure on average thresholds in each of the specified age groups (**Table 11.9**). In addition to age, sex, and race, occupational noise exposure is significantly associated with educational level, recreational noise exposure including firearms, and smoking. Accounting for these variables can significantly decrease the hearing loss attributable to occupational noise exposure (Agrawal, Niparko, & Dobie, 2010; Kavanagh, 1992, 2001).

Table 11.9   Average Auditory Thresholds (dB) at 0.5, 1, 2, and 3 kHz for Highly Screened (Database A) and Unscreened (Database B) Populations of Men Based on Table A.3 and Table B.1 of ISO-1999 (International Organization of Standardization, 1990)

Percentile	Age (Years)							
	30		40		50		60	
	A	B	A	B	A	B	A	B
90th	10.5	14.5	14	23.5	19.5	29	27	38
50th	1.25	4.2	3.25	7	6.75	10.5	11.25	14.5
10th	−6.5	−2.75	−5.25	−1.25	−3.5	0.25	−0.75	2.25

Special Compensation for Deafness in Combination with Other Disabilities

Occupational hearing loss can be presented jointly with heart problems, lung disease, and other ailments as a contributing factor in "omnibus" permanent total disability claims (Ginnold, 1979). Estimates of dual sensory impairments (legal blindness and hearing loss) across different age groups among veterans (Goodrich, 2002) are shown in **Fig. 11.3**, and age appears to be a significant contributor to dual sensory impairments.

Penalty for Lack of Use of Hearing Protection Devices

In some jurisdictions, a claim can be denied or a penalty may be assessed against any compensation if a worker willfully disregards requirements to wear HPDs.

Cost of Treatment

Attention should be paid to long-term rehabilitative needs, including continued provision and servicing of hearing aids or cochlear implants and

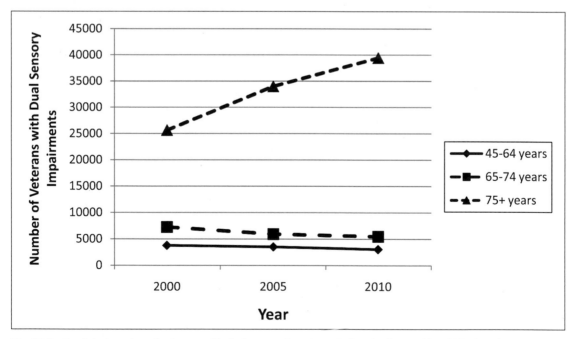

Fig. 11.3   Predicted number of veterans with dual sensory impairments (hearing loss and legal blindness) across different age groups; based on estimates provided by Goodrich (2002).

assistive listening devices, batteries needed to operate these devices, communication strategies training, auditory training, and speechreading training, as necessary. The costs for these services should include the average fees for services in the specific region and should be estimated for the rest of the worker's expected lifespan. As an example of eligibility for hearing aid–related costs, under 38 CFR §17.149, the VA provides hearing aids to veterans who receive VA healthcare services and who meet one or more of the following criteria:

- A minimal of 10% service-connected disability or combination of disabilities
- Former prisoner of war
- Receiving special benefits under 38 U.S.C. 1151 (tort claims)
- Receiving increased pensions based on the need for aid and assistance or because of being permanently housebound
- Hearing impairment due to another medical condition for which the veteran is receiving VA care, or which resulted from the treatment of such condition (e.g., ear surgery)
- A significant functional or cognitive impairment deduced by reduced activities of daily living, but not including normally occurring hearing impairment
- Hearing impairment so severe that hearing aids are necessary to permit active participation in any medical treatment
- Presence of a service-connected hearing disability rated as 0% (see example in **Table 11.7**) and thus noncompensable, if the hearing impairment contributes to a loss of communication ability

Other Factors

It is important to consider any other factors as required by the specific statute related to the claimant, including the following:

- Previous employment in a noisy environment and any award from previous employments.
- Improvement in hearing ability due to the use of hearing aids: A few jurisdictions allow any improvement from use of hearing aids to be considered in the calculation of awards. Some states specify that improvement with hearing aids should not be considered.

- Presence of a conductive element in the hearing loss based on bone conduction thresholds.
- Medical conditions: Consider conditions such as diabetes, cardiovascular problems, or head trauma that could cause elevation in thresholds (the elevation should be documented in audiograms obtained prior to employment).
- Ototoxic medications: Consider any current or previous use of ototoxic medications. For example, furosemide can cause a temporary elevation in threshold. The elevation can disappear after discontinuation of the medication. Aspirin can cause tinnitus that may disappear after discontinuation of the medication.
- Recreational and other noise exposure without the use of HPDs.

◆ Workers' Compensation Claims

In ideal workers' compensation systems, employees will not make any false claims of work-related injuries or will not exaggerate injuries, and employers would automatically pay for all work-related injury claims. In reality, determination of the fair amount of benefits can be difficult because of differences in compensability procedures across jurisdictions. Thus, there is a litigation industry built around each compensable industrial disability (Barth, 1984) and in practice, attorneys are usually involved. A checklist for preparing for workers' compensation claims is provided in the Appendix at the end of the chapter.

Procedures for Processing of Workers' Compensation Claims

A variety of procedures exist for processing workers' compensation claims, as follows:

- A government agency acts as an exclusive insurance carrier, which collects premiums from employers and investigates and pays claims. An example of this is the Federal Employee Compensation program (Ginnold, 1979).
- In North Dakota and Wyoming, employers can purchase insurance only from state funds (Clayton, 2003–2004).

- In Ohio, Washington, and West Virginia, employers must purchase insurance from the state fund or be approved to be self-insured (Clayton, 2003–2004).
- In most states, employers carry workers' compensation insurance with private insurance companies, which investigate, pay, or disputes claims. The workers' compensation agency monitors the insurance companies and evaluates any disputes between claimants and insurers. Employers are also permitted to insure themselves but must apply and meet the standards of the Worker's Compensation Act. Often, the largest employers choose this option to save insurance premiums and to better control claims (Clayton, 2003–2004; Ginnold, 1979).
- In many states, employers who employ fewer than three to five employees, farmers, and employers of private home owners with domestic servants are not required to purchase workers' compensation coverage.

Potential Advantage of Private Insurance Companies

One potential advantage of private insurance companies is that the competition among different insurance companies can result in lower premiums. Private insurance companies may also provide incentives to employers for enforcing stricter noise controls up to a degree, as lowering of noise levels below 75 dBA can eliminate the need of liability insurances for hearing loss.

Employer and Employee Responsibilities

Employers are often required to post notices informing employees to notify the employer about any injuries along with the name of the employer's carrier and the address and telephone number of the insurer or, if the employer is self-insured, the name, address, and telephone number of the person who can address claims or related enquiries. For example, Pennsylvania requires the following statement in the posted notices: "Remember, it is important to tell your employer about your injury." The term *impairment* is often defined as an anatomic or functional abnormality or loss that is a result of a permanent compensable injury.

Employees or their representatives are required to notify the employer and the workers' compensation agency of any work-related injuries. After an employee notifies the employer, the employer is expected to report the disability to the insurer and to the designated state agency along with a statement as to whether or not, on the basis of the information available, the employer disputes the worker's claims. The insurer can check the employer's report and, if there is no dispute, send a check to the worker.

When an employer or insurer disputes a worker's claim for NIHL, the employee can contest the claim by filing a petition with the workers' compensation agency. The agency then notifies the insurer. After evaluating the petition, the insurer might decide to pay the claim if it is not too large or if they feel it is well-documented and will not set a precedent for future litigations. If this does not occur, a hearing is scheduled. Before formal hearing occurs or is scheduled, the employee and/or attorney can agree on a settlement with the insurance company.

◆ Forensic Audiology

The application of audiology to legal issues is referred to as forensic audiology. Forensic audiologists may be involved in resolving disputes related to the determination of compensation for disability resulting from NIHL or fitness for service (see Chapter 12) following NIHL. The audiologist can assist as a special claims analyst in hearing loss claims. The audiologist may be called to testify for the defense or prosecution in civil or criminal courts, requested to serve as an advisor for the attorneys, or may be appointed as an expert.

Expert Audiological Witness

An expert witness is an individual who has more expertise than the court in a science related to the issues on trial. An audiologist who has performed detailed audiological evaluation of a patient who is seeking disability compensation or medical clearance for service is an expert witness. Another example of an expert witness is an audiologist who is asked to give an opinion about the validity of the hearing disability claim based on audiometric test data submitted as evidence by others. If the audiologist does not believe that he or she has the expertise to serve as an expert because of special expertise in other area(s) of audiology or because of a lack of sufficient familiarity with published opinion and research, the audiologist may recommend another person with greater expertise to serve as an expert witness (Schmitz, 1982).

Expert witnesses can lose their credibility if they serve exclusively as a witness for the defense or for the plaintiff; the unbiased nature of observations can be questioned in such cases (Vernon, 1996). For example, lawyers Spence and Spencer (1994) argued, "audiologists can be found to ascribe virtually any hearing loss to any cause for which they are paid to ascribe it." Vernon (1996) also noted that attorneys in the United States often ask expert witnessess to provide an opinion about the "medical" probability of an occurrence. Those who are not medical doctors, including audiologists, need to change the wording to state the probability of occurrence based on "audiologic" or "scientific" (not medical) testing while providing opinions in such cases.

It is important to negotiate any consultation fees before providing consultation to attorneys and testifying in the court. Because court trials can last for extended periods, the best approach is to charge fees for each time any consultation or any other court services are provided. If the liability insurance of the expert witness does not cover legal activities, it may be appropriate to ask the plaintiff or defendant to agree to pay for counsel and to cover the witness in case of a subsequent legal action based on accusations of malicious statements intended to harm a party (Dobie, 1993c).

Preparation for the Testimony

Properly prepared expert opinion can stimulate negotiations and can shorten the duration of the trial. The expert witness should be adequately familiar with any disputed issues related to the case, calibration records, noise exposure records, noise levels during audiometric testing, the qualifications and experience of individuals who determined audiometric thresholds, audiometric test records, and any other relevant history such as the availability and use of HPDs. Because patients receive compensation that is often based on the degree of hearing loss demonstrated during audiological evaluation, the possibility of exaggerated hearing

loss must be carefully considered. Objective data such as results of the auditory brainstem response tests can be very useful in such cases (Miller, Crane, Fox, & Linstrom, 1998). With reference to tinnitus, it is often necessary to explain to courts that the measured loudness of tinnitus has no correlation with the perceived severity of tinnitus.

Some lawyers use what is known as the electronic discovery process, which extracts, organizes, and preserves data from workstations, e-mail and other servers, personal digital assistants, and other electronic equipment for use in litigation. It is better to be aware of what the claimant may have stated in e-mails to various individuals including insurance agents, physicians, nurses, otolaryngologists, and audiologists.

Pretrial Meeting with the Attorney

During the pretrial meeting with the attorney, the audiologist can develop an outline for an orientation to the field of audiology and audiological testing suitable to the jury using nontechnical language. At this meeting, the audiologist can practice explaining the test results clearly and succinctly to individuals who have no expertise in audiology. The audiologist should prepare to refrain from making statements outside the area of expertise to minimize questions regarding credibility during cross-examination.

Direct Examination

During direct examination, the attorney who requested the audiologist to be the expert witness asks questions designed to demonstrate the expertise of the witness to the case and to present a clear and cohesive picture of the client's hearing ability. It is important for the audiologist to appear calm and self-assured without seeming arrogant. During direct examination, audiograms and other hearing data such as auditory brainstem responses can be used. Such records are admitted as evidence by the court and are referred to as exhibits.

Use of Visual Aids

Large displays of audiograms and noise exposure level maps can be used for the benefit of jurors if permitted by the court. Projection of PowerPoint slides, when possible, can allow flexibility in explaining the various parts and adding pertinent details as necessary. It is important to articulate all references made when pointing to different parts of the display so that the court transcripts are easy to understand at any later dates without the benefit of the visual aids.

Cross-Examination

During this portion of the trial, the opposing attorney has an opportunity to question the witness. The attorney may attempt to discredit the expert witness or to cast suspicion on the accuracy of the direct testimony. To achieve this goal, the attorney may anticipate the testimony of the expert witness and prepare to question areas that are debatable. A comprehensive pretrial preparation that produces a clear and nonquestionable testimony on direct examination can minimize the chance of cross-examination and can give confidence to the audiologist in answering any questions if the opposing attorney chooses to cross-examine.

Examples of Results of Compensation Claims Related to Noise-induced Injuries

Claim for Tinnitus due to Noise Exposure

In the state of Washington, the Board of Industrial Insurance Appeals (BIIA) is a separate state agency that operates independently from the Department of Labor and Industries and hears appeals on decisions made by the department in several areas, including workers' compensation. The Department of Labor and Industries had denied compensation for tinnitus to a claimant on the grounds that he did not have a compensable hearing loss. The claimant had operated chainsaws in the woods as an employee of a company. The BIIA reversed the order and remanded the claim to the department to accept the claim for occupational tinnitus and for noncompensable occupational hearing loss, and instructed the self-insured employer to provide benefits to which the claimant may be entitled including the payment of any medical bills incurred for reasonable treatment, testing, and diagnosis of hearing loss and tinnitus, including payment for hearing aids or masking devices if necessary and recommended by a physician.

The BIIA acknowledged the fact that the Department of Labor and Industries had been reluctant to recognize tinnitus as a compensable condition because of a perceived inability to objectively measure the degree of impairment. Based on the medical evidence, the BIIA concluded that the frequency and intensity of the tinnitus could be verified and measured (see Chapter 5), at least partly, in an objective manner. The BIIA also recommended a greater degree of standardization in evaluation of tinnitus, its causal relation to noise exposure, and its relative severity, to allow more consistency and fairness in settlement of claims of noise-induced tinnitus (see www.biia.wa.gov/SignificantDecisions/920602.htm).

This case is interesting because the BIIA also noted that an endless succession of adversarial cases and various otolaryngologists/forensic examiners called as witnesses by the defense are not sensible, efficient, or cost-effective approaches. The BIIA further pointed out that although such litigious procedures are lucrative to the medical expert witnesses and attorneys, they do not advance certainty and consistency desired by workers and employers.

Claim for Compensation Related to Hearing Loss from a Single Noise Exposure Incidence

In this case, a 71-year-old claimant contended that he sustained a compensable hearing loss due to a tire explosion while putting air in the tire. He was serving as a nonemergency medical transportation driver for his employer. One of the other employees testified and noted that before the tire explosion incident, the claimant usually spoke loudly and some instructions had to be repeated to him. This testimony and the employee's age suggested the possibility of previous hearing loss. The court ordered the employer to pay all medical and related treatment as the result of the claimant's hearing loss, together with continued, reasonably necessary medical treatment, including, but not limited to hearing aids (see www.awcc.state.ar.us/opinions/alj/2005/gi/harmon_winfred_f412552_20050519.pdf). It appears that any previous hearing loss may not have been as disabling as the hearing loss after the explosion.

The court in the context of this case noted that audiological evaluations by a trained audiologist are the best and most accurate scientific evaluations to test for hearing loss. This case is interesting because in many cases, hearing loss from a single explosion tends to be temporary or minimal, although impulse noise above

140 dB SPL can cause permanent acoustic trauma (National Institutes of Health Consensus Statement, 1990).

Failure to Establish Injury from Noise Exposure during Specific Employment

In this case, the claimant reported a constant, locust-like, whistle in his ears. There was no history of ear diseases, ear surgeries, or treatment of hearing loss. The tinnitus affected his ability to hear the television or radio, to talk on the telephone, and to hear conversations distinctly, particularly in noisy environments. At times, the ringing affected his ability to fall asleep.

Complicating factors in this case included non-occupational noise exposure including hunting and use of a chainsaw, and noise exposure from previous employment for 11 years without the use of HPDs. The court concluded that the claimant had failed to prove that his tinnitus was casually related to his employment with the particular employer. The claimant's claim for compensation was denied (see www.labor.mo.gov/LIRC/Forms/WC_Decisions/wcdec07/Hudson,%20Sidney.htm).

◆ Review Questions

1. Why is it necessary to have a workers' compensation policy for noise-induced injuries?
2. Discuss the factors you need to consider in determining eligibility for workers' compensation.
3. An employee who has worked for a company for 12 years claims that he has suffered from a NIHL due to exposure at work. The company does not have an HCP in place, and thus the employee was never provided with HPDs. You conducted dosimetry on 3 days; dosimetry showed that the mean TWA exposure of the employee was 73 dBA with the maximum dose of 74 dBA. Noise surveys completed on 3 days show that the highest peak levels are 82 dBC. How will you proceed in this case?
4. Calculate percentage impairment using the AAO/ACO (1979) procedure for auditory thresholds presented in **Table 11.7**.
   4a. Compare your answer to the answer you get from using the web-based calculator at the following website: www.occupationalhearingloss.com.
   4b. Compare your answer to that presented in **Table 11.7** using the VA procedure.

4c. Is the hypothetical veteran in **Table 11.7** eligible for receiving hearing aids from the VA?
5. Review the variables proposed by different investigators that can yield different percentage of hearing impairment for the same audiometric thresholds.
6. Discuss the various procedures that can be used in accounting for age-related hearing loss in workers' compensation cases.
7. What are the advantages and disadvantages of accounting for age-related hearing loss for workers' compensation cases? Under which special circumstances does accounting for age-related hearing loss appear to be appropriate?
8. Compare and contrast the various procedures for considering speech recognition scores in the calculation of percentage of hearing impairment.
9. Review the potential problems associated with awarding compensation for noise-induced tinnitus.
10. You are invited to serve as an expert witness for your patient who is eligible and has filed for workers' compensation. How will you prepare yourself before the trial?

References

Agrawal Y, Niparko JK, Dobie RA. (2010). Estimating the effect of occupational noise exposure on hearing thresholds: the importance of adjusting for confounding variables. *Ear Hearing.* 31(2):234–237.

Alberti PW, Morgan PP, Fria TJ, LeBlanc JC. (1976). Percentage hearing loss: various schema applied to large population with noise-induced hearing loss. In: Henderson D, Hamernick RP, Dosanjh DS, Mills JH, eds. *Effects of Noise on Hearing.* New York: Raven Press: 479–496.

American Academy of Ophthalmology and Otolaryngology. (1959). Guide for the evaluation of hearing impairment. *Trans Am Acad Ophthalmol Otolaryngol.* 63:236–238.

American Academy of Otolaryngology Committee on the Medical Aspects of Noise and American Council of Otolaryngology. (1979). Guide for the evaluation of hearing handicap. *JAMA.* 241(19):2055–2059.

American Medical Association. (1942). Tentative standard procedure for evaluating the percentage of useful hearing loss in medicolegal cases. *JAMA.* 119:1108–1109.

American National Standards Institute. (1997). *ANSI S3.5–1997 (R2007). American National Standard Methods for the Calculation of the Speech Intelligibility Index.* New York: American National Standards Institute.

American Speech-Language-Hearing Association Task Force. (1981). On the definition of hearing handicap. *ASHA.* 23(4):293–297.

Atherley GR. (1973). Noise-induced hearing loss: the energy principle for recurrent impact noise and noise exposure close to the recommended limits. *Ann Occup Hyg.* 16(2):183–194.

Axelsson A. (1996). How severe is his tinnitus and what is its prognosis? In: Reich GE, Vernon J, eds. *Proceedings of the Fifth International Tinnitus Seminar.* Portland, OR: American Tinnitus Association: 363–366.

Axelsson A, Coles R. (1996). Compensation for tinnitus in noise-induced hearing loss. In: Axelsson A, Borchgrevink HM, Hamernick RP, Hellstrom PA, Henderson D, Salvi RJ, eds. *Scientific Basis of Noise-Induced Hearing Loss.* New York: Thieme: 423–429.

Barth PS. (1984). A proposal for dealing with the compensation of occupational diseases. *J Legal Studies.* 13(3): 569–586. Available at: www.jstor.org/stable/724296. Accessed July 7, 2011.

Bureau of Labor Statistics. (2009). *Nonfatal Occupational Illnesses by Major Industry Sector and Category of Illness, 2008.* Washington, DC: U.S. Department of Labor.

Chuang WP. (1986). Tinnitus as suffering. *J Laryngol Otol Suppl.* 11:37–38.

Clayton A. (2003–2004). Workers' compensation: a background for Social Security professionals. *Soc Secur Bull.* 65(4):7–15. Available at: http://www.ssa.gov/policy/docs/ssb/v65n4/v65n4p7.html. Accessed July 7, 2011.

Committee on Hearing, Bioacoustics, and Biomechanics, National Academy of Sciences, National Research Council. (1975). *Compensation Formula for Hearing Loss. Report of Working Group 77.* Washington, DC: Committee on Hearing, Bioacoustics, and Biomechanics.

Corso JF. (1980). Age correction factor in noise-induced hearing loss: a quantitative model. *Audiology.* 19(3):221–232.

Danermark B, Cieza A, Gangé JP, et al. (2010). International classification of functioning, disability, and health core sets for hearing loss: a discussion paper and invitation. *Int J Audiol.* 49(4):256–262.

Davis H. (1948). The articulation area and the social adequacy index for hearing. *Laryngoscope.* 58(8): 761–778.

Davis H, Silverman SR. (1978). *Hearing and Deafness,* 4th ed. New York: Holt Reinhart and Winston.

Dejonckere PH, Coryn C, Lebacq J. (2009). Experience with a medicolegal decision-making system for occupational hearing loss-related tinnitus. *Int Tinnitus J.* 15(2): 185–192.

Dejonckere PH, Lebacq J. (2005). Medicolegal decision making in noise-induced hearing loss-related tinnitus. *Int Tinnitus J.* 11(1):92–96.

Department of Insurance and Finance of the State of Oregon. (1988). Worker's compensation division 35, Disability rating standards, Page 37. Available at: www.cbs.state.or.us/external/wcd/policy/rules/div_035/35_3-1988.pdf. Accessed July 7, 2011.

Department of Veterans Affairs. (1999). Schedule for rating disabilities; Diseases of the ear and other sense Organs. 38 CFR Part 4 RIN 2900-AF22, Final rule. Federal Register Tuesday May 11, 1999; 64(90):25202–25209.

Dobie RA. (1993a). Confidence intervals for hearing loss allocation estimates. *Ear Hear.* 14(5):315–321.

Dobie RA. (1993b). Diagnosis and allocation. In: Dobie RA. *Medical-Legal Evaluation of Hearing Loss.* New York: Van Nostrand Reinhold: 260–301.

Dobie RA. (1993c). The expert witness. In: Dobie RA. *Medical-Legal Evaluation of Hearing Loss.* New York: Van Nostrand Reinhold: 325–340.

Dobie RA. (1996). Estimation of occupational contribution to hearing handicap. In: Axelsson A, Borchgrevink HM, Hamernick RP, Hellstrom PA, Henderson D, Salvi RJ, eds. *Scientific Basis of Noise-Induced Hearing Loss.* New York: Thieme: 415–422.

Federal Employee Liability Act. (1908). Federal Employee Liability Act. 45 U.S.C. §§51–60.

Fowler EP. (1942). A method for measuring the percentage capacity for hearing speech. *J Acoust Soc Am.* 13: 373–382.

Fowler E P. (1947). The percentage of capacity to hear speech, and related disabilities. *Laryngoscope.* 57(2):103–113.

Gabriels P, Monley P, Guzeleva D. (1996). Noise exposed workers: Is tinnitus being ignored? In: Reich GE, Vernon J, eds. *Proceedings of the Fifth International Tinnitus Seminar.* Portland, OR: American Tinnitus Association: 373–380.

Gatehouse S. (1990). Determinants of self-reported disability in older subjects. *Ear Hear.* 11(5 Suppl):57S–65S.

Ginnold RE. (1979). *Occupational Hearing Loss: Workers Compensation Under State and Federal Programs.* Washington, DC: U.S. Environmental Protection Agency, Office of Noise Abatement and Control.

Giolas TG, Owens E, Lamb SH, Schubert ED. (1979). Hearing performance inventory. *J Speech Hear Disord.* 44(2):169–195.

Goodrich GL. (2002). Introduction. In: McMahon R, ed. *Visual Impairment and Blindness. Independent Study Course.* Washington DC: Veterans Health Administration. 7–8.

Griest SE, Bishop PM. (1996). Evaluation of tinnitus and occupational hearing loss based on 20-year longitudinal data. In: Reich GE, Vernon J, eds. *Proceedings of the Fifth International Tinnitus Seminar.* Portland, OR: American Tinnitus Association: 381–394.

Hardick EJ, Melnick W, Hawes NA, Pillion JP, Stephens RG, Perlmutter DJ. (1980). *Compensation for Hearing Loss for Employees Under the Jurisdiction of the U. S. Department of Labor: Benefit Formula and Assessment Procedures. Final Report for Contract No. J-9-E-90205.* Washington, DC: U.S. Department of Labor.

Hinchcliffe R. (2000). Effects of noise on hearing- aspects of assessment: guidelines for giving advice to expert witnesses. *J Audiological Med.* 9:1–18.

International Organization for Standardization. (1990). *ISO-1999. Acoustics: Determination of Occupational Noise Exposure and Estimation of Noise-Induced Hearing Impairment.* Geneva: International Organization for Standardization.

Johansson MS, Arlinger SD. (2002). Hearing threshold levels for an otologically unscreened, non-occupationally noise-exposed population in Sweden. *Int J Audiol.* 41(3):180–194.

Jones PH. (2007). Disability assessment in noise-induced hearing loss. In: Luxon LM, Prasher D, eds. *Noise and its Effects.* West Sussex, England: John Wiley & Sons, Ltd.: 232–257.

Kavanagh KT. (1992). Evaluation of patients with suspected occupational hearing loss. *J Am Acad Audiol.* 3:215–220.

Kavanagh KT. (2001). Evaluation of hearing handicaps and presbyacusis using World Wide Web-based calculators. *J Am Acad Audiol.* 12(10):497–505.

King PF, Coles RRA, Lutman ME, Robinson DW. (1992). *Assessment of Hearing Disability. Guidelines for Medicolegal Practice.* London: Whurr Publishers.

Kryter KD. (1973). Impairment to hearing from exposure to noise. *J Acoust Soc Am.* 53(5):1211–1234.

Kryter KD. (1998). Evaluating hearing handicap. *J Am Acad Audiol.* 9:141–146.

Mackenzie IJ. (1997). *Legislation and Compensation. Proceedings of WHO-PDH Informal Consultation on Prevention of Noise Induced Hearing Loss. Geneva 28–30 October 1997.* Geneva: World Health Organization.

Macrae JH. (1974). *Notes on the Procedure for Determining Percentage Loss of Hearing.* Sydney, Australia: Commonwealth Department of Health.

Macrae JH. (1988). *Improved Procedure for Determining Percentage Loss of Hearing.* National Acoustic Laboratories Report No. 118. Canberra, Australia: Department of Community Services and Health, Australian Government Publishing Service.

Macrae JH. (1991). *A Procedure for Determining Percentage Loss of Hearing of Clients with Abnormally Poor Speech Discrimination.* National Acoustic Laboratories Report No. 124. Canberra, Australia: Department of Community Services and Health, Australian Government Publishing Service.

Macrae JH, Brigden DN. (1973). Auditory threshold impairment and everyday speech reception. *Audiology.* 12(4):272–290.

Miller MH, Crane MA, Fox J, Linstrom C. (1998). Pseudohypacusis: Workers' compensation costs and professional implications. *Hear J.* 52(4):42–45.

National Acoustic Laboratories. (1976). *Procedure for Determining Percentage Loss of Hearing.* Sydney, Australia: National Acoustic Laboratories.

National Institutes of Health Consensus Statement. (1990). Noise and Hearing Loss. *Development Conference Consensus Statement.* Jan 22–24; 8(1):1–24.

Occupational Safety and Health Administration. (1983). 29 CFR 1910.95. Occupational noise exposure; hearing conservation amendment; final rule, effective 8 March 1983. *Federal Register.* 48:9738–9785.

Rawool VW. (2007). The aging auditory system, Part 3: Slower processing, cognition, and speech recognition. *Hear Review.* 14: 38, 43, 44, 46, 48. Available at: www.hearingreview.com/issues/articles/2007-09_02.asp. Accessed June 2010.

Rawool VW. (2008). Growing up noisy: The sound exposure diary of a hypothetical young adult. *Hear Review.* 15(5):30, 32, 34, 39–40.

Rawool VW, Colligon-Wayne LA. (2008). Auditory lifestyles and beliefs related to hearing loss among college students in the USA. *Noise Health.* 10(38):1–10.

Rawool VW, Kiehl JM. (2009). Effectiveness of informational counseling on acceptance of hearing loss among older adults. *Hear Review.* 16(6):14–22.

Robinson DW, Sutton GJ. (1979). Age effect in hearing - a comparative analysis of published threshold data. *Audiology.* 18(4):320–334.

Sabine PE. (1942). On estimating the percentage of loss of useful hearing. *Trans Am Acad Ophthalmol Otolaryngol.* 46:179–196.

Schmitz HD. (1982). The audiologist as an expert witness in court. In: Kramer MB, Armbruster JM, eds. *Forensic Audiology.* Baltimore: University Park Press: 45–55.

Sindhusake D, Mitchell P, Smith W, et al. (2001). Validation of self-reported hearing loss. The Blue Mountains Hearing Study. *Int J Epidemiol.* 30(6):1371–1378.

Snow WB. (1931). Audible frequency ranges of music, speech and noise. *J Acoust Soc Am.* 3(1.1):155–166.

Spence EB, Spencer CW Jr. (1994). Accrual of hearing loss actions under the FELA: the objective standard prevails. *Cumberland Law Review.* 24;113.

Thorne PR, Ameratunga SN, Stewart J, et al. (2008). Epidemiology of noise-induced hearing loss in New Zealand. *N Z Med J.* 121(1280):33–44.

U.S. Code Compensation For Work Injuries. (2008). Title 5 Part III Subpart G Chapter 81 (January 8, 2008) Available at: http://uscode.house.gov/download/pls/05C81.txt. Accessed July 2009.

U.S. Environmental Protection Agency. (1974). Information on Levels of Environmental Noise Requisite to Protect the Public Health and Welfare with an Adequate Margin of Safety. Washington, DC: U.S. Environmental Protection Agency.

Vernon J. (1996). Is the claimed tinnitus real and is the claimed cause correct? In: Reich GE, Vernon J, eds. *Proceedings of the Fifth International Tinnitus Seminar.* Portland, OR: American Tinnitus Association: 395–396.

Veterans Benefits Administration. (2008). Annual Benefits Report, Fiscal Year 2008. Washington, DC: Department of Veterans Affairs.

Walsh TE, Silverman SR. (1946). Diagnosis and evaluation of fenestration. *Laryngoscope.* 56:536–555.

World Health Organization. (2001). *International Classification of Functioning, Disability and Health – ICF.* Geneva: World Health Organization.

◆ Appendix A

Checklist for Addressing Workers' Compensation Claims

Claimant name:_____ Date: _____

1. List the condition(s) the employee claims to have suffered from:
   - ◆ NIHL
   - ◆ Noise-induced tinnitus
   - ◆ External or middle ear problems due to the use of HPDs
   - ◆ Any other

2. When did the employee first become aware of the condition?
   Date: _____

2a. Considering this date, is the claim within any statute of limitations?
   Yes _____ No _____ Not applicable in the jurisdiction _____

2b. Considering this date, has any waiting period expired?
   Yes _____ No _____ Not applicable in the jurisdiction _____

3. If there is a requirement of hazardous noise exposure within the jurisdiction, does the claimant's exposure meet this requirement?
   Yes _____ No _____ Not sure, no records of noise exposure _____
   Are measurements of noise exposure necessary? Yes _____ No _____

4. Is it highly possible that the specified condition partially or fully resulted during and because of the current employment? Yes _____ No _____

5. Is it highly likely that a particular event(s) or occurrence(s) partially or fully caused the condition claimed in question 1? Yes _____ No _____

6. Do the average hearing thresholds for the specified frequency exceed the low fence?
   Yes _____ No _____
   Note: If the response is "No," then the employee is not eligible for compensation for hearing loss; the employee may be eligible for compensation based on other factors such as tinnitus.

7. When did the claimant begin the current employment?
   Date:
   Duration of employment:
   Full-time: _____ Part-time: _____

8. Does the employer have an HCP in place?
   Yes _____ No _____
   Was the HCP in place since the beginning of the claimant's employment?
   If no, when did the HCP begin?
   Date: _____

9. Were HPDs, education, and training provided by the employer?
   Yes _____ No _____
   The type of HPD, if provided: _____

10. Did the employee use HPDs?

Yes _____ No _____ Not provided by the employer _____

If yes, how often did the employee use HPDs when in loud noise?

Most of the time (76 to 100% of the time) _____

Sometimes (75 to 26% of the time) ____ _____

Rarely (25% or less of the time) _____

11. If the employee does not or rarely uses HPDs, what are the reasons?

Ear problems or pain:

Hearing difficulties with use of HPDs:

Fear of not hearing warning signals:

12. Check all the factors that may have contributed to the total hearing loss based on case history (see case history form in the appendix of Chapter 4):

◆ Current employment (documented hazardous noise exposure; TWA or peak levels)
◆ Previous employment
◆ Medical history (specify)
◆ Conductive hearing loss (e.g., otosclerosis)
◆ Ototoxic medications
◆ Smoking
◆ Recreational noise exposure
◆ Other (specify): _____

13. Is it possible to distinguish the degree of hearing loss caused by any of the previous conditions based on previous audiological tests?

Yes _____ No _____

14. Is the employee receiving compensation for hearing loss from any of the previous employers?

Yes _____ No _____

15. What is the percentage of hearing impairment?

16. How much award can be recommended for the occupational NIHL based on auditory thresholds during current employment?

17. How much, if any, additional award can be recommended based on any of the following considerations?

◆ Tinnitus
◆ Exposure to industrial ototoxins
◆ Hearing aids and assistive devices
◆ Maintenance cost for hearing aids and assistive devices
◆ Replacement cost for hearing aids and assistive devices
◆ Aural rehabilitation

participation, and two measures of productivity. *J Occup Environ Med.* 47(4):343–351.

Canadian Standards Association. (2008). *Inclusive Design for an Aging Population* (B659–08). Mississauga, ON: Canadian Standards Association.

Casali JG, Robinson GS, Lee SE. (1998). *Role of Driver Hearing in Commercial Motor Vehicle Operation: An Evaluation of the FHWA Hearing Requirement.* Washington, DC: Federal Highway Administration.

Chisolm TH, Abrams HB, McArdle R. (2004). Short- and long-term outcomes of adult audiological rehabilitation. *Ear Hear.* 25(5):464–477.

Choi SW, Peek-Asa C, Sprince NL, et al. (2005, Oct). Hearing loss as a risk factor for agricultural injuries. *Am J Ind Med.* 48(4):293–301.

Coelho CB, Tyler R, Hansen M. (2007). Zinc as a possible treatment for tinnitus. *Prog Brain Res.* 166;279–285.

Cooke M. (2006). Policy changes and the labour force participation of older workers: evidence from six countries. *Can J Aging.* 25(4):387–400.

Cruickshanks KJ, Wiley TL, Tweed TS, et al. (1998). Prevalence of hearing loss in older adults in Beaver Dam, Wisconsin. The Epidemiology of Hearing Loss Study. *Am J Epidemiol.* 148(9):879–886.

Danermark B, Gellerstedt LC. (2004). Psychosocial work environment, hearing impairment and health. *Int J Audiol.* 43(7):383–389.

de Croon EM, Sluiter JK, Frings-Dresen MH. (2003). Need for recovery after work predicts sickness absence: a 2-year prospective cohort study in truck drivers. *J Psychosom Res.* 55(4):331–339.

Dishman RK, Berthoud HR, Booth FW, et al. (2006). Neurobiology of exercise. *Obesity (Silver Spring).* 14(3):345–356.

Enrico P, Sirca D, Mereu M. (2007). Antioxidants, minerals, vitamins, and herbal remedies in tinnitus therapy. *Prog Brain Res.* 166:323–330.

Eriksson-Mangold MM, Erlandsson SI. (1984). The psychological importance of nonverbal sounds. An experiment with induced hearing deficiency. *Scand Audiol.* 13(4):243–249.

Federal Motor Carrier Safety Administration. U S Department of Transportation. (2010). Federal Motor Carrier Safety Regulation (FMCSR). 49 CFR 391.41(b) (11) Qualification of drivers and longer combination vehicles (LCV) driver instructors: Subpart E - Physical qualifications and examinations, Physical qualifications for drivers. Available at: http://www.fmcsa.dot.gov/rules-regulations/administration/fmcsr/fmcsrruletext.aspx?reg=391.41. Accessed July 8, 2011.

Ficca G, Axelsson J, Mollicone DJ, Muto V, Vitiello MV. (2010). Naps, cognition and performance. *Sleep Med Rev.* 14(4):249–258.

Fok D, Shaw L, Jennings MB, Cheesman M. (2009). Towards a comprehensive approach for managing transitions of older workers with hearing loss. *Work.* 32(4):365–376.

Fornaro M, Martino M. (2010). Tinnitus psychopharmacology: A comprehensive review of its pathomechanisms and management. *Neuropsychiatr Dis Treat.* 6:209–218.

Forti S, Costanzo S, Crocetti A, Pignataro L, Del Bo L, Ambrosetti U. (2009). Are results of tinnitus retraining therapy maintained over time? 18-month follow-up after completion of therapy. *Audiol Neurootol.* 14(5):286–289.

Garinther GR, Peters LJ. (1990) *Impact of Communications on Armor Crew Performance: Investigating the Impact of Noise and Other Variables on Mission Effectiveness.* Army Research, Development, & Acquisition Bulletin (January/February):1–5.

Girard SA, Picard M, Davis AC, et al. (2009). Multiple work-related accidents: tracing the role of hearing status and noise exposure. *Occup Environ Med.* 66(5):319–324.

Goldberg RL, Spilberg SW, Weyers SG. (2002). Medical Screening Manual for California Law Enforcement. Chapter XII Hearing Guidelines. California Commission on Peace Officer Standards and Training (POST), Post S&E 2002-02, POST Media Distribution Center, Sacramento, California , USA. Available at: http://libcat.post.ca.gov/dbtw-wpd/documents/POST/56769727.pdf. Accessed July 8, 2011.

Goodman MF, Bents F, Tijerina L, Wierwille W, Lerner N, Benel D. (1997). *An Investigation of the Safety Implications of Wireless Communications in Vehicles: Report Summary.* Available at: www.nhtsa.dot.gov/people/injury/research/wireless/#rep. Accessed September 2010.

Goodrich GL. (2002). Introduction. In: McMahon R, ed. *Visual Impairment and Blindness. Independent Study Course.* Washington, DC: Veterans Health Administration: 7–8.

Grimby A, Ringdahl A. (2000). Does having a job improve the quality of life among post-lingually deafened Swedish adults with severe-profound hearing impairment? *Br J Audiol.* 34(3):187–195.

Günther VK, Schäfer P, Holzner BJ, Kemmler GW. (2003). Long-term improvements in cognitive performance through computer-assisted cognitive training: a pilot study in a residential home for older people. *Aging Ment Health.* 7(3):200–206.

Hallam R, Ashton P, Sherbourne K, Gailey L. (2006). Acquired profound hearing loss: mental health and other characteristics of a large sample. *Int J Audiol.* 45(12):715–723.

Hallberg LR, Barrenäs ML. (1994). Group rehabilitation of middle-aged males with noise-induced hearing loss and their spouses: evaluation of short- and long-term effects. *Br J Audiol.* 28(2):71–79.

Hawkins DB. (2005). Effectiveness of counseling-based adult group aural rehabilitation programs: a systematic review of the evidence. *J Am Acad Audiol.* 16(7):485–493.

Hazell JW, Williams GR, Sheldrake JB. (1981). Tinnitus maskers—successes and failures: a report on the state of the art. *J Laryngol Otol Suppl.* 4(4):80–87.

Health Technology Information Service. (2010). *Tinnitus Retraining Therapy: A Review of Clinical Effectiveness. Health Technology Assessment.* Ottawa, Ontario, Canada: Canadian Agency for Drugs and Technologies in Health.

Henry JA, Schechter MA, Zaugg TL, et al. (2006a). Clinical trial to compare tinnitus masking and tinnitus retraining therapy. *Acta Otolaryngol.* 126(556):64–69.

Henry JA, Schechter MA, Zaugg TL, et al. (2006b). Outcomes of clinical trial: tinnitus masking versus tinnitus retraining therapy. *J Am Acad Audiol.* 17(2):104–132.

Hilton M, Stuart E. (2004). Ginkgo biloba for tinnitus. *Cochrane Database Syst Rev.* (2):CD003852.

Holgers KM, Erlandsson SI, Barrenäs ML. (2000). Predictive factors for the severity of tinnitus. *Audiology.* 39(5):284–291.

Hutchinson KM, Alessio H, Baiduc RR. (2010). Association between cardiovascular health and hearing function: pure-tone and distortion product otoacoustic emission measures. *Am J Audiol.* 19(1):26–35.

Jastreboff PJ, Hazell JW. (1993). A neurophysiological approach to tinnitus: clinical implications. *Br J Audiol.* 27(1):7–17.

Jastreboff PJ, Hazell JW. (2004). *Tinnitus Retraining Therapy: Implementing the Neurophysiological Mode.* Cambridge: Cambridge University Press.

Jennings MB, Shaw L. (2008). Impact of hearing loss in the workplace: raising questions about partnerships with professionals. *Work.* 30(3):289–295.

Johnson JV, Hall EM. (1988). Job strain, work place social support, and cardiovascular disease: a cross-sectional study of a random sample of the Swedish working population. *Am J Public Health.* 78(10):1336–1342.

Johnson JV, Hall EM, Theorell T. (1989). Combined effects of job strain and social isolation on cardiovascular disease morbidity and mortality in a random sample of the Swedish male working population. *Scand J Work Environ Health.* 15(4):271–279.

Kahlbrock N, Weisz N. (2008). Transient reduction of tinnitus intensity is marked by concomitant reductions of delta band power. *BMC Biol.* 6:4.

Kaldo V, Levin S, Widarsson J, Buhrman M, Larsen HC, Andersson G. (2008). Internet versus group cognitive-behavioral treatment of distress associated with tinnitus: a randomized controlled trial. *Behav Ther.* 39(4):348–359.

Kaltenbach JA. (2009). Insights on the origins of tinnitus: An overview of recent research. *Hear J.* 62:26–31.

Karasek RA. (1979). Job demands, job decision latitude and mental strain: implications for job redesign. *Administrative Science Quarterly.* 24:285–308.

Kochkin S. (2010). MarkeTrak VIII: The efficacy of hearing aids in achieving compensation equity in the workplace. *Hear J.* 63(10), 19–24, 26, 28.

Kolkhorst FW, Smaldino JJ, Wolf SC, et al. (1998). Influence of fitness on susceptibility to noise-induced temporary threshold shift. *Med Sci Sports Exerc.* 30(2):289–293.

Kramer SE, Allessie GH, Dondorp AW, Zekveld AA, Kapteyn TS. (2005). A home education program for older adults with hearing impairment and their significant others: a randomized trial evaluating short- and long-term effects. *Int J Audiol.* 44(5):255–264.

Kramer SE, Kapteyn TS, Houtgast T. (2006). Occupational performance: comparing normally-hearing and hearing-impaired employees using the Amsterdam Checklist for Hearing and Work. *Int J Audiol.* 45(9):503–512.

Láinez MJ, Piera A. (2007). Botulinum toxin for the treatment of somatic tinnitus. *Prog Brain Res.* 166:335–338.

Laplante-Lévesque A, Hickson L, Worrall L. (2010). Factors influencing rehabilitation decisions of adults with acquired hearing impairment. *Int J Audiol.* 49(7):497–507.

Laplante-Lévesque A, Pichora-Fuller MK, Gagné JP. (2006). Providing an internet-based audiological counselling programme to new hearing aid users: a qualitative study. *Int J Audiol.* 45(12):697–706.

Li EP, Li-Tsang CW, Lee TK, Lee GW, Lam FC. (2006). Vocational rehabilitation program for persons with occupational deafness. *J Occup Rehabil.* 16(4):503–512.

Mace RL. (1998). Universal design in housing. *Assist Technol.* 10(1):21–28.

Mahncke HW, Connor BB, Appelman J, et al. (2006). Memory enhancement in healthy older adults using a brain plasticity-based training program: a randomized, controlled study. *Proc Natl Acad Sci USA.* 103(33): 12523–12528.

Martinez-Devesa P, Waddell A, Perera R, Theodoulou M. (2007). Cognitive behavioural therapy for tinnitus. *Cochrane Database Syst Rev.* (1);CD005233.

McGinnis C. (2001). Tinnitus self-help groups: How, and why, they work. *Hear J.* 54(11):50–52.

Melamed S, Fried Y, Froom P. (2004). The joint effect of noise exposure and job complexity on distress and injury risk among men and women: the cardiovascular occupational risk factors determination in Israel study. *J Occup Environ Med.* 46(10):1023–1032.

Milner CE, Cote KA. (2009). Benefits of napping in healthy adults: impact of nap length, time of day, age, and experience with napping. *J Sleep Res.* 18(2):272–281.

Mohren DC, Jansen NW, Kant IJ. (2010). Need for recovery from work in relation to age: a prospective cohort study. *Int Arch Occup Environ Health.* 83(5):553–561.

Nachtegaal J, Kuik DJ, Anema JR, Goverts ST, Festen JM, Kramer SE. (2009). Hearing status, need for recovery after work, and psychosocial work characteristics: results from an internet-based national survey on hearing. *Int J Audiol.* 48(10):684–691.

Neri G, De Stefano A, Baffa C, et al. (2009). Treatment of central and sensorineural tinnitus with orally administered Melatonin and Sulodexide: personal experience from a randomized controlled study. *Acta Otorhinolaryngol Ital.* 29(2):86–91.

Nondahl DM, Cruickshanks KJ, Dalton DS, et al. (2007). The impact of tinnitus on quality of life in older adults. *J Am Acad Audiol.* 18(3):257–266.

Occupational Safety and Health Administration. (2005). *Innovative Workplace Safety Accommodations for Hearing Impaired Workers.* Washington, DC: U.S. Department of Labor. Available at: www.osha.gov/dts/shib/shib072205 .html. Accessed on July 8, 2011.

Picard M, Girard SA, Simard M, Larocque R, Leroux T, Turcotte F. (2008). Association of work-related accidents with noise exposure in the workplace and noise-induced hearing loss based on the experience of some 240,000 person-years of observation. *Accid Anal Prev.* 40(5):1644–1652.

Rabinowitz PM, Sircar KD, Tarabar S, Galusha D, Slade MD (2005). Hearing loss in migrant agricultural workers. *J Agromedicine.* 10(4):9–17.

Rawool VW. (2007a). The aging auditory system, Part 1: Controversy and confusion on slower processing. *Hear Review.* 14(7): 14–19.

Rawool VW. (2007b). The aging auditory system, Part 2: Slower processing and speech recognition. *Hear Review.* 14 (8):36, 38, 40, 42, 43.

Rawool VW. (2007c). The aging auditory system, Part 3: Slower processing, cognition, and speech recognition. *Hear Review.* 14: 38, 43, 44, 46, 48. Available at: www. hearingreview.com/issues/articles/2007-09_02.asp. Accessed June 2010.

Rawool VW. (2010). "Auditory Thresholds in Quiet and Background Noise during a Visuo Spatial Task." Poster presentation at the 2010 MidWinter Meeting for the Association for Research in Otolaryngology, Anaheim, CA, February 6–10.

Rawool VW, Keihl JM. (2008). Perception of hearing status, communication, and hearing aids among socially active older individuals. *J Otolaryngol Head Neck Surg.* 37(1):27–42.

Rejali D, Sivakumar A, Balaji N. (2004). Ginkgo biloba does not benefit patients with tinnitus: a randomized placebo-controlled double-blind trial and meta-analysis of randomized trials. *Clin Otolaryngol.* 29(3):226–231.

Rikli RE, Edwards DJ. (1991). Effects of a three-year exercise program on motor function and cognitive processing speed in older women. *Res Q Exerc Sport.* 62(1):61–67.

Robinson S. (2007). Antidepressants for treatment of tinnitus. *Prog Brain Res.* 166:263–271.

Sauberman H. (1984). Report on Tinnitus Working Group of the Committee on Hearing, Bioacoustics and Biomechanics. Proceedings of the II International Tinnitus Seminar New York 10 and 11 June 1983. *J Laryngol Otol.* (Suppl 9):250–252.

Scarinci N, Worrall L, Hickson L. (2008). The effect of hearing impairment in older people on the spouse. *Int J Audiol.* 47(3):141–151.

Schaette R, König O, Hornig D, Gross M, Kempter R. (2010). Acoustic stimulation treatments against tinnitus could be most effective when tinnitus pitch is within the stimulated frequency range. *Hear Res.* 269(1–2):95–101.

Searchfield GD, Kaur M, Martin WH. (2010). Hearing aids as an adjunct to counseling: tinnitus patients who choose amplification do better than those that don't. *Int J Audiol.* 49(8):574–579.

Sherbourne K, White L, Fortnuni H. (2002). Intensive rehabilitation programmes for deafened men and women: an evaluation study. *Int J Audiol.* 41(3):195–201.

Signal TL, Gander PH, Anderson H, Brash S. (2009). Scheduled napping as a countermeasure to sleepiness in air traffic controllers. *J Sleep Res.* 18(1):11–19.

Sluiter JK, de Croon EM, Meijman TF, Frings-Dresen MH. (2003). Need for recovery from work related fatigue and its role in the development and prediction of subjective health complaints. *Occup Environ Med.* 60(Suppl 1):i62–i70.

Spielberg AR. (1998). On call and online: sociohistorical, legal, and ethical implications of e-mail for the patient-physician relationship. *JAMA.* 280(15):1353–1359.

Strayer DL, Johnston WA. (2001). Driven to distraction: dual task studies of simulated driving and conversing on a cellular phone. *Psychol Sci.* 12;463–466.

Swaen GM, Van Amelsvoort LG, Bültmann U, Kant IJ. (2003). Fatigue as a risk factor for being injured in an occupational accident: results from the Maastricht Cohort Study. *Occup Environ Med.* 60(Suppl 1):i88–i92.

Sweetow RW, Sabes JH. (2010). Effects of acoustical stimuli delivered through hearing aids on tinnitus. *J Am Acad Audiol.* 21(7):461–473.

Toppila E, Pyykkö I, Starck J. (2001). Age and noise-induced hearing loss. *Scand Audiol.* 30(4):236–244.

Trotter MI, Donaldson I. (2008). Hearing aids and tinnitus therapy: a 25-year experience. *J Laryngol Otol.* 122(10):1052–1056.

Tye-Murray N, Spry JL, Mauzé E. (2009). Professionals with hearing loss: maintaining that competitive edge. *Ear Hear.* 30(4):475–484.

United Nations. (1991). U.N. Principles for Older Persons. Adopted by the UN General Assembly (resolution 46/91) on 16 December 1991. United Nations Department of Public Information. DPI/1261/Rev.1—98–18895--September 1998--20M. Available at: http://www.un.org/NewLinks/older/99/principles.htm. Accessed July 9, 2011.

United Nations. (2002). Report of the Second World Assembly on Ageing. Madrid, 8-12 April 2002 A/CONF.197/9 United Nations publication, Sales No. E.02.IV.4, United Nations, New York. Available at: http://www.un-ngls.org/orf/pdf/MIPAA.pdf Accessed July 9, 2011.

U.S. Department of Defense. (2005). *Medical Standards for Appointment, Enlistment, or Induction in the Armed Forces* (DoD Instruction No. 6130.4). Washington, DC: U.S. Government Printing Office.

U.S. Equal Employment Opportunity Commission. (2007). *Questions and Answers about Deafness and Hearing Impairments in the Workplace and the Americans with Disabilities Act. Notice Concerning the Americans with Disabilities Act Amendments Act of 2008.* Washington, DC: U.S. Equal Employment Opportunity Commission.

van Amelsvoort LG, Kant IJ, Bültmann U, Swaen GM. (2003). Need for recovery after work and the subsequent risk of cardiovascular disease in a working population. *Occup Environ Med.* 60(Suppl 1):i83–i87.

van Veldhoven MJ, Sluiter JK. (2009). Work-related recovery opportunities: testing scale properties and validity in relation to health. *Int J Arch Occup Environ Health.* 82(9):1065–1075.

Vernon JA, Meikle MB. (2003). Masking devices and alprazolam treatment for tinnitus. *Otolaryngol Clin North Am.* 36(2):307–320, vii.

Viljoen DA, Nie V, Guest M. (2006). Is there a risk to safety when working in the New South Wales underground coal-mining industry while having binaural noise-induced hearing loss? *Intern Med J.* 36(3):180–184.

Wadley VG, Benz RL, Ball KK, Roenker DL, Edwards JD, Vance DE. (2006). Development and evaluation of home-based speed-of-processing training for older adults. *Arch Phys Med Rehabil.* 87(6):757–763.

Wayner DS, Abrahamson JE. (2001). *Learning to Hear Again. An Audiologic Rehabilitation Curriculum Guide,* 2nd edition. Latham, NY: Hear Again Publishing.

Chapter 13

Hearing Conservation in Educational Settings

It appears that there was a 31% increase in the prevalence of hearing loss among adolescents 12 to 19 years of age in 2005 and 2006 relative to the prevalence seen in 1988 and 1994 (Shargorodsky, Curhan, Curhan, & Eavey, 2010). Incorporation of prevention of noise-induced hearing loss (NIHL) in the health curricula taught in schools has been recommended (National Institutes of Health Consensus Statement, 1990). The need for such a program is obvious for several reasons:

- Children are frequently exposed to high noise levels (Rawool, 2008). A study in Australia found the use of personal stereos to be a significant risk factor for slight to mild sensorineural hearing loss among elementary school children (Cone, Wake, Tobin, Poulakis, & Rickards, 2010). Approximately 12 to 15% of school-aged children may have NIHL (Niskar, Kieszak, Holmes, Esteban, Rubin, & Brody, 2001).
- NIHL at an early age has the potential to accelerate age-related hearing loss later in life (Kujawa & Liberman, 2006).
- A critical need is apparent for promoting healthy hearing behaviors among young adults in college and occupational settings (Rawool & Colligon-Wayne, 2008).
- In the United States, among male youths who are 18 years old, construction labor is the second most common occupation during the school year and the most common summer occupation (U.S. Department of Labor, 2003), which can cause occupational noise exposure to students.

◆ Applicable Regulations/Standards

Individuals with Disabilities Education Act

Audiologists are required to create and administer programs for prevention of hearing loss and to guide children, parents, and teachers regarding hearing loss under the Individuals with Disabilities Education Act (34 CFR 300.34[c][1][iv and v]) (U.S. Department of Education, 2006).

American National Standards Institute (2010) Acoustical Guideline for Classrooms

The American National Standards Institute (ANSI) (2010; ANSI/ASA S12.60–2010/Part 1) standard has specified 35 dBA and 55 dBC as the maximum 1-hour averaged A-weighted and C-weighted steady background noise level in unoccupied and furnished core learning spaces (e.g., classrooms, instructional pods, group instruction rooms, conference rooms, libraries, speech clinics, offices used for educational purposes, and music rooms for instruction, practice, and performance) with volumes equal to or less than 20,000 ft^3. For core learning areas with volumes greater than 20,000 ft^3 and all ancillary (e.g., corridors, cafeterias, gymnasia, and indoor swimming pools) learning areas, the specified noise levels are 40 dBA and 60 dBC. The standard has also specified maximum reverberation time for sound pressure levels in octave bands with midband frequencies of 500, 1000, and 2000 Hz. These are 0.6 seconds for core learning areas with volumes less than 10,000 ft^3 and 0.7 seconds for areas with volumes in the range of 10,000 to 20,000 ft^3. The standard also specifies noise isolation design requirements.

In implementing strategies for controlling noise levels for prevention of hearing loss, the previously mentioned specifications should be considered. In general, noise and reverberation in classrooms and other learning spaces should be minimized to ensure good access to auditory information presented in such spaces to all students, including those with hearing loss. Annex C of the ANSI/ASA S12.60–2010/Part1 (ANSI, 2010) standard includes useful design guidelines for controlling reverberation in classroom and other learning spaces.

◆ Education Settings with Hazardous Noise

Aerobics or Physical Exercise Classes

Nassar (2001) noted average noise levels of 89 to 96 dBA in aerobics classes and temporary threshold shifts in participants immediately after attending a 1-hour class. Yaremchuk and Kaczor (1999) noted noise levels ranging from 78 to 106 dBA in aerobics classes, and only 21% of the readings were below 90 dBA. Our own discussion with an aerobics instructor revealed that she tried to set the music levels to 90 dBA because she believed it to be the safe exposure limit specified by the Occupational Safety and Health Administration (OSHA, 1983), which suggests a possible tendency to set the music to highest possible "safe" levels. In reality, noise levels created by students and instructors performing aerobics activities can increase the noise due to reverberation and other factors such as hard floors above and beyond the music levels. Considering the safety limit of 85 dBA specified by the National Institute of Occupational Safety and Health (1998) and the additional noise created by factors other than the music itself, the music should not be set beyond 80 dBA, and attempts should be made to set it lower than that.

Hunter Education

There appears to be a significant correlation between firearm use and hearing loss at 6000 Hz among students ranging in age from 10 to 20 years (Holmes, Kaplan, Phillips, Kemker, Weber, & Isart, 1997). Hunter education is provided in school programs in almost all states. The length of the training program can vary from of 10 to 28 hours. The majority of the programs include some instruction in hearing conservation and provide hearing protection devices (HPDs) during live fire aspects of practice. However, there are some programs that may not provide training or HPDs, and the training manuals may contain none or very little information about hearing conservation (Woodford & Lass, 1994). Both hunter educators and their students need to be well trained in the hearing conservation aspects of firearms (see Chapters 6 and 10).

Industrial Arts (Carpentry, Metal, Printing, Plumbing, Automotive, Welding, etc.)

Industrial arts classes can include teaching of fabrication of objects in wood and/or metal using various hand, machine, and power tools. Currently, both engineering and industrial technologies are included in such classes. Several other classes use machines or power tools that can produce hazardous sound levels as high as 122 dBA. The sound levels produced by a router can range from 95 to 100 dBA and those from a surface planer can range from 96 to 114 dBA (Lankford & West, 1993). Very high impulse sounds are also emitted in the shop during activities such as hammering of cold steel or chipping of welds (Woodford, Lawrence, & Bartrug, 1993). A pneumatic metal chipper in an automotive mechanic shop can emit sound levels in the range of 110 to 122 dBA (Plakke & Brown, 1984). Our measurements in a wood and metal workshop showed peak measurements of 128 dBA from a power-activated nailer. If several tools are operated at the same time, higher noise levels can be expected. Sound levels in school shops can contribute to temporary threshold shifts (Lankford & West, 1993) and even sensorineural hearing loss in the presence of other types of noise exposure (Woodford & O'Farrell, 1983). Instructors in these classes may not be as vigilant about wearing hearing protection as they are about wearing eye protection (Plakke, 1985). Superintendents or principles of technical vocational schools may not be completely aware of noise exposure levels (Allonen-Allie & Florentine, 1990) and the potential negative impact.

In Iowa, students and teachers in schools are required to use HPDs while participating in noisy activities in classes such as vocational or industrial arts shops and laboratories. In addition, teachers are responsible for ensuring that these requirements are met [Acts 1974 (65 G. A.) ch. 1168, 13].

Music Education

As stated in Chapter 9, musical instruments can produce sounds that are greater than 85 dBA, and the levels can vary depending on several factors. Mean sound levels during music practice can range from 87 to 95 dBA, and those generated by brass players are significantly higher than other instrument groups (Phillips & Mace, 2008). Hearing loss can occur in student musicians (Phillips, Henrich, & Mace, 2010). There is a relationship between exposure to the number of hours or instrumental practices and reports of impaired hearing and tinnitus among students enrolled in the school of music. A few students may stop practicing because of tinnitus and/or hearing problems (Hagberg, Thiringer, & Brandström, 2005).

The College of Music at the University of North Texas has a policy that requires labeling of music ensemble classes as "at-risk instructional settings." All ensemble instructors/directors and conductors are required to notify students about music-induced hearing loss and provide guidelines about safe exposure at the start of each semester. A model video shows how this goal can be achieved with live music demonstrations (www. unt.edu/untresearch/2007-2008/hearingvids. htm#unt). The website also has a model video for instructing fifth-grade students about music and NIHL. Students who major in music may be more likely to respond positively to education-based hearing conservation efforts (Chesky, Pair, Yoshimura, & Landford, 2009).

Agricultural Education

Agricultural workers are exposed to pesticides, organic dusts, gasoline fumes, excessive sun exposure, heat, mechanical injury, musculoskeletal trauma, injury from livestock, pathogens from animals and waste, noise, and vibration (Perry, 2003). There are numerous noise sources in agriculture including tractors, four-wheelers, all-terrain vehicles, dairy pumps, squealing pigs, skid steers (bobcats), rifles, chainsaws, radios inside tractor cabs, mechanical silo elevators, grain dryers, and wood splitters. Farmers have significantly greater high-frequency hearing loss compared with control populations (Marvel, Pratt, Marvel, Regan, & May, 1991). Up to 80% of farmers have a hearing loss using the criteria of thresholds above 20 dB hearing level at any one frequency and approximately 10% report tinnitus. Besides noise, smoking is one of the risk factors for increased prevalence of hearing loss among farmers (Carruth, Robert, Hurley, & Currie, 2007). Self-reported hearing loss and younger age are risk factors for at least one severe farm injury (Hwang, Gomez, Stark, St. John, May, & Hallman, 2001), and hearing aid use and young age are risk factors for animal-related injuries (Sprince, Park, Zwerling, et al., 2003), suggesting that younger age and hearing loss together can increase the risk of agricultural injuries. Exposure to noise increases the risk of injury in farmers with hearing loss (Choi, Peek-Asa, Sprince, et al., 2005).

Many children are expected to work on their family farms at a very young age; in some rural areas in some countries, families may not even send their child to school during busy farm work seasons such as harvesting. Boys may begin to operate tractors alone around the age of 11 years and girls may begin to do so around the age of 12 years, although some children may begin much earlier at the age of 5 years (Browning, Westneat, & Szeluga, 2001). Some children can get very high noise doses exceeding the OSHA (1983) action levels of 85 dBA time weighted average (TWA; Lander, Rudnick, & Perry, 2007). Students who work on farms are more likely to suffer from hearing loss than the general population (Broste, Hansen, Strand, & Stueland, 1989; Renick, Crawford, & Wilkins, 2009).

Organophosphate pesticides have been identified as potentially ototoxic (U.S. Army Center for Health Promotion and Preventive Medicine, 2003). In addition to noise, exposure to insecticides or pesticides, especially organophosphates, may contribute to hearing loss in farmers (Hoshino, Pacheco-Ferreira, Taguchi, Tomita, & Miranda Mde, 2008). Hearing loss in farmers is significantly associated with a history of spraying crops in the preceding year (Beckett, Chamberlain, Hallman, et al., 2000). Because of the possibility of hearing loss from noise, pesticides, solvents, and vibration, the hearing conservation program for agricultural students needs to be comprehensive and needs to address all these aspects. In addition, risk factors such as smoking need to be discussed, and strategies for preventing and minimizing smoking addiction need to be implemented. Because there are several other safety hazards in agriculture (Perry, 2003), the hearing conservation program can be offered as part of the overall safety training in formats such as farm safety camps (Lankford, DeLorier, & Meinke, 2000), with sufficient care to ensure that the hearing conservation component is not lost in the midst of other obvious safety hazards such as tractor injuries. Three informative brochures are readily available for informing students about hearing safety from farm noise:

1. *They're Your Ears, Protect Them: Hearing Loss Caused by Farm Noise is Preventable* (Department of Health and Human Services [National Institute of Occupational Safety and Health] Publication No. 2007–175). Available at www.cdc.gov/niosh/docs/2007-175/pdfs/2007-175.pdf.
2. *Have You Heard? Hearing Loss Caused by Farm Noise is Preventable. Young Farmers' Guide for Selecting and Using Hearing Protection* (Department of Health and Human Services [National Institute of Occupational Safety and Health] Publication No. 2007–176). Available at: www.cdc.gov/niosh/docs/2007-176/pdfs/2007-176.pdf.

Both these flyers were developed by the National Institute of Occupational Safety and Health in the Department of Health and Human Services at the Centers for Disease Control and Prevention.

3. *Noise and Hearing in the Farming Community.*

This third flyer is available from the National Hearing Conservation Association (www.hearingconservation.org).

Extracurricular Activities

Sporting events and dances held during activities such as proms can produce noises that are hazardous. Daneneberg, Loos-Cosgrove, and LoVerde (1987) obtained pure tone air conduction thresholds of students (12 to 17 years) and adults (37 to 43 years) before and after a school

dance. All students but one and all teachers but one showed worsening of hearing following exposure. Fifteen of the nineteen students and all the adults that experienced the threshold shift also experienced slight tinnitus.

Noise levels at sports events such as hockey games can range from 100 to 103 dBA with peak levels of 120 dBA (Hodgetts & Liu, 2006). The current author guided a graduate student at West Virginia University (Lily Hughes) to perform dosimetry at a tailgating event before a big football game and again at the actual game. The levels at the tailgating event ranged from 65 to 104.1 dBA with a peak of 143.4 dB sound pressure level (SPL). During a period of 1 hour and 13 minutes, the student wearing the dosimeter received a dose of 29.69% (81.1 dBA TWA) using the OSHA (1983) criteria. The levels at the football game ranged from 68.3 to 124.8 dBA with peak levels recorded at 138.6 dB SPL. Within a period of 4 hours and 11 minutes (from entering the stadium until leaving it), the student received a noise dose of approximately 101.2% (90 dBA TWA). The levels can be expected to be higher near the cheering and band sections.

Part-time Work within Education Settings

Students who work at university entertainment venues can get exposed to sounds exceeding 90 dBA and can suffer from temporary thresholds shifts (Sadhra, Jackson, Ryder, & Brown, 2002).

◆ Hearing Education Curricula/ Campaigns

Several campaigns/curricula have been developed over the years to increase the awareness of NIHL and hearing conservation strategies. Some of these curricula are discussed subsequently.

Dangerous Decibels (www.dangerousdecibels.org)

This campaign is designed to decrease NIHL and tinnitus by changing knowledge, attitudes, and behaviors of school-aged children. Several organizations are involved in the project including the Oregon Hearing Research Center at Oregon Health & Science University, the Oregon Museum of Science and Industry, the School of

Community Health at Portland State University, the Portland Veterans Affairs National Center for Rehabilitative Auditory Research, and the American Tinnitus Association. The sources of dangerous sounds, the impact of exposure to dangerous sounds, and the ways of protecting hearing from dangerous sounds are three components that are included in all of the activities within the Dangerous Decibels campaign.

Key features of the campaign include the following:

◆ A 12-component, 2000-square-feet, permanent exhibit at Oregon Museum of Science and Industry. The exhibit covers topics such as physics of sound, normal anatomy and physiology of hearing, NIHL and tinnitus (simulations), indicators of hazardous noise levels, and an interactive education on the selection of HPDs and hearing health. For example, the exhibit titled "Save Your Ears" inserts the visitor in several virtual scenarios and asks the visitor to evaluate the potential danger of the noise exposure and determine an appropriate hearing conservation strategy.
◆ Interactive lively activities on the Internet based on eight of the museum exhibits.
◆ A 45-minute classroom presentation for children in kindergarten through 12th grade and training for adults and high school students in presenting the program in classrooms.
◆ An educator resource guide and DVD.
◆ Epidemiologic and effectiveness evaluation research conducted on all of the above.

Don't Lose the Music (www.dontlosethemusic.com)

This campaign takes a pop culture approach to preventing NIHL among individuals in the age range of 18 to 30 years. It has several helpful promotional flyers and materials, including a flyer titled "Like it Loud?" that provides tips on minimizing a "noise hangover," and a report of research conducted on 16- to 30-year-old music fans.

U.S. Environmental Protection Agency (www.epa.gov/air/noise/ochp_noise_ middleschool_book.pdf)

The U.S. Environmental Protection Agency has a 16-page booklet designed for middle school

students to help them to keep their hearing health. It is titled *Say What? Play It Safe With Your Ears. Play It Safe With Your Health*. It has brief information about hearing conservation in an easy-to-understand format along with a quiz and some interacting activities such as puzzles.

Health Promotion in Schools of Music Project (www.unt.edu/hpsm)

This project is developed by the Performing Arts Medicine Association (www.artsmed.org) in collaboration with the University of North Texas and addresses hearing, vocal, neuromusculoskeletal, and mental health issues of musicians. They have four recommendations listed at their website including adopting a health promotion framework, offering a course on occupational health to all music majors, informing students about hearing loss as part of ensemble-based classes, and assisting students through active engagement with health care resources.

It's a Noisy Planet. Protect Their Hearing (www.noisyplanet.nidcd.nih.gov)

This campaign, launched by the National Institute of Deafness and Communication Disorders (NIDCD) in 2008, is designed to increase awareness among parents of children ages 8 to 12 years (tweens) about the causes and prevention of NIHL. With this information, parents and other caregivers are expected to instill healthy hearing habits in children that could minimize the possibility of NIHL. NIDCD is focusing its campaign on the parents and tweens because children begin to become independent in their attitudes and habits related to their health at this age. They also are beginning to develop their own listening, leisure, and work habits. Thus, this age provides an ideal opportunity to parents for promoting healthy hearing habits. Parents can access information in English and Spanish about NIHL, tips on how to encourage their children to adopt healthy hearing habits, and other measures they can take to protect their child's hearing at the Noisy Planet website. This website also contains information for tweens including interactive games about noise and hearing. NIDCD is also collaborating with other agencies such as 4-H, which is a positive youth development organization designed to empower children to achieve their full potential. 4-H and the Noisy Planet campaign are planning to develop materials for a rural audience that will be distributed through 4-H program's extensive network.

It's How You Listen That Counts (www.earbud.org)

This campaign is sponsored by the House Ear Institute and is designed for older children and young adults, ages 12 to 22 years. This campaign has a wide audience with involvement of the MTV Network, MTV.com, and five Yahoo! sites. The campaign website and its educational spot have reached a large audience (9 million) (House Ear Institute, 2006).

Know Noise® (www.sightandhearing.org/products/knownoise.asp)

This is a comprehensive hearing conservation program for children in grades 3 to 6. It includes a 13-minute video featuring music and two characters called Brenda and Luke who travel in the ear and give dramatic examples of how noise affects hearing. It also includes a curriculum with a 140-page teacher's manual including 26 standard lesson plans, related learning activities, technical information, local and national resources, and supplemental articles. In addition, two audiotapes featuring an "unfair" hearing test and ear plugs are also included.

Listen to Your Buds (www.listentoyourbuds.org)

This campaign is developed by the American Speech-Language-Hearing Association and is designed for children in the age range of 5 to 10 years.

Noise Education Section of the Environmental Protection Department of the Government of the Hong Kong Special Administrative Region (www.epd.gov.hk/epd/noise_education/young/eng_young_html/m5/m5.html)

This website is designed to provide information to young children. The website has five sections describing the nature of noise and the common types of environmental noises. The interesting feature is that the principles of controlling noise including source, path, or receiver control, and procedures for tackling noise including planning, abatement, control, and teamwork have been incorporated in the website. The site includes pictorial and interactive demonstrations of use of buffer zones, noise barriers, and absorptive materials to reduce traffic noise and use of good quality glazing and air conditioning to reduce noise in classrooms. Additionally, it includes tips on reducing pet noise, music, and other noises in the neighborhood.

NoiseOFF Teacher's Guide (http://noiseoff.org/document/teachers.guide.pdf)

This guide contains content for two different levels. Level 1 is for elementary and high school students and includes short units about the nature of sound, the human ear, noise pollution, decibel, and ways of protecting hearing. Level 2 is for high school students and is designed to stimulate critical thinking about noise pollution, civics, human health, and the environment, and includes questions such as, "Why has noise pollution become so prevalent in society?"

Operation Bang (http://militaryaudiology.org/site/resources/be-aware-of-noise-generation/)

Because most states requires hearing screenings for fifth graders and because it is easier to motivate children at this age, this program is designed for fifth graders. It is a 3-hour curriculum that can be offered over 3 days. The first hour is spent on the basic anatomy and physiology of the ear and basic information about sounds and noise. The second hour is spent on providing students with experiences with hazardous noises. The third hour is devoted to hearing appreciation, which includes experience with the effects of noise on hearing and the significance of conserving hearing. Educators are expected to repeat two basic concepts throughout the execution of the curriculum: the ways to protect hearing (reducing noise level, moving away from the sound source and covering ears) and to recognize hazardous noise using the 3-ft rule (If you have to increase your voice level to be heard above noise at arm's length, then the noise is dangerously loud). Two condensed versions of the curricula are available; one for second and third graders and another for fourth and fifth graders.

Sound and Hearing (www.standards.dfes. gov.uk/schemes2/secondary_science/ sci08l/?view=activities)

This site provides a teaching unit related to sound and hearing with several activities, related objectives, and outcomes. The site can be very useful to teachers who wish to be well informed about sound and hearing and wish to incorporate hearing conservation concepts in their science curricula.

Sound Sense: Save Your Hearing for the Music (www.soundsense.ca/)

The Sound Sense website has sections for teachers, children, and parents, including an essay contest. The section for teachers provides information about a curriculum developed by the Hearing Foundation of Canada that has been piloted and evaluated with sixth-grade students. It is designed to comply with the local injury prevention/health curriculum for grade 6 and to help students in grades 4 to 7 understand the dangers of loud music. It includes a lesson plan for teachers and a 10-minute video featuring the animated characters Spike and his sidekick Mike, who interact with a band.

WISE EARS!®
(www.nidcd.nih.gov/health/wise)

The WISE EARS! campaign was launched in 1999 jointly by NIDCD and the National Institute for Occupational Safety and Health. The objectives of the campaign were to educate the general public about risks of NIHL and to motivate the public to take actions against NIHL. As part of the campaign, free bilingual educational materials including multimedia presentations were developed and distributed. These materials can be downloaded through the campaign website. The section for children and teachers features student and teacher activities and two bookmarks titled, "How Loud is Too Loud?" and "Ten Ways to Recognize Hearing Loss." The site contains useful information for children, including activities and video clips. A video clip is available for children from grades 3 to 6 called, "I Love What I Hear." A middle school curriculum supplement titled, "How Your Brain Understands What Your Ears Hear" is available for seventh and eighth graders.

The campaign's visibility in the general population appears to be low based on lack of notice in recent media coverage. The materials developed through the campaign are used by several organizations but may be too broad for being specifically useful or effective for all populations (Blessing, 2008).

◆ Effectiveness of Hearing Education Programs

Effectiveness of the PROjectEAR Campaign in Austria

A study examined the effect of a hearing education campaign on the music listening practices of 1757 Austrian high school students through a survey completed before and one year after the campaign. The campaign (PROjectEAR) consisted of four 45-minute sessions distributed across 3 days and included various approaches to make the topic of hearing conservation attractive to the best possible extent. It included multimedia presentations with films and audio samples, demonstrations of ear protection devices and hearing aids, role play, creative group work such as drafting postcards and a webpage, and a discussion with an individual suffering from tinnitus or hearing loss. The campaign was not effective in reducing loud music exposure, but the number of students taking regeneration breaks while at the discotheque increased slightly from 70 to 76%. Also after the campaign, a larger number of students wanted the music levels at the discotheque to be reduced (Weichbold & Zorowka, 2007).

Effectiveness of the Dangerous Decibels Outreach Educational Program

The Dangerous Decibels 35-minute outreach educational program covers topics such as the physics of sound, mechanisms of hearing, the damaging effects of loud sounds on hearing, impact of hearing loss, and hearing loss prevention strategies. The effectiveness of the program has been evaluated on fourth- and seventh-grade students using experimental and comparison groups. The results show that the 35-minute intervention was effective in improving knowledge and attitudes, although attitudes improved to a lesser degree. Before the program, 15% of the seventh-grade participants indicated that they would use HPDs at a loud concert. This percentage increased significantly after the program, but only to 44%, suggesting room for improvement. Long-term retention of attitudes was only apparent in the fourth-grade students (Griest, 2008; Griest, Folmer, & Martin, 2007).

Long-term Effectiveness of Training to Industrial Technology Teachers

Plakke (1991) found a need to improve the effectiveness of hearing conservation training provided to industrial technology (arts) teachers following the implementation of a hearing conservation program that included teacher guides, materials, and workshops.

Effectiveness of Hearing Conservation Program for Agricultural Students

Berg and colleagues (2009) reported the results of a study designed to provide a hearing conservation program for students who were enrolled in grades 7 to 9 at the time of recruitment, were active participants in farm work, and were enrolled in schools with an active vocational agricultural program. The conservation program comprised classroom instruction, distribution of HPDs, direct mailings, measurement of noise levels at the student's home, and annual audiometric monitoring. The control group received only annual audiometric monitoring. Students in the experimental group reported more frequent use of HPDs, but there was a lack of evidence of decreased amount of NIHL in the experimental group that could be either due to inflated reports about the use of HPDs following training or lack of correct use of HPDs.

Effectiveness of other School-based Interventions for Students

Many studies have shown the short-term effectiveness of hearing conservation programs on kindergarten, elementary, middle school, and high school students by comparing performance on pre- and post-training questionnaires (Bennett & English, 1999; Blair, Hardegree, & Benson, 1996; Chermak, Curtis, & Seikel, 1996; Chermak & Peters-McCarthy, 1991; Lass, Woodford, Lundeen, et al., 1987; Lerman, Feldman, Shnaps, Kushnir, &

Ribak, 1998; Lukes & Johnson, 1998; Scrimgeour & Meyer, 2002). These studies show that immediately following training, students show better knowledge about hearing conservation practices. For example, Chermak, Curtis, and Seikel (1996) evaluated the effectiveness of a school-based intervention using pre- and post-test questionnaires. The participants were 48 fourth-grade students who showed improvement in both knowledge and intention to use protective behaviors following the two 1-hour sessions separated by 1 week. Scrimgeour and Meyer (2002) evaluated the effectiveness of an interactive education program titled "Ears for Listening, Voice for Speaking" (ELVS) by presenting it to 66 kindergarten students. Comparison of pre- and post questionnaires suggested a statistically significant increase in the students' knowledge following participation in the ELVS program. The limitations of many of these studies include the lack of control or comparison groups and lack of determination of long-term retention and impact.

◆ Recommended Program for Prevention of Hearing Loss within Education Settings

A comprehensive hearing conservation program should have all the following components for hearing loss prevention specified by OSHA (1983) and described throughout this book:

◆ *Noise measurement:* Identify the sources of noise that are potentially hazardous and conduct measurements (see Chapter 2).
◆ *Noise control:* New machinery can be bought with "quiet" specifications, as stated in Chapter 3. Old equipment can be modified or retrofitted to be quieter. In addition, noise exposure can be controlled by locating students away from noise sources and restricting the hours of exposure. Strategies for reducing loud music exposure are discussed in Chapter 9. The best strategy for preventing hearing loss is to control the noise. There are many barriers to the use of HPDs, and HPDs should be considered a last option for hearing conservation (Chesky, Pair, Yoshimura, & Landford, 2009).
◆ *Audiological monitoring and follow-up procedures:* In many states, children in

some grades (e.g., grades 1 through 3, 7, and 11) are required to undergo hearing screenings. In addition to this, children who conduct noisy activities (e.g., performing in school bands or working on farms) should undergo air conduction audiometry on an annual basis, and the frequencies of 3000 and 6000 Hz should be included in such testing. When a hearing loss or a significant hearing threshold shift (15 dB or greater) is apparent on any audiogram, the audiogram should be repeated to confirm the threshold shift after reinstructing the child. If the threshold shift persists, parents should be informed, and a full audiological evaluation should be scheduled. Along with the results of hearing screenings, parents should be also informed or reminded about NIHL and prevention strategies. Brochures such as "Crank it Down: Noise, Hearing Loss, and Children" available from the American Academy of Audiology (www.audiology.org) or the National Hearing Conservation Association (www.hearingconservation.org) and weblinks to campaigns such as It's a Noisy Planet. Protect Their Hearing (www.noisyplanet.nidcd.nih.gov) can be used for this purpose.

- *HPDs:* Those children who are participating in classes with hazardous noise exposure should be fitted with appropriate HPDs (see Chapter 6). Younger children playing or practicing music can be fitted with the Baby Blues earplug (see Chapter 9).
- *Training and motivating school personnel and students:* Teachers and administrators need to be knowledgeable about NIHL and hearing conservation; training to teachers and administrators can be provided as part of an annual in-service training program. This will allow them to take appropriate measures to conserve hearing in the presence of hazardous noise. It will also allow teachers to incorporate the knowledge in courses they teach. The knowledge-based component to educators and students should include the following elements:
  - ◇ Basic understanding of how we hear
  - ◇ Significance of the hearing sense or the ability to hear
  - ◇ Impact of hearing loss including educational and social implications for individuals and society

- ◇ Treatment of hearing loss
- ◇ Limitations of hearing aids and why protection of hearing is the best strategy
- ◇ Hazardous sounds and how to recognize excessively loud sounds including music (if you have to speak loudly to be heard above noise approximately 3 feet away, the noise is too loud); examples of sources of loud sounds: band classes, toys, firearms, motorboats, all-terrain vehicles, etc
- ◇ The auditory and nonauditory effects of loud sounds and other ototoxins (see Chapters 1 and 10)
- ◇ Temporary and permanent hearing loss and the relationship between them
- ◇ Signs and symptoms of temporary hearing loss including tinnitus
- ◇ Nonauditory advantages of reducing noise exposure including reduction in stress, anxiety, headaches, and annoyance
- ◇ Strategies for protecting hearing:
  - ◆ Controlling the source of noise
  - ◆ Increasing distance from the noise source
  - ◆ Using HPDs whenever around loud noise inside and outside the educational setting, including any occupational and recreational settings (see Chapter 10)
  - ◆ Using fingers for short bursts of noise (e.g., firecrackers) or when unprepared with HPDs
  - ◆ Avoiding potentially ototoxic recreational drugs including smoking (see Chapter 1)
  - ◆ Minimizing exposure to other ototoxins such as pesticides
  - ◆ Adopting a healthy lifestyle including a balanced healthy diet (e.g., vegetables and fruits that are rich in antioxidants) and physical exercise, which may improve blood supply to the inner ear (Alessio & Hutchinson, 2004)

Promoting Application of Knowledge to Behavior

Studies have shown that even though students have knowledge about hearing conservation, they may not adopt protective behaviors. This observation applies to a wide range of students from young elementary students (Chen, Huang, & Wei, 2009) to college students (Rawool & Colligon-Wayne, 2008). Thus, it is important to use strategies for promoting the use of behaviors that can conserve hearing, including the following strategies:

♦ Allowing students to listen to simulations of hearing loss and tinnitus may be an important strategy for promoting protective behaviors (Rawool & Colligon-Wayne, 2008). Many websites are available for demonstrating the simulation of hearing loss, including the website of the Better Hearing organization (www.betterhearing.org/hearing_loss/hearing_loss_simulator/index.cfm). Tinnitus can be demonstrated by presenting tonal or wideband or narrowband noise stimuli using a simple audiometer. A disk with simulation for hearing loss and tinnitus can also be ordered from the National Acoustic Laboratories in Australia (www.nal.gov.au/dvd-cd-report_tab_tinnitus-simulation-cd.shtml).

♦ Allowing students to select cosmetically appealing or "cool" HPDs may be important (Rawool & Colligon-Wayne, 2008).

♦ Set maximum levels of 80 dBA during extracurricular events such as dances and classes such as aerobics. Noise controls can be implemented to achieve this goal.

♦ Use peer pressure: Train class monitors and other students to request to turn the volume down when music is audible from a personal music player played by another student (Ferrari & Chan, 1991). For example, the Ida Institute has created an educational cartoon card for the purpose of giving it to individuals who are spotted listening to loud music with a simple message: "Loud music destroys your hearing." The website also has a short video clip modeling the intended effect of spreading the message. Schools could hold competitions for creating similar written messages/cartoons for handing out to individuals who listen to loud music.

♦ Post signs near elevators or other key places (entrance of sports and entertainment venues) to remind students about the potential dangers of exposure to loud sounds (Ferrari & Chan, 1991).

♦ Post signs near all classes, laboratories, and other facilities where hazardous noise exposure is likely to occur.

♦ Make HPDs readily available in settings where hazardous noise exposure is likely to occur and provide incentives or reinforcement (e.g., tokens that can be accumulated and exchanged later for gift certificates) for correct use.

♦ Invite a person with NIHL from the community to discuss how the loss was acquired, the impact of the hearing loss, and limitations of hearing aids. Provide students an opportunity to ask questions.

♦ Offer smoking cessation clinics for those who need them.

Delivery of Instruction

Research suggests that although hearing and hearing conservation concepts are taught in most schools, the effectiveness of methods and materials used to teach these concepts are questionable (Frager, 1986). There are several educational materials and curricula that are readily available. Instructors can use these as a starting point. However, the curricula need to be tailored to meet the specific characteristics of students in terms of the current cultural context and related interests, age, school grade, and cultural diversity. Students can quickly lose interest if older videos with outdated hairstyles, fashion trends, or background music are shown. Use of the available materials without consideration to student characteristics can be expected to lead to ineffective outcomes. Also, teachers are encouraged to create their own lesson plans, which may lead to more effective learning. Teachers may improve their knowledge base about sounds, noise, and hearing if they create the lessons themselves, perhaps by collaborating with audiologists and their students. Such a comprehensive knowledge base is necessary for teaching the class in an effective and interactive fashion, for answering any questions students may have, and for dispelling any misconceptions students may have.

Ongoing Evaluation of the Effectiveness of the Hearing Conservation Program

It is important to perform ongoing evaluations of the effectiveness of the hearing conservation program so that any deficient components of the program can be modified to improve effectiveness. The strategies for performing evaluations should include the following:

♦ Assessment of knowledge: A questionnaire-based evaluation of student's knowledge about NIHL and hearing protective behaviors (85% competency should be expected).

◆ Assessment of skills and behaviors: On-site observations of venues, teachers, and students in settings where hazardous noise exposure is likely to occur (e.g., music education). Sample questions that can be addressed during such observations include:
  ◇ Are warning signs about hazardous noise exposure clearly visible?
  ◇ Are HPDs readily available?
  ◇ Are HPDs available in different sizes and variety?
  ◇ Are HPDs used by teachers and students?
  ◇ Are HPDs inserted or placed correctly?
  ◇ If HPDs are not being used, what are the potential barriers?
  ◇ Are other protective behaviors such as not starting all machines at the same time or moving away from a noise source used?
  ◇ Can anything more be done to further control noise in the environment?
◆ Noise monitoring: Measurement of noise levels at events such as school dances or aerobics classes to ensure that the safety noise limit of 85 dBA is implemented correctly and is followed.

Review Questions

1. Why is it important to implement hearing conservation programs in educational settings?
2. Describe the regulations or standards that can apply to hearing conservation and noise control efforts in educational settings.
3. Why may music ensemble classes be labeled as "at-risk instructional setting" for hearing loss? (Hint: Refer to Chapter 9).
4. Describe two types of extracurricular activities within education settings where exposure to hazardous noise can occur. What can you do to reduce the risk of hearing loss during these activities?
5. Why is it necessary to include a hearing conservation program within agricultural education? Suggest five strategies to control noise exposure during agricultural activities.
6. Name and describe the two education campaigns about NIHL launched by NIDCD.
7. Summarize the effectiveness of hearing conservation education in school settings including successes and failures.
8. Develop a plan for a comprehensive hearing conservation program for a school in your area.
9. Plan an in-service training session for school administrators and teachers on hearing conservation and prepare appropriate presentation materials. Discuss strategies for assessing the short-term and long-term effectiveness of your in-service training session.
10. How will you evaluate the effectiveness of a hearing conservation program in a school setting?

References

Alessio H, Hutchinson K. (2004). Exercise promotes hearing health. *Hear Review.* Available at: www.hearingreview.com/issues/articles/2004-04_04.asp. Accessed August 2010.

Allonen-Allie N, Florentine M. (1990). Hearing conservation programs in Massachusetts' vocational/technical schools. *Ear Hear.* 11(3)237–240.

American National Standards Institute. (2010). *Acoustical Performance Criteria, Design Requirements, and Guideline for Schools: ANSI/ASA S12.60–2010/Part1.* New York, NY: American National Standards Institute.

Beckett WS, Chamberlain D, Hallman E, et al. (2000). Hearing conservation for farmers: source apportionment of occupational and environmental factors contributing to hearing loss. *J Occup Environ Med.* 42(8): 806–813.

Bennett JA, English K. (1999). Teaching hearing conservation to school children: comparing the outcomes and efficacy of two pedagogical approaches. *J Educational Audiol.* 7:29–33.

Berg RL, Pickett W, Fitz-Randolph M, et al. (2009, Dec). Hearing conservation program for agricultural students: short-term outcomes from a cluster-randomized trial with planned long-term follow-up. *Prev Med.* 49(6): 546–552.

Blair JC, Hardegree D, Benson PV. (1996). Necessity and effectiveness of a hearing conservation program for elementary students. *J Educational Audiol.* 4:12–16.

Blessing P. (2008). Wising up about noise-induced hearing loss: An evaluation of WISE EARS! A national campaign to prevent noise-induced hearing loss. *Sem Hear.* 29;94–101.

Broste SK, Hansen DA, Strand RL, Stueland DT. (1989). Hearing loss among high school farm students. *Am J Public Health.* 79(5):619–622.

Browning SR, Westneat SC, Szeluga R. (2001. Tractor driving among Kentucky farm youth: results from the farm family health and hazard surveillance project. *J Agric Saf Health.* 7(3):155–167.

Carruth A, Robert AE, Hurley A, Currie PS. (2007). The impact of hearing impairment, perceptions and attitudes about hearing loss, and noise exposure risk patterns on hearing handicap among farm family members. *AAOHN J.* 55(6):227–234.

Chen H, Huang M, Wei J. (2009). Elementary school children's knowledge and intended behavior toward hearing conservation. *Noise Health.* 11(42):54–58.

Chermak GD, Curtis L, Seikel JA. (1996). The effectiveness of an interactive hearing conservation program for elementary school children. *Lang Speech Hear Serv Sch.* 27:29–39.

Chermak GD, Peters-McCarthy E. (1991). The effectiveness of an educational hearing conservation program for elementary school children. *Lang Speech Hear Serv Sch.* 22:308–312.

Chesky K, Pair M, Yoshimura E, Landford S. (2009). An evaluation of musician earplugs with college music students. *Int J Audiol.* 48(9):661–670.

Choi SW, Peek-Asa C, Sprince NL, et al. (2005). Hearing loss as a risk factor for agricultural injuries. *Am J Ind Med.* 48(4):293–301.

Cone BK, Wake M, Tobin S, Poulakis Z, Rickards FW. (2010). Slight-mild sensorineural hearing loss in children: audiometric, clinical, and risk factor profiles. *Ear Hear.* 31(2):202–212.

Daneneberg M, Loos-Cosgrove M, LoVerde M. (1987). Temporary hearing loss and rock music. *Lang Speech Hear Serv Sch.* 18:250–266.

Ferrari JR, Chan LM. (1991). Interventions to reduce high-volume portable headsets: "turn down the sound"! *J Appl Behav Anal.* 24(4):695–704.

Frager AM. (1986). Toward improved instruction in hearing health at the elementary school level. *J Sch Health.* 56:166–169.

Griest S. (2008). Evaluation of a hearing-loss prevention program. *Sem Hear.* 29:122–130.

Griest SE, Folmer RL, Martin WH. (2007). Effectiveness of "Dangerous Decibels," a school-based hearing loss prevention program. *Am J Audiol.* 16(2):S165–S181.

Hagberg M, Thiringer G, Brandström L. (2005). Incidence of tinnitus, impaired hearing and musculoskeletal disorders among students enrolled in academic music education—a retrospective cohort study. *Int Arch Occup Environ Health.* 78(7):575–583.

Hodgetts WE, Liu R. (2006). Can hockey playoffs harm your hearing? *CMAJ.* 175(12):1541–1542.

Holmes AE, Kaplan HS, Phillips RM, Kemker FJ, Weber FT, Isart FA. (1997). Screening for hearing loss in adolescents. *Lang Speech Hear Serv Sch.* 28:70–76.

Hoshino AC, Pacheco-Ferreira H, Taguchi CK, Tomita S, Miranda Mde F. (2008). Ototoxicity study in workers exposed to organophosphate. *Braz J Otorhinolaryngol.* 74(6):912–918.

House Ear Institute. (2006). Teens tune-in to novel hearing conservation outreach campaign. *Hear Health.* 22;19.

Hwang SA, Gomez MI, Stark AD, St John TL, May JJ, Hallman EM. (2001). Severe farm injuries among New York farmers. *Am J Ind Med.* 40(1):32–41.

Kujawa SG, Liberman MC. (2006). Acceleration of age-related hearing loss by early noise exposure: evidence of a misspent youth. *J Neurosci.* 26(7):2115–2123.

Lander LI, Rudnick SN, Perry MJ. (2007). Assessing noise exposures in farm youths. *J Agromedicine.* 12(2):25–32.

Lankford JE, DeLorier J, Meinke D. (2000). Farm safety camp: hearing loss prevention. *Spectrum (Lexington, Ky.).* 17(4):6–9.

Lankford JE, West DM. (1993). A study of noise exposure and hearing sensitivity in a high school woodworking class. *Lang Speech Hear Serv Sch.* 24:167–173.

Lass NJ, Woodford CM, Lundeen C, et al. (1987). A hearing-conservation program for a junior high school. *Hear J.* 40(11):32–40.

Lerman Y, Feldman Y, Shnaps R, Kushnir T, Ribak J. (1998). Evaluation of an occupational health education program among 11th grade students. *Am J Ind Med.* 34(6):607–613.

Lukes E, Johnson M. (1998). Hearing conservation. Community outreach program for high school students. *AAOHN J.* 46(7):340–343.

Marvel ME, Pratt DS, Marvel LH, Regan M, May JJ. (1991). Occupational hearing loss in New York dairy farmers. *Am J Ind Med.* 20(4):517–531.

Nassar G. (2001). The human temporary threshold shift after exposure to 60 minutes' noise in an aerobics class. *Br J Audiol.* 35(1):99–101.

National Institutes of Health Consensus Statement. (1990). Noise and Hearing Loss. *Development Conference Consensus Statement.* Jan 22–24; 8(1):1–24.

National Institute for Occupational Safety and Health. (1998). *Preventing Occupational Hearing Loss: A Practical Guide* (Publication No. 96–110). Washington, DC: U.S. Department of Health and Human Services Publication.

Niskar AS, Kieszak SM, Holmes AE, Esteban E, Rubin C, Brody DJ. (2001). Estimated prevalence of noise-induced hearing threshold shifts among children 6 to 19 years of age: the Third National Health and Nutrition Examination Survey, 1988–1994, United States. *Pediatrics.* 108(1):40–43.

Occupational Safety and Health Administration. (1983). 29 CFR 1910.95. *Occupational Noise Exposure; Hearing Conservation Amendment; Final Rule, effective 8 March 1983. Federal Register.* 48:9738–9785.

Perry MJ. (2003). Children's agricultural health: traumatic injuries and hazardous inorganic exposures. *J Rural Health.* 19(3):269–278.

Phillips SL, Henrich VC, Mace ST. (2010). Prevalence of noise-induced hearing loss in student musicians. *Int J Audiol.* 49(4):309–316.

Phillips SL, Mace ST. (2008). Sound level measurements in music practice rooms. *Music Performance Res.* 2;36–47.

Plakke BL. (1985). Hearing conservation in secondary industrial arts classes: a challenge for school audiologists. *Lang Speech Hear Serv Sch.* 16:75–79.

Plakke BL. (1991). Hearing conservation training of industrial technology teachers. *Lang Speech Hear Serv Sch.* 22:134–138.

Plakke BL, Brown J. (1984). *A Guide for Iowa Industrial Arts Teachers for the Prevention of Hearing Loss.* Des Moines, IA: Iowa Department of Public Instruction, Special Education Division.

Rawool VW. (2008). Growing up noisy: The sound exposure diary of a hypothetical young adult. *Hear Review.* 15(5):30, 32, 34, 39–40.

Rawool VW, Colligon-Wayne LA. (2008). Auditory lifestyles and beliefs related to hearing loss among college students in the USA. *Noise Health.* 10(38):1–10.

Renick KM, Crawford JM, Wilkins JR 3rd. (2009). Hearing loss among Ohio farm youth: a comparison to a national sample. *Am J Ind Med.* 52(3):233–239.

Sadhra S, Jackson CA, Ryder TJ, Brown MJ. (2002). Noise levels and hearing loss amongst student employees in a university guild: a pilot study. *Ann Occup Hyg.* 46:455–463.

Scrimgeour K, Meyer SE. (2002). Effectiveness of a hearing conservation and vocal hygiene program for kindergarten children. *Special Serv Sch.* 18;133–150.

Shargorodsky J, Curhan SG, Curhan GC, Eavey R. (2010). Change in prevalence of hearing loss in US adolescents. *JAMA.* 304(7):772–778.

Sprince NL, Park H, Zwerling C, et al. (2003). Risk factors for animal-related injury among Iowa large-livestock farmers: a case-control study nested in the Agricultural Health Study. *J Rural Health.* 19(2):165–173.

U.S. Army Center for Health Promotion and Preventive Medicine. (2003). *Just the Facts. . . Occupational Ototoxins (Ear Poisons) and Hearing Loss* (Pub No. 51–002–0903). Aberdeen Proving Ground, MD: U.S. Army Center for Health Promotion and Preventive Medicine.

U.S. Department of Education. (2006). Assistance to states for the education of children with disabilities and preschool grants for children with disabilities; final rule (34 CFR parts 300 and 301). *Federal Register.* 71: 46540–46845.

U.S. Department of Labor. (2003).. *Employment Experience of Youth During the School Year and Summer.* Washington, DC: U.S. Department of Labor.

Weichbold V, Zorowka P. (2007). Can a hearing education campaign for adolescents change their music listening behavior? *Int J Audiol.* 46(3):128–133.

Woodford CM, Lass NJ. (1994). Hearing conservation in hunter education programs. *Am J Audiol.* 3;8–10.

Woodford CM, Lawrence LD, Bartrug R. (1993). Hearing loss and hearing conservation practices in rural high school students. *J Agricult Ed.* 77–83.

Woodford CM, O'Farrell ML. (1983). High frequency loss of hearing in secondary school students. An investigation of possible etiologic factors. *Lang Speech Hear Serv Sch.* 14:22–28.

Yaremchuk KL, Kaczor JC. (1999). Noise levels in health club settings. *Ear Nose Throat J.* 78:54–57.

Chapter 14

Future Trends in Hearing Conservation

Hearing conservation is an evolving area of expertise, and some strategies for improving implementation of hearing conservation are being investigated. Some of these strategies are presented in the current chapter.

◆ Active Noise Reduction Headphones for Audiometry

Low-frequency background noise can limit the accuracy of threshold determination in occupational settings, especially when young workers have very good sensitivity at the time of baseline audiograms. Low-frequency background noise can interfere with testing even with the use of insert earphones in a single-wall booth (Lankford, Perrone, & Thunder, 1999). Use of active noise reduction technology in audiometric headphones may reduce noise levels in the frequencies below 1500 to 2000 Hz and may allow the determination of more accurate thresholds at low frequencies in the presence of minimal background noise. Active noise-reducing headphones contain a reference or probe microphone to measure incoming background noise that is inverted by 180 degrees by a computer chip or controller. A speaker within the headphones emits this out-of-phase sound to cancel or actively minimize the incoming sound. There is also an error-checking microphone that attempts to further attenuate remaining sounds (Bromwich, Parsa, Lanthier, Yoo, & Parnes, 2008).

◆ Pharmacological/Surgical Strategies for Preventing Hearing Loss

Although hearing protection devices can be useful in reducing hazardous noise exposure, the use of hearing protection devices is problematic for many reasons, as presented in Chapters 6 and 9. In the future, pharmacological agents and other approaches could assist in the prevention of noise-induced and ototoxic hearing loss and/or correction of such hearing loss.

Pharmacological Agents

The nature of the damage that occurs after noise exposure can be temporary for several days or weeks after noise exposure (Fredelius, 1988). If an attempt is made to restore hair cells during this critical period, cell death can be prevented. Several different mechanisms are implicated in hearing loss resulting from exposure to hazardous levels of noise or ototoxins. Thus, several pharmacological agents are being investigated to address each of the underlying mechanisms.

Antiapoptotics

One obvious way of preventing noise-induced hearing loss (NIHL) is to prevent or minimize hair cell apoptosis or the process of programmed cell death. Disruption of mitogen-activated protein kinase cell death signaling can be achieved by administering D-JNK-1, which inhibits c-Jun N-terminal kinase (JNK) (Eshraghi, Wang, Adil, et al., 2007; Pirvola, Xing-Qun, Virkkala, et al., 2000;

Wang, Van De Water, Bonny, de Ribaupierre, Puel, & Zine, 2003). Src protein tyrosine kinase inhibition impacts several apoptosis pathways, resulting in prevention of NIHL (Harris, Hu, Hangauer, & Henderson, 2005). Blocking a critical step in apoptosis through intracochlear perfusion of caspase-3 and caspase-9 inhibitors can prevent cisplatin-induced ototoxicity (Wang, Ladrech, Pujol, Brabet, Van De Water, & Puel, 2004).

Antioxidants

Some possible mechanisms for NIHL include metabolic exhaustion of cells along with glycogen depletion and ischemia, possibly due to changes in the cochlear microcirculation (Spoendlin, 1962). Free radicals including reactive oxygen species (ROS) and reactive nitrogen species (RNS) are generated in the cochlea under normal metabolic conditions and are neutralized by antioxidants naturally present in the body, including enzymes that are active in glutathione metabolism, superoxide dismutases, and catalase. Hazardous noise exposure can increase the energy demands of hair cells, leading to overproduction of ROS and causing initial temporary hair cell trauma; if the overproduction of ROS/RNS continues, it can lead to permanent hair cell loss (Yamashita, Jiang, Schacht, & Miller, 2004). Other environmental factors that worsen cochlear oxidative stress and reduce blood flow include toxins such as toluene, smoking, and hyperlipidemia (see Chapter 1). Because of the role of oxidative stress in many types of acquired hearing loss, antioxidants appear to be ideal in preventing hearing loss.

N-acetyl-cysteine (NAC) is a broad spectrum antioxidant that can scavenge hydrogen peroxide and hydroxyl radicals. It may also inhibit lipid peroxidation or breaking down of lipid molecules by ROS and free radicals. NAC (1200 mg/d for 14 days) appears to prevent noise-induced temporary thresholds shifts in some workers who are exposed to occupational noise (Lin, Wu, Shih, et al., 2010). Sodium salicylate in combination with NAC is also effective in reducing noise-induced cochlear damage in chinchillas (Coleman, Huang, Liu, Kopke, & Jackson, 2010). Hearing loss in chinchillas induced by exposure to hazardous broadband noise can be minimized by administration of 4-hydroxy-PBN, which is a major metabolite of phenyl *N*-tert-butylnitrone (spin trapping agent of free radical species), along with the antioxidant

NAC 4 hours or longer after the noise exposure (Choi, Chen, Vasquez-Weldon, Jackson, Floyd, & Kopke, 2008). D-methionine (D-met) also appears to have direct and indirect antioxidant effects and may offer protection from carboplatin-, cisplatin-, aminoglycoside-, and hazardous noise (Campbell, Meech, Klemens, et al., 2007). D-Met reduces noise-induced oxidative stress and the associated permanent threshold shifts in the inner ear of the mouse (Samson, Wiktorek-Smagur, Politanski, et al., 2008).

Glutamatergic Neurotransmission Blockers

The most likely neurotransmitter at the synapse between the inner hair cells and afferent neurons is glutamate. Intense noise exposure may lead to excessive release of glutamate, which can bind to the postsynaptic receptors and lead to neuronal degeneration. Use of the glutamatergic neurotransmission blocker riluzole (Ruel, Wang, Pujol, Hameg, Dib, & Puel, 2005; Wang, Dib, Lenoir, et al., 2002) and glutamate receptor antagonist caroverine (Chen, Ulfendahl, Ruan, Tan, & Duan, 2004) can minimize NIHL in guinea pigs.

Metabolites

Metabolites such as cobalamin (vitamin B_{12}) are helpful in stabilizing neural activity and can improve vascular endothelial function (Chambers, Ueland, Obeid, Wrigley, Refsum, & Kooner, 2000). Poor vitamin B_{12} and folate status appear to be associated with age-related hearing loss (Houston, Johnson, Nozza, et al., 1999). Among Army personnel, B_{12} deficiency is found more frequently among those who suffer from NIHL and tinnitus compared with those with normal hearing or just NIHL (Shemesh, Attias, Ornan, Shapira, & Shahar, 1993). Temporary threshold shifts at 3 and 4 kHz measured 2 minutes after the end of a narrowband noise exposure of 112 dB sound pressure level centered at 3 kHz are significantly lower when cobalamin is administered to increase the B_{12} serum levels to more than 2350 pg/mL (Quaranta, Scaringi, Bartoli, Margarito, & Quaranta, 2004).

Neurotrophic Growth Factors

Neurotrophic agents such as T-817MA that also reduce oxidative stress can minimize noise-induced auditory thresholds shifts and hair cell death in guinea pigs (Yamashita, Shiotani, Kanzaki, Nakagawa, & Ogawa, 2008). Delivery of neurotrophins either through a device or through gene therapy can improve the survival of spiral ganglia following hair cell loss and can improve the effectiveness of cochlear implants in animal models (Fransson, Maruyama, Miller, & Ulfendahl, 2010). Use of coated or impregnated electrodes has been suggested for short-term delivery of neurotrophins to the cochlea (Staecker & Garnham, 2010).

Vasodilators

Noise exposure can reduce the blood supply to the cochlea to 70% (Thorne & Nuttall, 1987). Thus, agents that can improve blood flow can be expected to minimize the related ischemia-induced hearing loss. An increase in extracellular magnesium is associated with vasodilation of the arterioles, precapillary sphincters, and venules (Altura, Altura, Gebrewold, Ising, & Günther, 1992). Magnesium can protect against NIHL (Attias, Sapir, Bresloff, Reshef-Haran, & Ising, 2004; Joachims, Babisch, Ising, Günther, & Handrock, 1983), and the administration of magnesium is quick and easy with relatively minimum side effects (Attias, Weisz, Almog, et al., 1994).

Gene Therapy

Recent studies have identified genes that may make some individuals more susceptible to noise-induced (*CT, KCNE1*) or drug-induced (*12S rRNA*) hearing loss (Konings, Van Laer, Pawelczyk, et al., 2007). For example, the *HSP70, PCDH15,* and *MYH14* genes appear to be NIHL susceptibility genes (Konings, Van Laer, Michel, Pawelczyk, et al., 2009; Konings, Van Laer, Wiktorek-Smagur, et al., 2009). Heat shock proteins (HSPs) are a group of proteins that are expressed in cells under physiological and pathological circumstances. They assist in the synthesis, folding, assembly, and intracellular transport of many proteins. HSPs are induced in the cochlea after auditory overstimulation (Samson, Sheeladevi, Ravindran, & Senthilvelan, 2007). Induction of Hsp70 appears to have the potential to prevent aminoglycoside-induced hearing loss (Taleb, Brandon, Lee, Harris, Dillmann, & Cunningham, 2009).

Because of the involvement of genetic factors in increasing susceptibility to NIHL, a promising future strategy for preventing NIHL is gene therapy. The introduction of atonal homolog 1 (*Atoh-1*) or *Math-1*, a gene involved in the regulation of development of hair cells (Bermingham, Hassan, Price, et al., 1999), spiral ganglion neurons, and accessory auditory nuclei (Maricich, Xia, Mathes, et al., 2009) in experimental animals appears to stimulate hair cell regrowth and hearing recovery (Izumikawa, Minoda, Kawamoto, et al., 2005), but the presence of differentiated supporting cells in the cochlea is necessary for adequate function (Izumikawa, Batts, Miyazawa, Swiderski, & Raphael, 2008). The *Atoh-1*–induced hair cells are functional when the *Atoh-1* gene is overexpressed in a developing cochlea (Gubbels, Woessner, Mitchell, Ricci, & Brigande, 2008). Further research is necessary to prevent the accompanying growth of supernumerary hair cells, which is associated with profound hearing loss.

Stem Cell–based Therapies

Stem cells have the ability to develop into different cell types depending on their origin and environmental cues. The inner ear of mice appears to have its own endogenous stem cells, and those cells can differentiate in vitro into hair cell–like cells (Li, Roblin, Liu, & Heller, 2003). Stem cells from various sources can be guided to develop into different cell phenotypes (Beisel, Hansen, Soukup, & Fritzsch, 2008; Li, Roblin, Liu, & Heller, 2003; Li, Corrales, Edge, & Heller, 2004; Raphael, Kim, Osumi, & Izumikawa, 2007). A protocol has been developed for the use of mouse embryonic stem and induced pluripotent stem cells. These stem cells can be directed to become ectoderm capable of responding to otic-inducing growth factors. The ensuing otic progenitor cells are subjected to varying differentiation conditions, one of which can advance the organization of the cells into epithelial clusters containing hair cell–like cells with stereociliary bundles that are capable of responding to mechanical stimulation with currents that are similar to transduction currents in immature hair cells (Oshima, Shin, Diensthuber, Peng, Ricci, & Heller, 2010). Additional research is necessary to guide the development of two types of hair cells, the outer and the inner hair cells in the entire cochlea starting from base to apex.

Review Questions

1. Discuss a potentially useful strategy for obtaining accurate low-frequency thresholds in the presence of minimal background noise.
2. List the antiapoptotic drugs that might be useful in minimizing NIHL.
3. Discuss the potential role of antioxidants in minimizing NIHL.
4. List the antioxidants that appear to be successful in minimizing noise-induced or drug-induced hearing loss.
5. Discuss the potential role of glutamatergic neurotransmission blockers in minimizing NIHL.
6. Review the connection between the metabolite B_{12} and NIHL.
7. Discuss the potential role of neurotrophic growth factors in hearing preservation.
8. How can vasodilators be used in minimizing NIHL?
9. Review recent findings related to gene therapy for recovery from hearing loss.
10. How can stem cells be potentially used to treat hearing loss? What are the current limitations to stem cell–based therapies?

References

Altura BM, Altura BT, Gebrewold A, Ising H, Günther T. (1992). Noise-induced hypertension and magnesium in rats: relationship to microcirculation and calcium. *J Appl Physiol.* 72(1):194–202.

Attias J, Sapir S, Bresloff I, Reshef-Haran I, Ising H. (2004). Reduction in noise-induced temporary threshold shift in humans following oral magnesium intake. *Clin Otolaryngol Allied Sci.* 29(6):635–641.

Attias J, Weisz G, Almog S, et al. (1994). Oral magnesium intake reduces permanent hearing loss induced by noise exposure. *Am J Otolaryngol.* 15(1):26–32.

Beisel K, Hansen L, Soukup G, Fritzsch B. (2008). Regenerating cochlear hair cells: quo vadis stem cell. *Cell Tissue Res.* 333(3):373–379.

Bermingham NA, Hassan BA, Price SD, et al. (1999). Math1: an essential gene for the generation of inner ear hair cells. *Science.* 284(5421):1837–1841.

Bromwich MA, Parsa V, Lanthier N, Yoo J, Parnes LS. (2008). Active noise reduction audiometry: a prospective analysis of a new approach to noise management in audiometric testing. *Laryngoscope.* 118(1):104–109.

Campbell KC, Meech RP, Klemens JJ, et al. (2007). Prevention of noise- and drug-induced hearing loss with D-methionine. *Hear Res.* 226(1–2):92–103.

Chambers JC, Ueland PM, Obeid OA, Wrigley J, Refsum H, Kooner JS. (2000). Improved vascular endothelial function after oral B vitamins: An effect mediated through reduced concentrations of free plasma homocysteine. *Circulation.* 102(20):2479–2483.

Chen Z, Ulfendahl M, Ruan R, Tan L, Duan M. (2004). Protection of auditory function against noise trauma with local caroverine administration in guinea pigs. *Hear Res.* 197(1–2):131–136.

Choi CH, Chen K, Vasquez-Weldon A, Jackson RL, Floyd RA, Kopke RD. (2008). Effectiveness of 4-hydroxy phenyl N-tert-butylnitrone (4-OHPBN) alone and in combination with other antioxidant drugs in the treatment of acute acoustic trauma in chinchilla. *Free Radic Biol Med.* 44(9):1772–1784.

Coleman J, Huang X, Liu J, Kopke R, Jackson R. (2010). Dosing study on the effectiveness of salicylate/N-acetylcysteine for prevention of noise-induced hearing loss. *Noise Health.* 12(48):159–165.

Eshraghi AA, Wang J, Adil E, et al. (2007). Blocking c-Jun-N-terminal kinase signaling can prevent hearing loss induced by both electrode insertion trauma and neomycin ototoxicity. *Hear Res.* 226(1–2):168–177.

Fransson A, Maruyama J, Miller JM, Ulfendahl M. (2010). Post-treatment effects of local GDNF administration to the inner ears of deafened guinea pigs. *J Neurotrauma.* 27(9):1745–1751.

Fredelius L. (1988). Time sequence of degeneration pattern of the organ of Corti after acoustic overstimulation. A transmission electron microscopy study. *Acta Otolaryngol.* 106(5–6):373–385.

Gubbels SP, Woessner DW, Mitchell JC, Ricci AJ, Brigande JV. (2008). Functional auditory hair cells produced in the mammalian cochlea by in utero gene transfer. *Nature.* 455(7212):537–541.

Harris KC, Hu B, Hangauer D, Henderson D. (2005). Prevention of noise-induced hearing loss with Src-PTK inhibitors. *Hear Res.* 208(1–2):14–25.

Houston DK, Johnson MA, Nozza RJ, et al. (1999). Age-related hearing loss, vitamin B-12, and folate in elderly women. *Am J Clin Nutr.* 69(3):564–571.

Izumikawa M, Batts SA, Miyazawa T, Swiderski DL, Raphael Y. (2008). Response of the flat cochlear epithelium to forced expression of Atoh1. *Hear Res.* 240(1–2):52–56.

Izumikawa M, Minoda R, Kawamoto K, et al. (2005). Auditory hair cell replacement and hearing improvement by Atoh1 gene therapy in deaf mammals. *Nat Med.* 11(3):271–276.

Joachims Z, Babisch W, Ising H, Günther T, Handrock M. (1983). Dependence of noise-induced hearing loss upon perilymph magnesium concentration. *J Acoust Soc Am.* 74(1):104–108.

Konings A, Van Laer L, Michel S, et al. (2009). Variations in HSP70 genes associated with noise-induced hearing loss in two independent populations. *Eur J Hum Genet.* 17(3):329–335.

Konings A, Van Laer L, Pawelczyk M, et al. (2007). Association between variations in CAT and noise-induced hearing loss in two independent noise-exposed populations. *Hum Mol Genet.* 16(15):1872–1883.

Konings A, Van Laer L, Wiktorek-Smagur A, et al. (2009). Candidate gene association study for noise-induced hearing loss in two independent noise-exposed populations. *Ann Hum Genet.* 73(2):215–224.

Lankford JE, Perrone DC, Thunder TD. (1999). Ambient noise levels in mobile audiometric testing facilities: compliance with industry standards. *AAOHN J.* 47(4):163–167.

Li H, Corrales CE, Edge A, Heller S. (2004). Stem cells as therapy for hearing loss. *Trends Mol Med.* 10(7):309–315.

Li H, Roblin G, Liu H, Heller S. (2003). Generation of hair cells by stepwise differentiation of embryonic stem cells. *Proc Natl Acad Sci USA.* 100(23):13495–13500.

Lin CY, Wu JL, Shih TS, et al. (2010). N-Acetyl-cysteine against noise-induced temporary threshold shift in male workers. *Hear Res.* 269(1–2):42–47.

Maricich SM, Xia A, Mathes EL, et al. (2009). Atoh1-lineal neurons are required for hearing and for the survival of neurons in the spiral ganglion and brainstem accessory auditory nuclei. *J Neurosci.* 29(36): 11123–11133.

Oshima K, Shin K, Diensthuber M, Peng AW, Ricci AJ, Heller S. (2010). Mechanosensitive hair cell-like cells from embryonic and induced pluripotent stem cells. *Cell.* 141(4):704–716.

Quaranta A, Scaringi A, Bartoli R, Margarito MA, Quaranta N. (2004). The effects of 'supra-physiological' vitamin B12 administration on temporary threshold shift. *Int J Audiol.* 43(3):162–165.

Pirvola U, Xing-Qun L, Virkkala J, et al. (2000). Rescue of hearing, auditory hair cells, and neurons by CEP-1347/KT7515, an inhibitor of c-Jun N-terminal kinase activation. *J Neurosci.* 20(1):43–50.

Raphael Y, Kim YH, Osumi Y, Izumikawa M. (2007). Non-sensory cells in the deafened organ of Corti: approaches for repair. *Int J Dev Biol.* 51(6–7):649–654.

Ruel J, Wang J, Pujol R, Hameg A, Dib M, Puel JL. (2005). Neuroprotective effect of riluzole in acute noise-induced hearing loss. *Neuroreport.* 16(10):1087–1090.

Samson J, Sheeladevi R, Ravindran R, Senthilvelan M. (2007). Stress response in rat brain after different durations of noise exposure. *Neurosci Res.* 57(1):143–147.

Samson J, Wiktorek-Smagur A, Politanski P, et al. (2008). Noise-induced time-dependent changes in oxidative stress in the mouse cochlea and attenuation by D-methionine. *Neuroscience.* 152(1):146–150.

Shemesh Z, Attias J, Ornan M, Shapira N, Shahar A. (1993). Vitamin B12 deficiency in patients with chronic-tinnitus and noise-induced hearing loss. *Am J Otolaryngol.* 14(2):94–99.

Spoendlin H. (1962). Ultrasound features of the organ of Corti in normal and acoustically situated animals. *Annals Otol Rhinol Laryngol.* 71:657–677.

Staecker H, Garnham C. (2010). Neurotrophin therapy and cochlear implantation: translating animal models to human therapy. *Exp Neurol.* 226(1):1–5.

Taleb M, Brandon CS, Lee FS, Harris KC, Dillmann WH, Cunningham LL. (2009). Hsp70 inhibits aminoglycoside-induced hearing loss and cochlear hair cell death. *Cell Stress Chaperones.* 14(4):427–437.

Thorne PR, Nuttall AL. (1987). Laser Doppler measurements of cochlear blood flow during loud sound exposure in the guinea pig. *Hear Res.* 27(1):1–10.

Wang J, Dib M, Lenoir M, et al. (2002). Riluzole rescues cochlear sensory cells from acoustic trauma in the guinea-pig. *Neuroscience.* 111(3):635–648.

Wang J, Ladrech S, Pujol R, Brabet P, Van De Water TR, Puel JL. (2004). Caspase inhibitors, but not c-Jun NH2-terminal kinase inhibitor treatment, prevent cisplatin-induced hearing loss. *Cancer Res.* 64(24):9217–9224.

Wang J, Van De Water TR, Bonny C, de Ribaupierre F, Puel JL, Zine A. (2003). A peptide inhibitor of c-Jun N-terminal kinase protects against both aminoglycoside and acoustic trauma-induced auditory hair cell death and hearing loss. *J Neurosci.* 23(24):8596–8607.

Yamashita D, Jiang HY, Schacht J, Miller JM. (2004). Delayed production of free radicals following noise exposure. *Brain Res.* 1019(1–2):201–209.

Yamashita D, Shiotani A, Kanzaki S, Nakagawa M, Ogawa K. (2008). Neuroprotective effects of T-817MA against noise-induced hearing loss. *Neurosci Res.* 61(1):38–42.

Index

Note: Page numbers followed by *f* and *t* indicate figures and tables, respectively.

A

AAO. *See* American Academy of Otolaryngology
ABR. *See* auditory brainstem response
absenteeism, reduced, noise control and, 52
absorption chambers, 61, 62*f*
absorption coefficients, 58, 60*t*
absorptive silencers, 54–55, 55*f*
Accident Compensation Corporation
  (New Zealand), 242
accidents
  noise and, 9
  reducing, noise control and, 52
  risk of, for workers with hearing loss, 269
accommodations, 270, 275
accountability, in training, 180
ACO. *See* American Council of Otolaryngology
Acoustical Guideline for Classrooms,
  283–284
acoustic calibrators, 37, 40, 42*f*, 43
acoustic component, of tinnitus, 276
acoustic crosstalk, checking for, 84
acoustic enclosures, 58, 60*f*
  maintaining and servicing, 62
  materials for, 58, 60*t*
  ordering, 58
acoustic pipe lagging, 56–57, 56*f*
acoustic radiations
  infrasonic, 45
  ultrasound, 45–46, 46*f*
  upper sonic, 45–46, 46*f*
acoustic reflex decay, 106, 112, 113*f*, 130, 131*f*

acoustic reflex testing, 112–114
  applications of results, 113–114
  in auditory dyssynchrony, 122*t*
  in auditory neuropathy, 113, 122*t*
  in auditory processing disorders, 122*t*
  in nonorganic hearing loss, 113–114, 114*f*
  in retrocochlear pathologies, 113
  in sensory hearing loss, 122*t*
  in temporal processing, 129–130, 129*f*, 131*f*
acoustic reflex thresholds (ARTs), 112–114, 113*f*
acoustic shock, 57
  in call center operators, 14
  definition of, 14
acoustic shock limiters, 57
acoustic test fixture, 155–156
acoustic treatments, 61, 230
ACS 100 Software, 85
action with reflection, in learning, 179
active hearing protection devices, 141
active job, 266
active noise cancellation, 56
active noise reduction (ANR), 145
active noise reduction headphones, 296
activity limitation, 243
ADA. *See* Americans with Disabilities Act
additive effects, 10
administrative control, 63
aerobics classes, 284
Aero Technologies, 165
AFFD. *See* auditory fitness for duty
affective involvement, in training, 179